3D Printing in Biomedical Engineering

3D Printing in Biomedical Engineering

Aviraj Chandrahauns Chavan

ARCLER
PRESS

www.arclerpress.com

3D Printing in Biomedical Engineering

Aviraj Chandrahauns Chavan

Arcler Press
4164 Lakeshore Road
Burlington, ON L7L 1A4
Canada
www.arclerpress.com
Email: orders@arclereducation.com

ISBN: 978-1-77956-974-5 (Hardcover)

ABOUT THE AUTHOR

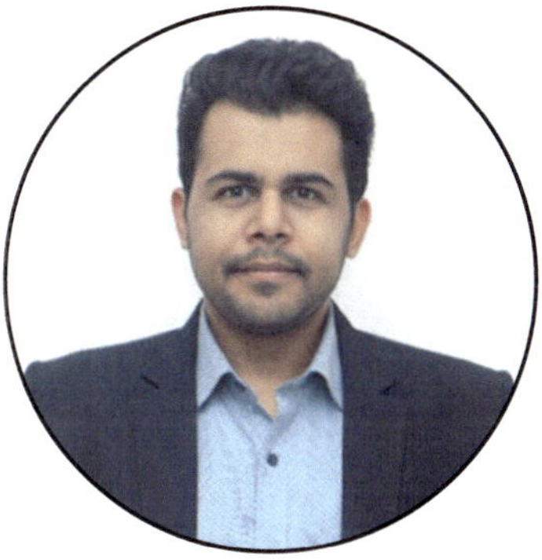

Aviraj Chandrahauns Chavan is a management professional with a strong foundation in operations, complemented by a deep passion for continuous learning and creative expression. He holds a Master of Management Studies (MMS) in Operations from Welingkar Institute of Management Studies, Mumbai, and a Bachelor's degree in Mechanical Engineering from Mumbai University. He is pursuing Ph. D in Management studies from Jamnalal Bajaj Institute of Management Studies, University of Mumbai.

With hands-on experience at organizations such as MAHYCO and Radhakrishna Foodland Pvt. Ltd., Aviraj has worked extensively across demand forecasting, supply planning, material resource planning, and inventory optimization. In his role as Senior Executive – Supply Chain Planning, he was responsible for managing critical supply and inventory operations, including forecasting and planning. His work has involved employing efficient supply models, handling transport, and warehouse management projects to reduce lead times and improve serviceability. His ability to blend data-driven strategies with real-time operational insights has consistently delivered measurable improvements in supply chain performance. He is known for his analytical mindset, adaptability, and a clear communication style.

TABLE OF CONTENTS

LIST OF FIGURES

PREFACE

The last couple of decades have seen a revolution in biomedical engineering that has revolutionized the practice of medicine as well as healthcare delivery. One of the most groundbreaking of these innovations is three-dimensional (3D) printing, which has evolved from being an experimental curiosity into one of the fundamental tools of contemporary medicine. What was once the stuff of science fiction—making personalized prosthetics, printing living tissue, or creating intricate medical devices with unmatched accuracy—can now be done. The value of 3D printing is not just in its accuracy but also in its ability to make medical solutions patient-specific, thus taking the principles of personalized medicine a step further. With healthcare transitioning to patient-centric models, this technology is a strong facilitator, unlocking new opportunities in treatment, diagnostics, and rehabilitation.

Interestingly, 3D printing in biomedical engineering also raises significant material, ethical, regulatory specification, and access issues. The development of biocompatible materials that may safely interact with human tissue, the capability to scale tissue engineering to meaningful levels, and the assurance of printed organs or devices' safety for clinical use are some of the major challenges confronting researchers and practitioners. These challenges notwithstanding, they also reflect the vast potential of the technology. In bringing engineering design, material science, and medical practice together, 3D printing offers a platform for interdisciplinarity. From making accessible, cost-effective surgical models that advance medical education to the printing of implants that enhance patients' quality of life, its applications demonstrate how innovation can be a direct response to human health.

The book *3D Printing in Biomedical Engineering* has been designed to introduce a systematic and comprehensive study of the new discipline. The book introduces basic ideas about 3D printing and discusses advanced applications in the biomedical sector as well. Every chapter is devoted to separate topics encompassing the topic from technical fundamentals and material science to advanced applications such as tissue engineering and organ printing. With technical specificity balanced against everyday relevance, the book aims to aid students, researchers, and practitioners alike by defining concepts clearly and simply. It focuses on the achievements secured to date as well as possibilities yet to be realized, offering the reader a path to understand the contribution of the technology to medicine's future.

Chapter 1 provides an introduction to 3D printing in biomedical engineering. This encompasses the historic development of additive manufacture, the basic principles of the technology, and its application in medicine. It points out the distinction between traditional production methods and additive ones, and the reasons why 3D printing has had such a profound impact within the biomedical field.

Chapter 2 covers the fundamentals of additive manufacturing processes. In this chapter, one is presented with the fundamental processes that make 3D printing possible, including stereolithography, selective laser sintering, fused deposition modeling, and other common processes. The chapter covers the differences among these processes, their strengths and limitations, and what considerations impact their use in biomedical devices.

Chapter 3 presents materials for 3D printing in biomedicine. It highlights the polymers, metals, ceramics, and bio-inks suitable for biomedical applications and their mechanical and biological properties. Specific focus is laid on biocompatibility, biodegradability, and the difficulty of developing new materials suitable for implants, scaffolds, and tissue engineering.

Chapter 4 explores design and modeling for biomedical devices. It explains how advanced computer-aided design (CAD) tools are used to create models of patient-specific devices and implants. The chapter also considers simulation techniques, optimization methods, and design strategies to improve the precision and performance of 3D-printed biomedical products.

Chapter 5 discusses tissue engineering and bioprinting. In chapter 5, the significance of 3D printing in scaffold and tissue construct fabrication to support cell growth and regeneration is emphasized. The chapter educates readers on techniques of bioprinting, the incorporation of living cells into structures printed, and how such processes contribute to regenerative medicine and drug testing platforms.

Chapter 6 discusses 3D printing of prosthetics and implants. The subject varies from customized implants being designed to accommodate patient anatomy to improving outcomes in orthopedics, dentistry, and reconstructive surgery. It also covers developing prosthetic limbs that are light, cost-effective, and specifically designed to accommodate particular patients' needs.

Chapter 7 is dedicated to organ and soft tissue printing. Very much still in research phases, this represents one of the most ambitious applications of 3D printing. The chapter looks at developments toward printing functioning organs, the scientific challenges in replicating vascularization and organ complexity, and the potential of organ replacement therapies.

Chapter 8 discusses medical devices and surgical planning. It demonstrates how 3D printing is used to create anatomical models for pre-surgical planning to achieve greater precision in complex surgeries. The chapter also recognizes printed surgical guides, dental aligners, and other devices that improve training as well as clinical performance.

Chapter 9 discusses microfluidics and lab-on-a-chip devices. This fast-growing technology demonstrates how 3D printing is able to create small systems for diagnostics, drug testing, and biological research. The chapter shows examples of uses of how lab-on-a-chip technology is being developed to offer faster, cheaper, and more accurate point-of-care testing.

Chapter 10 provides an overview of trends and emerging technologies. It maps out the directions of future biomedical 3D printing, including hybrid manufacturing, artificial intelligence, and advances in bio-inks and organ printing. It also touches on ethical and regulatory aspects, citing such concerns as patient safety, intellectual property, and global access.

This book is intended for an audience of readers that covers undergraduate and graduate students in the field of biomedical engineering, medical students interested in learning the use of engineering in medicine, and scientists in the subject matter of material science, biology, and engineering. It is also a practitioner's guide for surgeons and clinicians who would like to know how 3D printing is going to be used in clinical practice, whether in designing implants, planning surgeries, or testing tissue growth. Additionally, medical device company professionals and regulatory agents will find the book helpful because it speaks not just of technical potential but of broader implications of adopting the technology. Through the provision of a balance between basic material and real-world applications, the book is a reference as well as an inspiration to those working to shape the future of biomedical engineering.

CHAPTER 1

INTRODUCTION TO 3D PRINTING IN BIOMEDICAL ENGINEERING

Contents

INTRODUCTION

The three-dimensional (3D) printing revolution has ignited revolutionary change in a wide range of fields, including the field of biomedical engineering. The new manufacturing method is founded upon the process of objects being built layer by layer, making possible unprecedented customization and fast prototyping. The ability to create intricate designs tailored precisely to the specific needs of individual patients is a remarkable breakthrough in medical treatment. As opposed to traditional manufacturing techniques that require significant time and cost investments, 3D printing makes it possible to produce customized medical solutions at a fraction of the cost and much quicker turnaround. The technology is revolutionizing not only the production logistical side but also enhancing patient care through the provision of customized healthcare solutions previously unavailable. As a result, it is essential to highlight the central role 3D printing will perform in revolutionizing medical engineering practices in the years to come (Branch et al., 2015). Investigating further the biomedical applications of 3D printing offers an impressive array of applications that continues to increase. From dental implants and prosthetic limbs to organ and tissue bioprinting, the potential of 3D printing to address the wide range of needs in healthcare is overwhelming. Evidence indicates that synthetic polymers and hydrogels are already applied in 3D printing to print scaffolds facilitating tissue engineering. Among the most prominent studies, the fabrication of a honeycomb scaffold of hyaluronic acid, gelatin, and alginate for regenerative use was reported, utilizing a calcium chloride bath as the cross-linker (Macwan et al., 2018). Not only does the technique impart better mechanical strength, but it also promotes cell growth within an optimal environment, a sign of the huge potential of 3D-printed constructs in regenerative medicine. Therefore, with the introduction of new technologies, the implications for more advanced treatment modes are increasingly deep. With a glimpse of the future in mind, the introduction of 3D printing into biomedical engineering is poised to unleash unprecedented potential. In addition to the development of the technology, advances in materials science, including biocompatible and biodegradable materials, will continue to expand the range of potential applications. 3D printing has the potential to print surgery tools, drug delivery systems, and even living tissue to implant organs. Ongoing research and development on these technologies have the promise to break through current limitations and provide solutions to complex medical issues. Additionally, coupling machine learning and artificial intelligence with 3D printing processes has the potential to make them even more accurate and efficient and allow for even more personalized medicine. Through fostering continued dialogue and collaboration among engineers, physicians, and scientists, the full potential of 3D printing in biomedical engineering can be achieved, ultimately improving patient care and health care delivery worldwide (Branch et al., 2015).

Definition of 3D Printing

The process is also known as additive manufacturing and involves a wide range of methods used to manufacture three-dimensional objects from computer data. The process operates by constructing layers of material, often plastic, metal, or bio-compatible substances, in the process of creating intricate structures that would otherwise be impossible with traditional manufacturing processes. As a disruptive process, 3D printing supports the creation of highly complex and custom-made components with the potential for rapid prototyping and efficient manufacturing processes. By employing techniques such as selective laser sintering or fused deposition modeling, 3D printing not only conserves material but also improves the velocity and effectiveness of production. It is particularly valuable in a broad spectrum of applications, from biomedical engineering to fields where precision and tailored solutions are paramount. In biomedical engineering alone, the potential applications of 3D printing extend far beyond mere production.

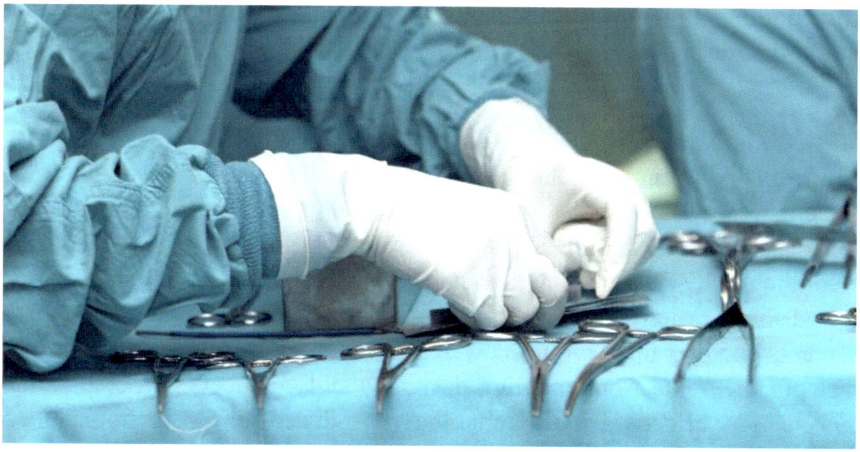

Figure 1.1. The ability to produce patient-specific models for surgical planning enhances the accuracy and outcomes of various medical procedures.

Source: https://advancementsinoncology.com/wp-content/uploads/2024/06/surgery_dreamstime_xxl_7465323-1280x640.jpg.

This technology allows for the creation of highly personalized medical devices, implants, and even tissue scaffolds that can be tailored to the specific anatomy of an individual patient. The ability to print patient-specific models for surgical planning enhances the accuracy and success of many medical procedures. Furthermore, the use of smart materials, as discussed in recent studies, introduces a new dimension of functionality for 3D-printed products. For example, bio-responsive hydrogels or organic thin film electronic devices could lead to intelligent healthcare products, such as smart bandages sensitive to physiological wound microenvironment changes (Oliver et al., 2009). Such technology can be seen as evidence of the potential for patient care transformation via adaptive and customized medical solutions, offered by the combination of 3D printing and biomedical engineering. The future of 3D printing in biomedical applications is promising, with continuous improvement in material technology and science. With researchers exploring the potential of different biomaterials, from those that have interaction and response capabilities, new product development is highly augmented. Industry 4.0 and the emergence of smart manufacturing emphasize the integration of these advanced materials in support of decentralized production meeting the current needs of healthcare (Dehghanghadikolaei et al., 2019). It not only improves production efficiency but also improves sustainability through waste material minimization and enabling localized manufacturing. As technology improves in 3D printing, its application in biomedical engineering is bound to grow, and maybe even more novel solutions to reduce the challenges of intricate health issues and improve the benefits for patients globally (Figure 1.1).

Brief History of 3D Printing Technology

The history of 3D printing technology stretches back to the 1980s, a revolutionary decade that laid the groundwork for what would go on to revolutionize several industries, including biomedical engineering. The initial successful method, stereolithography, was invented by Charles Hull in 1983. Hull's innovation allowed the creation of complex 3D models by curing photopolymer resins in layers, opening up a whole new realm of rapid prototyping and product development. Aside from enabling designers and engineers to visualize their concepts more effectively, this technology introduced staggering time and cost reductions to the production process. As 3D printing progressed, its application diversified with the possibility of uses outside traditional manufacturing and giving way to future expansion in medical use, thus creating a base for the future expansion of the field of biomedical engineering. The following decades saw the expansion of 3D printing by the development of various technologies like Selective Laser Sintering (SLS) and Fused Deposition Modeling (FDM). These advances drastically changed the availability and accessibility of 3D printing, inspiring its application across numerous industries. Open-source 3D printers in the early 2000s allowed people and small companies to experiment with this technology, fostering an environment of innovation and creativity. At the same time, research institutions began exploring 3D printings applications in medical fields, particularly in prosthetics and modeling organs. The realization that 3D printing could potentially reduce organ rejection rates by creating patient-specific implants marked a transformative moment in biomedical engineering. This shift underscored the technology's promise in improving patient outcomes, allowing researchers and clinicians to envision a future where personalized medical solutions could become the norm. As the 2010s progressed, 3D printing technology entered a new phase marked by increased sophistication and integration into clinical settings. This period witnessed major input from cross-disciplinary collaboration, particularly among researchers, healthcare experts, and engineers. Advanced developments involved bioprinting, where living cells could be deposited to fabricate bioengineered organs and tissues, pushing the boundaries of regenerative medicine. Organizations like the Boston University Photonics Center embarked on pioneering studies in developing new materials and processes to further enhance 3D printing technology, evident in effective programs focused on the intersection of photonics and biomedical applications (N/A, 2016). Most significantly, all of these advances necessitated an intensive examination of the biological and mechanical interfacing of 3D-printed objects, as outlined in neuromechanical accounts that emphasize the complex interactions between engineered and biological structures (Santello et al., 2017). Such integration of technological progress and research reaffirmed 3D printings fundamental contribution to rewriting the remit of modern medicine and biomedical engineering (Figure 1.2).

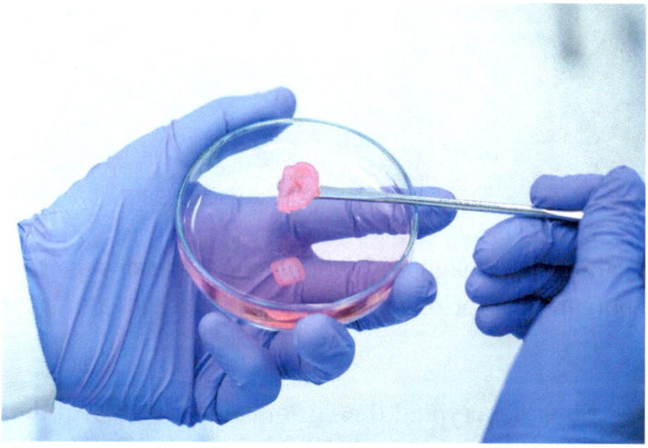

Figure 1.2. Cutting-edge advancements included bioprinting, which enabled the deposition of living cells to create bioengineered tissues and organs, advancing the field of regenerative medicine.

Source: https://www.cellink.com/wp-content/uploads/2022/08/The-Ear-Image-3D-bioprinting-ears.jpg.

Overview of its Applications in Various Fields

The revolution of 3D printing has revolutionized much, but above all biomedical engineering, whose uses span from tailored medical devices to printing organs and tissues. In prosthetics, for instance, 3D printing enables the creation of tailored-fit devices that enhance users' comfort and functionality. This personalized technique not only improves the patients experience but also promotes an increased sense of autonomy and quality of life. Practitioners can produce intricate designs that were previously unattainable with conventional methods by utilizing additive manufacturing techniques, culminating in the production of intricate parts as well as highly personalized products. The revolution that is brought forth by 3D printing extends into surgical planning, where real anatomy models are used for preoperative diagnosis and thus reduce risks in real procedures.

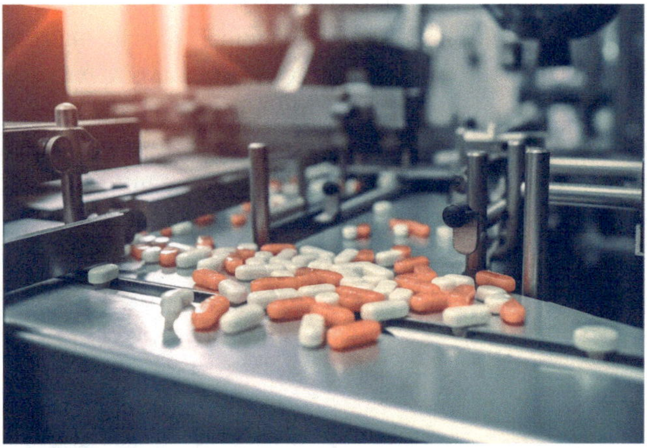

Figure 1.3. The ability to design and manufacture oral dosage forms on demand exemplifies the potential 3D printing holds in enhancing treatment compliance and effectiveness.

Source: https://encrypted-tbn0.gstatic.com/images?q=tbn:ANd9GcT_L-vb81zzFOjj5lzL0ItHG5z_PCuUEk1DLWEjvlxCiIXTxTaExd3yy_bfaR1rlklbNeY&usqp=CAU.

Furthermore, the convergence of 3D printing with regenerative medicine is a critical milestone, particularly with bioprinting tissues and organs. Through employing bio-inks derived from living cells, researchers can print structures similar to the natural tissues, which enables pathways for drug testing and transplantations without depending solely on animal models. It not only contributes to an understanding of human biology but also provides scope for creating patient-specific therapies and treatments. The ability to print tissues at will, functionally, can significantly alleviate organ shortages and provide patients with customized forms of care. As the evolution of industry 4.0 continues, the crossroads between smart manufacturing and bioprinting unlock new horizons for sustainable approaches and creative biomedical technologies that signal the state-of-the-art technology of the healthcare industry against different health complexities (Dehghanghadikolaei et al., 2019). Additionally, the business uses of 3D printing are further applied to pharmaceutical drug development, and there it shows the ability to tailor drug dosages and forms to specific needs. This tailor-made approach is especially valuable in pediatrics and geriatrics, where a one-size-fits-all dosage form is not adequate for the unique requirements of different patient groups. The on-demand construction and production of oral dosage forms represent the kind of value that 3D printing can bring to treatment compliance and efficacy. Aside from drugs, additive manufacturing techniques are also being explored for the production of intricate drug delivery systems capable of delivering drugs at controlled rates. Thus, the consequences of 3D printing in biomedical engineering not only bridge missing links in existing medical treatments but also require a more responsive healthcare system, accelerating advancements on many fronts, including the economic and environmental spheres engaged in the production of drugs and medical devices (Ewart et al., 2019) (Figure 1.3).

1.1. FUNDAMENTALS OF 3D PRINTING TECHNOLOGY

The evolution of 3D printing technology has revolutionized various industries, among them biomedical engineering being a particular special favorite. This process, otherwise referred to as additive manufacturing, allows for the layer-by-layer fabrication of objects directly from digital models. The great control of the final shape and structure of printed material has aided the development of customized implants, prosthetics, and medical devices that precisely address individual patient needs. One illustration of this technology is in the creation of ankle-foot orthoses (AFOs), where uniform structures allow for testing of stiffness and stress distribution integral to patient mobility and comfort. Such innovations not only augment the performance of medical devices but also their effortless integration into dominant clinical procedures, constituting a paradigm shift towards personalized medicine in medicine. Further accentuating the universality of 3D printing technology, its uses extend into tissue engineering and regenerative medicine. Bone graft substitutes, normally lifelines in cases of severe bone defects, are prime examples of the way 3D printing can contribute to breakthrough advances in biocompatible materials. The integration of scaffolds produced by rapid prototyping techniques makes it possible to design structures that mimic the natural architecture of bone to trigger cellular activities required for regeneration. These scaffolds possess some necessities such as porosity and mechanical properties similar to native tissue that are essential for enhancing vascularization and cell migration. Optimization of such scaffolds through the application of finite element analysis in association with advanced imaging techniques enables scaffolds to be tailored to meet the functional and mechanical needs of the native biological microenvironment and thereby enhance the possibility of successful clinical results (Jung et al., 2016). While technology in 3D printing is improving, its principles as a basis for the integration of methods into biomedical engineering remain essential to its application. The precision offered by digital fabrication opens up new possibilities in design and deployment of medical solutions. Moreover, the verification processes that are used in ensuring that devices made with 3D printing meet rigorous clinical requirements are of the utmost importance. Using AFOs, for example, finite element model construction can quantify such attributes as stiffness and position them in relation to patient-specific requirements (Beule et al., 2019). This considered care not only guarantees patient well-being but allows for the production of new designs that standard manufacturing cannot provide. The intersection of technology and personalized medicine holds forth the promise of a new era when 3D printing becomes the central focus of biomedical engineering solutions (Figure 1.4).

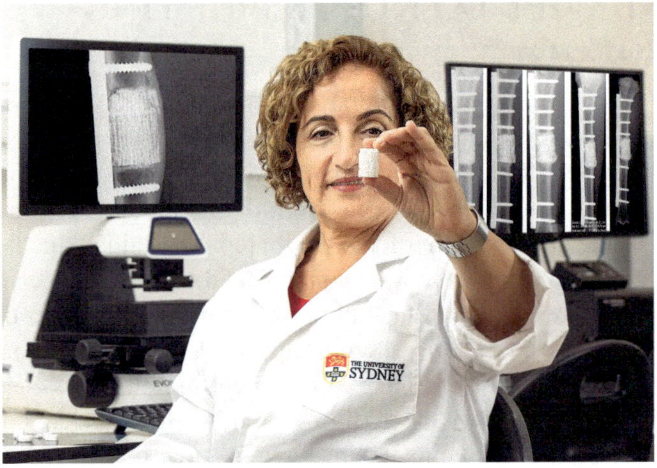

Figure 1.4. Bone graft substitutes, often critical in cases of severe bone defects, exemplify how 3D printing can foster innovations in biocompatible materials.

Source: https://createdigital.org.au/wp-content/uploads/2020/06/create-online-mag-hala-zreiqat-featured.jpg.

1.1.1. Explanation of Additive Manufacturing

Additive manufacturing (AM), or 3D printing, is a paradigm shift in production technologies, particularly in biomedical engineering. By and large, AM is the sequential additive creation of three-dimensional objects from digital models by layers, which grants unprecedent design freedom. Such a characteristic is particularly valuable in biomedical applications, where geometrical complexity and custom geometries can be decisive for the performance of medical devices, prosthetics, and tissue scaffolds. As a result, AM not only enhances the ability of manufacturing complex parts but also ensures an innovation-friendly culture for product development towards truly personalized medicine addressing individual patient needs (Dehghanghadikolaei et al., 2019). The integration of AM within the industry 4.0 scheme further increases its effect in biomedical engineering. With the advent of smarter manufacturing systems and novel information technologies, AM enables decentralized production. Decentralization enables rapid prototyping, which results in accelerated development cycles and reduced time-to-market for new biomedical devices.

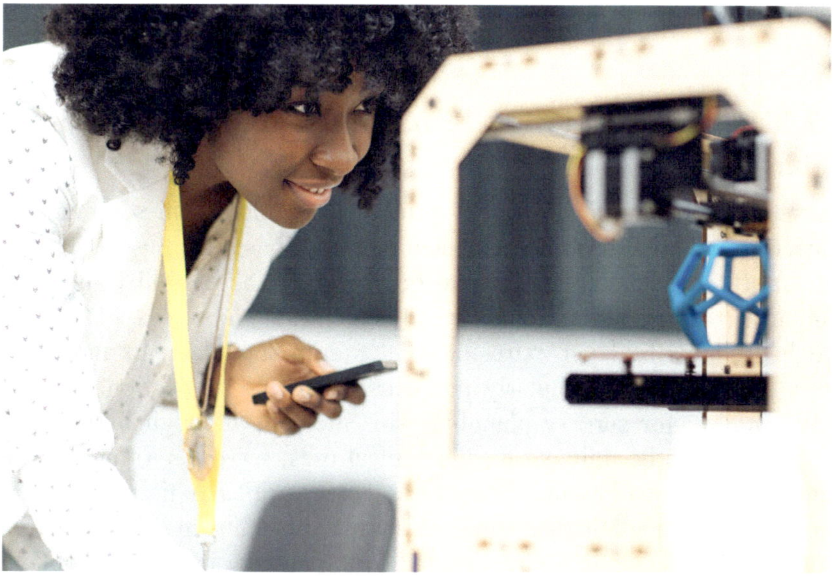

Figure 1.5. With the advent of smarter manufacturing systems and advanced information technologies, AM contributes to a more decentralized approach to production.

Source: https://www.ibm.com/content/dam/connectedassets-adobe-cms/worldwide-content/stock-assets/getty/image/others/8b/a8/8ba88b83-19d7-4a64-9806c1343ff604e8.jpg/_jcr_content/renditions/cq5dam.web.1280.1280.jpeg.

The technology also leads to massive material savings and reduced waste, enabling greater sustainability in manufacturing (Dehghanghadikolaei et al., 2019). These characteristics become all the more pertinent when considering the ever-growing high expectations of efficient and customized solutions in the healthcare industry, redefining AM as an intrinsic component of modern biomedical engineering processes. Moreover, the versatility of AM is also relevant to its potential for hybrid processing modes, which can enhance the quality and performance of biomedical components. For example, as demonstrated in recent studies, the combination of additive and subtractive processes allows complex molding inserts to be manufactured with improved surface finishes and performance for particulate injection molding (PIM) procedures. Hybridization of such processes not only precludes defect development associated with AM when working with challenging materials like titanium but demonstrates the kind of innovation that is possible through hybrid solutions. With the progression of biomedical engineering, exploration into these methods shows necessity in overcoming specific challenges in order to maximize on the advantages that additive manufacturing has to offer (Figure 1.5).

1.1.2. Types of 3D Printing Technologies used in Biomedical Engineering

There are a number of various 3D printing technologies in the biomedical engineering field that have unique benefits for various uses. Fused Deposition Modeling (FDM) stands out for its affordability and accessibility and is most commonly used in producing anatomical models and prototypes. FDM is done through the layer-by-layer extrusion of thermoplastic filaments into desired shapes, which could particularly prove useful in the production of patient-specific models for surgery planning. This method, although limited in the materials that can be imitated for biomedical uses, serves as a foundation for ongoing exploration of complex structures that are critical in tissue engineering and regenerative medicine, as stipulated in recent studies in the field (Chia et al., 2015). Selective Laser Sintering (SLS) is another significant technology applied in biomedical engineering, particularly due to its ability to manage a variety of materials including metals and polymers. It involves the use of a laser to join powdered materials together, layer by layer, to form solid objects. SLS is crucial in producing high-strength components of orthopedic implants and customized prosthetics due to its precision and strength. Besides, it allows for the development of scaffolds imitating the natural tissue architecture to allow cell growth and integration. SLS's ability to work with a variety of material compositions has potential in enhancing the biocompatibility of implants, thus addressing major challenges in patient-specific therapy and the construction of tissue engineering (Dehghanghadikolaei et al., 2019). Stereolithography (SLA) is another essential 3D printing technology that has gained popularity in biomedical engineering because of its unrivaled resolution and rapid prototyping. The process operates through photopolymerization, where the liquid resin is hardened by an illumination source to form solid shapes. SLAs high resolution is particularly helpful when creating extremely detailed designs, such as models for dental restorations or complex vascular structures. Moreover, the use of biomaterials with SLA can enable the creation of devices that closely mimic the human tissue properties. As such, studies keep advancing the materials and processes applied in SLA for creating complex organs and tissue constructs hitherto impossible, thereby developing the regenerative medicine field (Chia et al., 2015) (Figure 1.6).

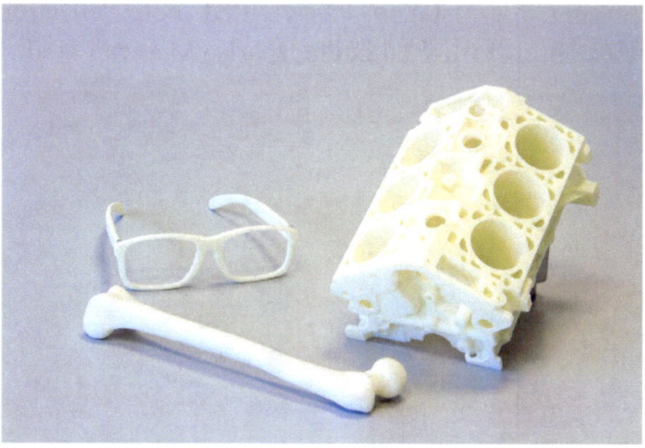

Figure 1.6. Selective laser sintering (SLS) represents another significant technology utilized in biomedical engineering, particularly for its ability to work with a variety of materials, including metals and polymers.

Source: https://www.ineo.es/images/2019/09/10/technologies-laser-sintering-sls-applications-glasses-bones-part.jpg.

1.1.3. Materials Commonly used in Biomedical 3D Printing

The material discovery in biomedical 3D printing reveals an extensive range of synthetic and natural polymers that are especially formulated for specific applications in regenerative medicine and tissue engineering. Poly-lactide (PLA) ranks among the top material due to its extreme popularity owing to its biodegradability and biocompatibility. PLAs flexibility makes it suitable to develop scaffolds that ensure structural support for cell culture as well as induce tissue integration. Furthermore, the creation of PLA formulations, including its blending with a variety of additives, has made it possible to enhance the mechanical properties of the scaffolds, as well as their applications in numerous applications in biomedical engineering fields. These developments facilitate the enhanced cell growth and proliferation, which enhance the scaffolds' ability to support living tissues, an important feature in constructing functional tissues for transplantation and repair. In addition, hydrogels have also been of particular interest in 3D printing within the field of biomedical applications due to their tunability and high-water content. Hyaluronic acid, gelatin, and alginate are common substances utilized in the formation of hydrogels, which form a biological environment that is favorable to cell growth and differentiation. Existing studies have demonstrated the effectiveness of chemically cross-linking such polymers into mechanically stable scaffolds without compromising porosity for the diffusion of nutrients and cell migration. Calcium chloride bath-induced cross-linking, for instance, has yielded increased structural stability compared to their non-cross-linked counterparts (Macwan et al., 2018).

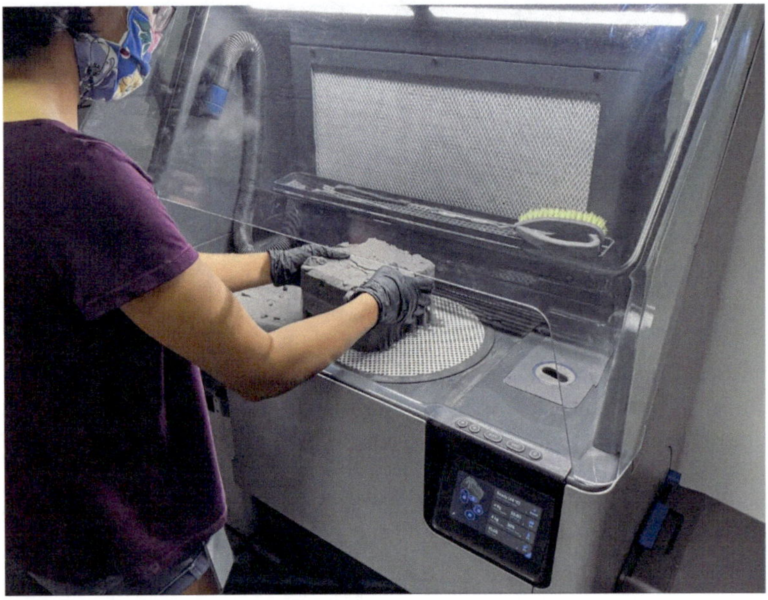

Figure 1.7. Materials such as hyaluronic acid, gelatin, and alginate are commonly employed in the fabrication of hydrogels, providing a biological environment conducive to cell growth and differentiation.

Source: https://img.facfox.com/imgs/2021/08/a939f50108a824e8.png.

This method depicts the adaptability of hydrogels to be designed for various tissue engineering tasks, ranging from organ regeneration to intraocular implant design, which depicts the pliability of materials in 3D printing. Furthermore, the insertion of cutting-edge materials such as carbon nanotubes into typical 3D printing scaffolds has provided new avenues for scaffold designing. Through the incorporation of these nanomaterials, the scaffolds' mechanical strength and electrical conductivity have been enhanced by researchers, thereby providing a suitable environment for cell attachment and growth. Not only does this procedure provide the physical requirements for scaffolding but also functionalizability of the scaffolds for drug release and gene delivery applications. For example, recent breakthroughs in poly-amidoamine dendrimers have revealed that they can make localized gene regulation possible, activate cell growth, and effective transfection of human cells (Abbaszadeh et al., 2018). These breakthroughs exhibit the ongoing evolution of materials used in biomedical 3D printing, an illustration of the fields commitment to improving healthcare treatment using engineered tissue constructs (Figure 1.7).

1.2. APPLICATIONS OF 3D PRINTING IN BIOMEDICAL ENGINEERING

The last few years have witnessed 3D printing introduce a paradigm shift in the field of biomedical engineering by enabling the production of very personalized medical appliances and prosthetics tailored to patients. The technology enables the production of complex geometries that are hard, if not impossible, to fabricate with traditional manufacturing methods. The emphasis on patient-customization has found its way into improved outcomes in a wide variety of applications, from orthopedic hardware to dental appliances. Furthermore, leveraging the rapid prototyping ability, engineers can quickly iterate design from clinical feedback with significantly reduced development time and cost. The ability to design medical solutions that are specific to the individual anatomy of every patient not only enhances functionality but also results in higher acceptability and satisfaction among patients, thus encouraging better healthcare practices overall. The other main application of 3D printing within biomedical engineering is the generation of bioprinted organs and tissue for transplantation and research purposes. This new method is centered on stacking living cells to create intricate tissue structures, potentially solving the continuing lack of available organ donors. With the aid of sophisticated printing methods, scientists have been able to create numerous types of tissue, from skin and cartilage to even vascular systems. Significantly, employing bioinks—substances that are capable of sustaining cell viability—is possible due to the formation of functional tissues that mimic natural anatomical features. Specifically, the use of bioprinting cannot just transform regenerative medicine but also facilitate drug testing by doing away with the use of animal models and rendering preclinical studies more meaningful. This development shows how 3D printing technologies are poised to take its place in future trends in personalized medicine, where patients will eventually be provided with tissues that are specifically designed for them. Moreover, the intersection of biomechanics and 3D printing has led to immense advances, particularly in making surgical models and preoperative planning. With the help of 3D printed models derived from the imaging information of patients, surgeons can better understand complex anatomical structures and can make accurate preoperative planning, thus helping in enhancing the accuracy of surgeries. These touch; patient-specific models promote more familiarity with the surgical area and can then decrease intraoperative operations and complication rates. The usability of 3D printing even facilitates the production of surgical guides that ensure suitable implant and other device placement. These advancements indicate the revolutionary potential of additive manufacturing, as aided by its alignment with trends towards industrial development (Dehghanghadikolaei et al., 2019). With continued development, continued research into incorporating new materials and methods has the promise to achieve more value in various arenas in the field of biomedical engineering (Farahi et al., 2010).

1.2.1. Custom Prosthetics and Orthotics

The development of 3D printing technology has significantly impacted the scope of biomedical engineering, especially in custom prosthetic and orthotic design and fabrication. The conventional design and production of such devices tended to be very time-consuming with little scope for customization, leading to the creation of devices that sometimes were not well-suited to the individual requirements of the patient. 3D printing, in contrast, enables the production of tailored devices specifically to accommodate the unique anatomy and functional requirements of each user. Such customization, apart from enhancing comfort, also optimizes the devices' overall performance during rehabilitation and normal use. Therefore, patients are more likely to utilize their devices, resulting in greater therapy compliance and overall outcomes. The integration of computational modeling and 3D printing techniques has also optimized the production of ankle-foot orthoses (AFOs) with the advantage of providing a platform for valid quantification and examination of design variables. In a recent investigation, it was demonstrated how application of advanced computer modeling software coupled with 3D printing resulted in a framework for examination of the stiffness of the ankle in several AFO designs and optimized their efficiency as well as conformity to patient needs. By utilizing finite element (FE) modeling, researchers can simulate the stresses and distributions that are experienced by natural movement and allow the creation of AFOs that offer more support for dynamic function. Model validation was encouraging, demonstrating the tremendous potential of 3D printing in the manufacturing process as well as the overall design of custom orthotics to develop more patient-specific solutions (Beule et al., 2019). Additionally, the cost-effectiveness of 3D printing has become a critical advantage, such that customized prosthetic solutions are made affordable to large groups of people. Traditional methods of fabrication are usually associated with outlandish prices, rendering them inaccessible to many who require such devices. By using additive manufacturing techniques, as demonstrated in a case study involving a prosthetic clinic, customized devices were produced at significantly reduced costs—up to 56% less than their similar traditional laminated counterparts. Not only cost savings but also extremely high levels of patient satisfaction, as the example demonstrates, shows the viability of 3D printed prosthetics as a viable solution for individuals requiring customized assistive devices. Enhanced accessibility not only promotes health equity but also encourages creative applications of technology within the biomedical sciences, revealing the revolutionary power of 3D printing in patient rehabilitation and care (Day et al., 2018) (Figure 1.8).

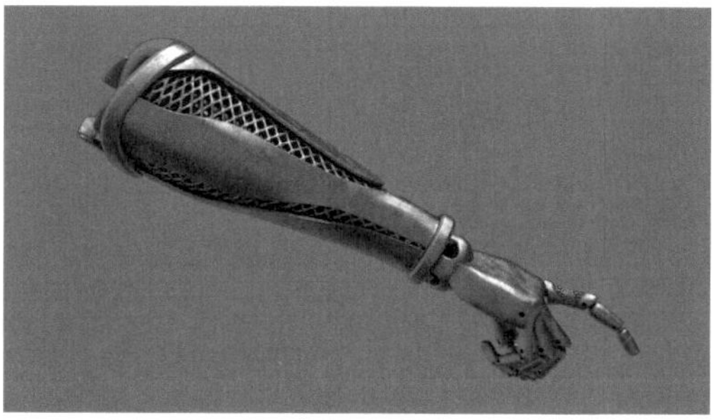

Figure 1.8. 3D printing, however, enables the production of tailored devices that match the unique anatomical and functional requirements of each user.

Source: https://www.ntop.com/_next/image/?url=https%3A%2F%2Fcdn.sanity.io%2Fimages%2Fg5181r9i%2Fproduction%2Fdda9a87c554468c86295989d075bad743dc30db6-1999x1125.png%3Fq%3D75%26fit%3Dclip%26auto%3Dformat&w=3840&q=80.

1.2.2. Bioprinting of Tissues and Organs

The advent of bioprinting represents a landmark moment in the coming together of biomedical engineering and regenerative medicine. Making use of extremely sophisticated 3D printing technologies, researchers can now print out complex tissue structures that closely mirror the structure and function of human organs. This is achieved through tactical layer-by-layer building of bioinks made up of living cells and biocompatible materials. As the tissues are developed, the cellular elements begin to arrange themselves in well-defined patterns, allowing for increased cell interaction and growth. Advances in this area not only have the potential to create beneficial tissue for transplantation but also enable the creation of more accurate models for drug discovery and disease research, potentially ending the use of animal models on a vast scale and improving pharmaceutical development with efficiency. One of the critical aspects of bioprinting is the employment of pluripotent stem cells, such as human embryonic stem cells (hESCs) and induced pluripotent stem cells (hiPSCs). They have the potency to differentiate into a variety of specialized cell types needed to construct complex tissue structures.

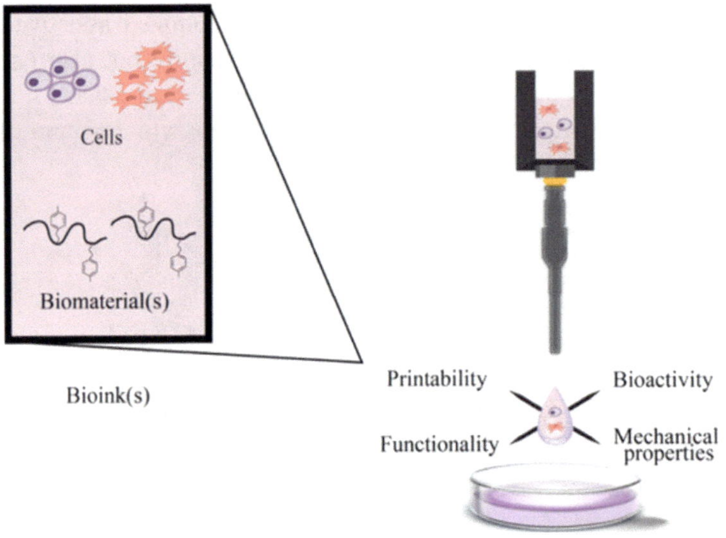

Figure 1.9. Nanogels, offer an innovative approach to enhancing the biocompatibility and functionality of bioinks used in bioprinting.

Source: https://www.mdpi.com/polymers/polymers-17-00917/article_deploy/html/images/polymers-17-00917-g005-550.jpg.

The use of stem cells takes advantage of their potential to generate functional tissues with characteristics akin to native organs. Existing research has proven the feasibility of producing functional tissues such as hepatic, cardiac, and vascular tissues through bioprinting techniques. The effectiveness of these uses, however, requires overcoming monumental challenges such as maintaining the viability of cells throughout printing and having sufficient vascularization in printed tissues to support long-term survival. These developments reflect both the promise and the complexities of bioprinting research, necessitating continued investigation and refinement within the field. The incorporation of nanotechnology into the bioprinting process still expands the range and possibility of 3D-printed organs and tissues. Nanogels, for instance, introduce an innovative way of increasing the biocompatibility and functionality of bioinks used in bioprinting. These architectures are produced by spanning nanoscopic micelles within a water-based system in which hydrophilic and hydrophobic payloads can be strategically loaded in support of tissue engineering and regenerative care. As the demand increases for highly engineered biomaterials that are personalized and provided to address particular requirements, the use of 3D printing within the fabrication process of nanogels is increasing (Cho et al., 2018). Their integration into bioprinted models also promises enormous potential for greater therapeutic efficacy and the delivery of a wider range of biological materials, expanding the applications of regenerative medicine and paving the way for more complex treatments tailored to individual patients (Figure 1.9).

1.2.3. Development of Surgical Models and Tools

The fast pace of development of surgical devices and models is highly influenced by the development in 3D printing technology. With this new technology, it becomes feasible to create highly accurate, patient-specific anatomical models with the potential to enhance preoperative planning and intraoperative navigation. With the utilization of imaging modality-derived information such as computed tomography (CT) data and magnetic resonance imaging (MRI) data, 3D printing has the capability to generate replicas of complex anatomical structures. Consequently, surgeons are provided with a better vision of the surgical landscape and can anticipate potential complications. These custom models not only improve surgery outcomes but also serve as a valuable tool in educating up-coming medical practitioners, hence enhancing the quality of care provided to patients. Furthermore, the use of new materials by 3D printing is transforming the fabrication of surgical equipment. Biocompatible material technological advancements, including nanogels, enhance the functionality of surgical instruments by increasing their functional properties. For example, use of nanomaterials enhances drug delivery systems that are critical in surgery, which results in delivery of treatment at the site with minimal side effects on the body as a whole. Use of 3D-printed equipment made from advanced materials can lead to lighter, yet more efficient equipment, improving maneuverability and reducing the fatigue on surgical teams. As the biomedical field moves towards personalized medicine, the ways to personalize instruments appropriate to the individual patient's specifications will undoubtedly revolutionize the practice of surgery. The Fourth Industrial Revolution, Industry 4.0, emphasizes the revolutionary capability of 3D printing, thereby highlighting its significance in the field of biomedical engineering. With additive manufacturing (AM) advancing every day, decentralized forms of production are enabled by it, which facilitate quick prototyping and efficient ways of utilizing resources with less wastage. This capability is in line with greater emphasis on sustainability in healthcare. The development of novel materials and technology opens up the potential scope of usage of AM for surgery from customized implants to surgical models that enhance clinical workflows. As further research in this field continues to develop, applications of 3D printing for surgical instruments and models suggest not only improved outcomes for patients but also the broader trajectory towards more efficient and sustainable medical practices (Cho et al., 2018; Dehghanghadikolaei et al., 2019).

1.3. ADVANTAGES OF 3D PRINTING IN HEALTHCARE

3D printing technology has transformed healthcare to a great extent through rapid prototyping of medical devices and tailor-made solutions according to unique patient needs. It is possible to produce highly personalized prosthetics and implants that can be designed according to the unique anatomy of the patient. For instance, 3D printing enables the production of patient-specific anatomical models that are accessible to surgeons for use during preoperative planning, improving surgery accuracy and results. Through 3D printing, design and manufacturing time is reduced compared to traditional manufacturing methods, thereby allowing health practitioners to deploy solutions faster, providing timely interventions that ultimately enhance patient care and safety. Apart from personalized implants and surgical instruments, 3D printing also holds promise in tissue engineering and regenerative medicine. With bio-ink made from living cells, researchers and physicians can print tissue structures that may be used to replace human organs. The technology provides the potential to make organ models for drug testing and disease research and decrease animal testing. Furthermore, the convergence of novel materials, like those in organic thin film electronic devices and bio-responsive hydrogels, shows the promise for 3D printing to lead to breakthrough applications for assistive healthcare. Such breakthroughs can potentially involve smart bandages that can track a wound and release medication based on it, a revolutionary leap in responsive patient care (Oliver et al., 2009). The economic contribution of 3D printing to the healthcare industry should not be downplayed, given that it provides channels for cost minimization of manufacturing medical devices and waste reduction. Traditional manufacturing involves huge overheads, lengthy production time, and huge material wastage. In contrast, 3D printing promotes on-demand manufacturing that eliminates inventory costs and logistics costs associated with global supply chains. By embracing a hybrid approach that supports additive manufacturing with traditional processes such as injection molding, healthcare institutions can optimize their workflow, leading to efficiency in operations. Through a series of case studies, the incorporation of 3D printing in medical procedures makes a niche platform for innovation, disrupts prototyping constraints, and promotes environmentalism in the domain of biomedical engineering (Ewart et al., 2019) (Figure 1.10).

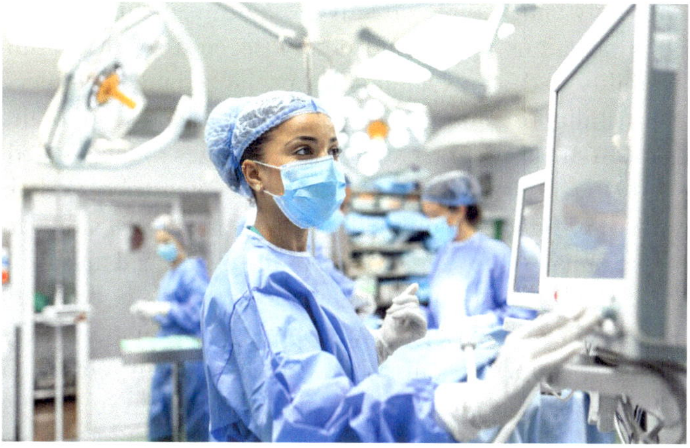

Figure 1.10. As 3D printing reduces design and production times compared to traditional manufacturing methods, healthcare providers can deploy solutions more rapidly, providing timely interventions that ultimately enhance patient care and safety.

Source: https://nota3d.com/wp-content/uploads/2023/07/healthcare-3D-print-pic-1080x675.jpg.

1.3.1. Personalization of Medical Devices

The history of biomedical devices has increasingly been centered on personalization, enabling customized therapies that are tightly tailored to the anatomy and specific requirements of patients. Personalization not only increases the effectiveness of medical treatments but also improves patient outcomes and satisfaction. 3D printing is now a revolutionary technology in biomedical engineering that provides unprecedented flexibility in the creation of customized medical devices. Unlike traditional manufacturing methods that are prone to rely on standard designs, 3D printing allows patient-specific devices, such as implants and prosthetics, to be designed to fit exactly each patient's unique anatomical features. This trend towards customization marks the value placed on patient-centered care in modern medicine where devices can now be optimized for better integration into a patient's life as well as body. One stark illustration of the personalization in medical device fabrication through 3D printing is that of fabrication of tailored stent grafts. One recent technique outlines the employment of a multi-robot system specifically to fabricate such customized stents. Such a system takes the form of a modular setup involving various modules, including a mandrel module with patient-specific geometry. By being individually designed to meet the particular requirements of each patient, such stents not only enhance the effectiveness of treatment but also minimize the risk of complications that would otherwise be associated with ill-fitting devices. The ability to design such highly specialized medical interventions is proof of the possibility of improved patient outcomes and proof of the immense advancements that 3D printing technology contributes to the biomedicine field (Hu et al., 2017). The use of extremely sophisticated robots combined with 3D printing also introduces additional personalization of healthcare devices. For instance, the bimanual sewing module of the mentioned multi-robot system relies on a learning-by-demonstration approach, accurately replicating human hand-sewing to achieve highly precise manufacturing of stents. Through this method, the robots can synchronize immaculately, again reproducing human capabilities but with precision. With this, the employment of robot systems in manufacturing paves the way for flexible production, enabling more varieties of customized products to accommodate the various needs of patients. In the long run, the technology not only streamlines the manufacturing process but also introduces new benchmarks for personalization in the development of medical devices (Chunmin et al., 2016).

1.3.2. Reduction in Production Costs and Time

The application of 3D printing technology in biomedical engineering has transformed production processes radically with significant time and cost reductions. Traditionally, manufacturing medical devices involved a significant amount of machining and prototyping stages with accompanying high labor and material waste costs. 3D printing eliminates all these challenges using additive manufacturing with little material waste and the ability to create complex designs that were unattainable previously. As noted, the increased design ability that 3D printing offers facilitates the production of highly tailored products made to meet the specific patient needs and also speed up the entire manufacturing process. Through efficient optimization of the process from design to manufacturing, 3D printing not only reduces costs associated with traditional manufacturing but also reduces the time taken to bring new biomedical products to market (Dehghanghadikolaei et al., 2019). In addition, the speeding up of prototyping stages plays a significant role in the evolution of new biomedical devices. Traditional development processes typically require multiple cycles to result in optimal structure and performance, creating long periods of time with increasing costs. On the other hand, 3D printing facilitates quick prototyping, and this permits designers and engineers to design and test several iterations in a short time and effectively. This cycle of iteration allows for quicker decision-making and instant feedback, which is crucial in a discipline where accuracy and effectiveness play such a critical role. Research has shown that using a combination of additive and subtractive methods of manufacturing can improve the quality of production without compromising on cost-effectiveness. By combining these techniques, companies can further enhance the improvement process, reflecting how 3D printing significantly minimizes time and money spent otherwise normatively needed to design a product in biomedical engineering (Ewart et al., 2019). Additionally, the decentralized nature of production processes offered through 3D printing enables further cost and time savings. Traditional production in most cases utilizes older centralized manufacturing plants that may be distant from end users, which increases shipping distances and costs. With 3D printing, localized production is a possibility where production facilities produce necessary biomedical components on location whenever there is need. This not only saves on transportation costs but also responds to emergent medical needs with fast turnaround times. Also, as the technology is utilized to enhance supply chains and propel innovation in the usage of materials, 3D printing is directly impacting how the economics of biomedical manufacturing are being changed. Thus, organizations in the sector can more effectively control resources, and that results in improved patient care and industry advancement overall (Dehghanghadikolaei et al., 2019).

1.3.3. Enhanced Patient Outcomes and Satisfaction

The use of 3D printing technology in biomedical engineering has significantly transformed the care of patients for improved outcomes and satisfaction levels. Through enabling the creation of tailored medical devices, implants, and prosthetics that match a patient, 3D printing is central to achieving personalized healthcare solutions. Through facilitating the proper fit and performance of medical interventions, customization raises the confidence and comfort levels of patients. Greater satisfaction is experienced as patients receive devices better aligned with their specific anatomical and functional needs, often leading to shorter recovery times and overall improved health. The ability to generate personalized, patient-specific solutions gives a sense of investment and engagement in their own treatment, and therefore greater overall satisfaction with medical care. Furthermore, the rapid prototyping aspect in 3D printing facilitates iterating medical models and devices for surgical planning or training.

This allows health experts to be capable of visualizing complex anatomies and developing more precise intervention plans. Based on the laydown in current research studies, the use of 3D-printed anatomical models has shown to significantly enhance preoperative knowledge of complex patient cases, and consequently surgical success. By minimizing the risk factors associated with procedures through better planning and execution, 3D printing has a direct impact on improved patient outcomes. As a result, medical professionals are given the tools necessary to provide personalized care, which ultimately results in higher rates of patient satisfaction and faith in the health care system, a reflection of the profound impact of 3D technology on the practice of medicine (Ewart et al., 2019). Additionally, the ability of 3D printing to save costs and time in manufacturing is paramount in enhancing patient satisfaction. By streamlining the manufacturing process of medical devices and accessories, hospitals are able to provide timely intervention to patients, thus eliminating complications related to delays. This efficiency in production, coupled with the option to add superior materials to ensure greater biocompatibility, results in devices that not only perform better but also meet changing patient needs more closely. As more patient-centered healthcare emerges, emphasis on effective and efficient care delivery becomes greater, paving the way for improved health outcomes. The intersection of cost-effectiveness and patient satisfaction addresses the transformative potential of 3D printing in biomedical engineering, combining health service objectives with the ultimate goal of optimizing patient care (Phelps et al., 2004) (Figure 1.11).

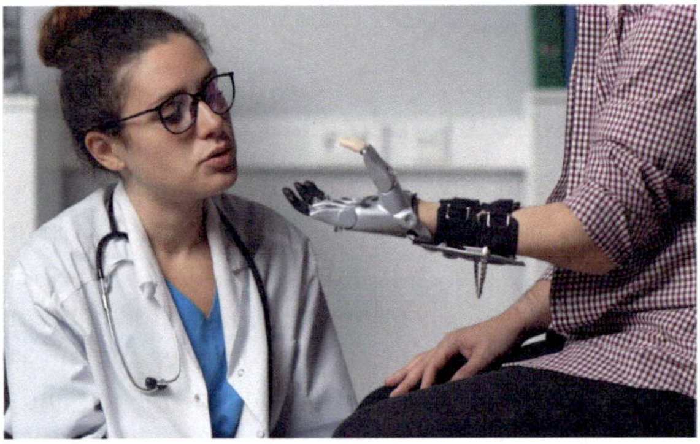

Figure 1.11. By enabling customized medical devices, implants, and prosthetics tailored to individual patients, 3D printing plays a critical role in achieving personalized healthcare solutions.

Source: https://edstechnologies.com/wp-content/uploads/2024/12/freepik__expand__12679.png.

1.4. CHALLENGES AND LIMITATIONS OF 3D PRINTING

Despite the widespread advancements in 3D printing technology, various challenges and limitations stifle the application of 3D printing in the biomedical industry on a wide scale. One of the main challenges is the regulatory mechanism that controls bio-printed goods and materials. Legal guidelines for the clearing of 3D-printed biomedical products are poorly outlined in most regions, opening doors to potential risks to innovation and use. Regulations fall behind technology advancements, creating uncertainties which impact the commercialization pace of life-saving products. Further, the heterogeneity in the mechanical characteristics and biocompatibility of 3D-printed materials makes validation processes more challenging because manufacturers must establish that printed devices meet rigorous requirements for safety before use in clinical settings. Thus, resolving such regulatory issues becomes key to incorporating 3D printing into standard biomedical practice, with a pressing need for collaborative effort from regulatory bodies, scientists, and industry actors. Moreover, scalability remains a significant problem in 3D printing technology development for biomedical purposes. Even though 3D printing allows for the fabrication of customized solutions with matching parameters in individual patients, such processes are limited in terms of throughput and speed. Such processes as Fused Deposition Modeling and Stereolithography, while useful in the prototype, may not be sufficient to scale up rapidly to print large quantities of detailed structures needed for production of certain medical devices on a large scale. It requires not just technological innovation but also tweaking of material consistency and resolutions of prints to transition from prototype to bulk production. These limitations must be overcome to allow 3D printing to move from specialist use to mainstream application in the healthcare industry, particularly in areas like tissue engineering and organ transplantation where demand is opening up at a rapid rate. Also, the materials allowable for 3D printing in healthcare are still relatively fewer than those in traditional manufacturing processes. While new biocompatible materials have been made accessible with the evolution of technology in recent years, these material features do not closely resemble natural tissue's sophisticated mechanical and biological functions. As noted in ongoing studies, it remains challenging to produce structures involving complex 3D microarchitectures by means of 3D printing techniques to construct functionally relevant tissues and organs. Additionally, material used for 3D printing tends to have flow variability and bonding characteristics that impact the mechanical performance of resulting products. Hence, extensive research and development of new materials that can provide the required biological properties and meet regulatory standards is crucial in order to address these issues, allowing 3D printing to realize its full potential in the field of biomedical engineering (Chia et al., 2015; Dehghanghadikolaei et al., 2019).

1.4.1. Regulatory and Ethical Considerations

The arrival of 3D printing technology in biomedical engineering brings in a whole gamut of regulatory and ethical considerations that are the requirement for right development. Among the top regulatory challenges is how to classify 3D printed biomedical devices. Regulatory institutions, such as the FDA, will need to create comprehensive frameworks that can create space for the particular nature of these devices, ranging from prosthetics to bioprinted tissues. This requires a knowledge of how the current regulations are to be implemented and what modifications need to be made for maintaining safety and efficacy. The personalized aspect of 3D printed devices complicates approval since standardization becomes impossible in the presence of tailor-made therapies. There has to be clear guidelines to promote innovation while ensuring patient safety and public trust in these emerging technologies. Ethics also play a role with the use of 3D printing technology in medicine. The ability of bioprinting human tissue brings into question the ethics of creating life-like constructs. Concerns with consent, ownership of the bioprinted tissue, and the potential for exploitation among vulnerable populations must be addressed. With the technology ongoing, the establishment of ethical standards is imperative to prevent misuse and maintain patients' rights. Moreover, the disparities among socioeconomic groups may widen, and this may lead to ethical dilemmas over access to innovative biomedical technologies. All the stakeholders, including researchers, clinicians, and policymakers, will need strong discussion to be able to effectively overcome the obstacles, providing equitable access and equitable practices in applying this groundbreaking technology. The governing of the technology must also address the dimension of handling data and privacy for 3D printing in medical centers. As these technologies collect and make use of large volumes of patient information for personalization and improvement, the threat of data breaches and misuse exists. It is critical to have robust data protection safeguards in place in maintaining patients' confidentiality and trust. The regulatory bodies must develop guidelines that address both physical and digital aspects of 3D printing, focusing on safeguarding patient information, informed consent, and ethical handling of biologically derived materials. Balancing innovation with ethics and compliance with regulations will play a vital role in seamlessly integrating 3D printing in the healthcare model eventually developing a safe and fair environment for the creation of medical technology (Kumar et al., 2023; Miura et al., 2017) (Figure 1.12).

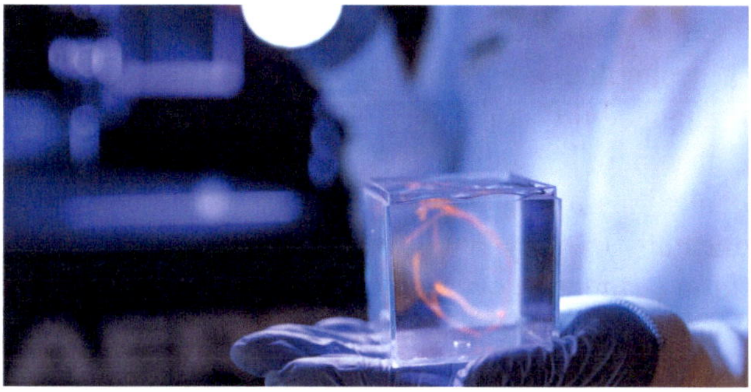

Figure 1.12. The ability to bioprint human tissues opens up debates regarding the moral implications of creating life-like structures.

Source: https://engineering.stanford.edu/sites/default/files/styles/card_1900x950/public/media/image/tfoe_bioprinting_0.jpg?h=0f4230fa&itok=SpcnsWfr.

1.4.2. Technical Limitations and Material Constraints

The evolution of 3D printing in biomedical engineering, although revolutionary, is severely handicapped by a collection of technical and material constraints. Among the primary challenges is a materials availability for application in medicine. Unlike traditional manufacturing methods, which rely on a broad spectrum of metals and polymers, 3D printing materials are normally limited to a few polymers and composites that may not possess the mechanical properties or biocompatibility required in such critical applications as implants or prosthetics. Besides that, the demand for materials that can perfectly mimic the mechanical properties of biological tissues is another constraint, and current materials could result in integration failure or side effects within the human body. Reports assert that the development of new materials demands that innovation must overcome these constraints to unlock the full potential of additive manufacturing in the medical industry (Dehghanghadikolaei et al., 2019). Another significant limitation pertains to the fidelity and resolution of the 3D printing technologies themselves. The layer-by-layer buildup process can influence surface finish and dimension integrity of the printed components. In the biomedical application, where accuracy is of paramount significance, danger from dimensional errors is compounded to include effects on function and patient outcomes. For instance, during the production of customized implants, minute deviations from the desired design may create misfits, and thus complications emanating during procedures on the operating table. This is clearly evident in complex geometries often required for anatomical compatibility, as depicted in a number of studies indicating problems on the MESO-scale features and complex cross-sections during manufacturing operations (Ewart et al., 2019). Therefore, continued advancement of technologies used in 3D printing is crucial to further improving the utilitarian applicability of this technology in biomedical engineering. Additionally, sustainability and access to 3D printing technologies present additional complexities to material constraints. As the industry transitions to more environmentally friendly practices, the environmental impact of materials used in 3D printing cannot be overlooked. The challenge is not only to identify biocompatible and effective materials, but also to manufacture them sustainably. The limitations of such constraints extend beyond the issues of the environment but directly affect the economic viability of 3D printing operations. For instance, studies on affordable alternatives often involve compromising quality or performance (Dehghanghadikolaei et al., 2019). Bridging these technical limitations by driving innovation in developing sustainable materials is the linchpin of the future of biomedical engineering 3D printing where improved patient outcomes and better healthcare solutions are achieved.

1.4.3. Cost Implications for Widespread Adoption

The introduction of quick 3D printing technology in biomedical engineering has witnessed new patient-specific solutions but implementing it on a large scale is very costly. The cost of purchasing 3D printing machines, materials, and medical staff training may be very expensive at first. For healthcare institutions, the significant cost of acquiring and maintaining sophisticated printers may deter shifting from traditional manufacturing methods. Moreover, ensuring that 3D printing is compatible with existing workflows entails not only infrastructure changes but also the likelihood of lost time in the transition period. Long-term cost-benefit considerations remain pertinent, with lower costs of production and better patient outcomes potentially having upfront financial expenses recovered over time. When stakeholders balance these considerations, financial projections will be the primary consideration determining whether to adopt or not adopt this new technology. Apart from installation costs, running costs also contribute significantly to assessing the feasibility of universal application of 3D printing in biomedical procedures. The varying cost of biocompatible materials used in 3D printing processes varies with market demands and supply levels, thereby influencing budgeting among health institutions. In addition, the requirement for trained personnel to operate and monitor the printing operations also contributes to the financial complexity, which necessitates training programs that are time-and-cost-intensive. Compliance expenses to regulatory standards may also be considerable, as products need to meet rigorous testing prior to their clinical application. Therefore, while 3D printing has numerous uses in personalized medicine, the cost of operation at present must be carefully scrutinized by medical facilities that aim to incorporate these technologies in a sustainable manner. The costs could extend to the overall healthcare system as well because the deployment of 3D printing affects the economics of caring for patients. For instance, tailor-made prosthetics and implants created through 3D printing have the ability to enhance treatment outcomes by allowing quicker recovery and reduced future healthcare costs (Ast et al., 2020). Although this transition is expected to create a short-term surge in expenditures with regard to the purchase and installation of necessary technologies. Also, effective reimbursement policies for 3D-printed medical devices need to be instituted to enable healthcare practitioners to recoup costs and encourage innovation. Finally, as the medical industry weighs the efficacy of 3D printing technologies, the linkage between initial cost and aggregate long-term cost savings will dictate their position as a pillar in biomedical engineering (Bini et al., 2020) (Figure 1.13).

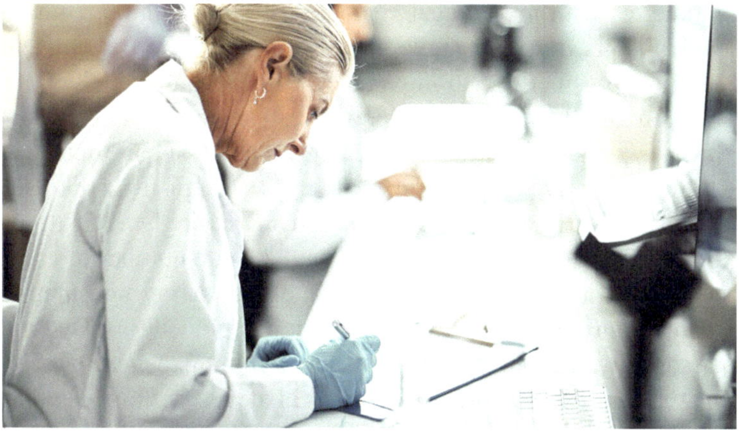

Figure 1.13. Costs associated with compliance to regulatory standards can also be considerable, as products must meet rigorous testing before they can be used clinically.

Source: https://www.scilife.io/hubfs/A-Guide-to-Accelerating-Your-Regulatory-Submissions.jpg.

1.5. CASE STUDIES IN 3D PRINTING APPLICATIONS

The application of 3D printing technology in biomedical engineering has also come a long way through a wealth of case studies documenting its revolutionary potential. A key domain is the development of low-cost molds for particulate injection molding (PIM). Using the synergy between additive and subtractive manufacturing techniques, researchers have created prototype molds that effectively demonstrate the feasibility of using complex geometries in medical devices. The project brought to the fore the strengths and weaknesses of different modes of production, revealing areas such as the finish on the surface and part removal defect when an individual uses blends of titanium metal. The above case outlines how technology in combination with methodology can optimize product development and reduce costs, ultimately making advanced biomedical application more affordable for manufacturers and medical care providers (Ewart et al., 2019). In addition, additive manufacturing trends reflect Industry 4.0 goals where smart systems and information technologies converge to redefine how production is conducted. In particular, 3D printing is a bedrock for innovation in this system since it facilitates the creation of mechanically advanced parts that can be developed to meet exact patient specifications. For instance, tissue engineering case studies illustrate how bioprinting can design scaffold structures with mechanical characteristics that mimic natural tissues. These developments not only make prototyping easier but also enhance the customization of prosthetics and implants and thus enhance patient outcomes. The application of 3D printing in biomedical engineering is the future of medicine where personalized therapy becomes progressively more viable and efficient with innovative production techniques (Dehghanghadikolaei et al., 2019). Sustainability is also emerging as an increasingly crucial parameter for biomedical uses of 3D printing. There have been a number of case studies that have indicated reducing material wastage and energy consumption with additive manufacturing over traditional subtractive procedures. By on-demand production capacity, medical systems are able to minimize environmental costs of manufacturing and distribution of medical devices. Greater concern for environmental stewardship also manifests through efforts toward the utilization of biodegradable printing materials. As identified by various studies, this attempt enhances the confidence that 3D printing not only facilitates technological development but also ensures a sustainable future in biomedical areas as an integral element of modern engineering practices (Dehghanghadikolaei et al., 2019).

1.5.1. Successful Implementation in Orthopedic Surgery

The integration of 3D printing technology in orthopedic surgery has been a breakthrough, highly enhancing procedural efficacy, and patient outcomes. The technology allows for the individualization of implants based on the anatomy of the patient, hence making successful surgery more likely. Patient-specific imaging data can be utilized to create customized implants for better fit and alignment, two aspects that are very vital in the longevity and functionality of orthopedic procedures. Along with that, the ability to produce scaffolds that can mimic natural bone tissue allows for improved integration of the implant into the biological tissue with reduced recovery time and increased overall patient satisfaction. The success of 3D printing technology is not just a surgery breakthrough in terms of accuracy but also a step towards patient-centered care in orthopedics that underscores the significance of innovation in achieving maximum surgical success. In addition to custom implant fabrication, 3D printing is also applied in preoperative planning and education. Surgeons are able to create accurate physical replicas of their patient's anatomy, allowing for thorough preoperative assessment and enhanced visualization of complex cases.

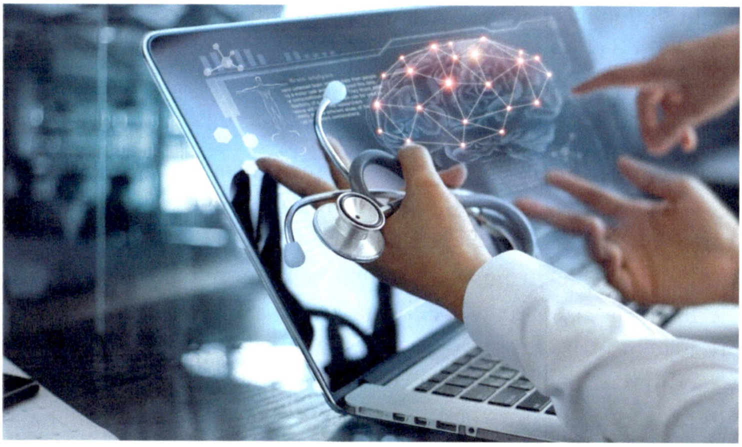

Figure 1.14. Personalized implants derived from patient-specific imaging data can improve fit and alignment, which are critical factors in the longevity and functionality of orthopedic interventions.

Source: https://physiciansgroupllc.com/wp-content/uploads/2024/01/Neurosurgery-1.webp.

This advanced planning helps reduce intraoperative complications because surgeons are able to plan individualized surgeries according to the specific needs of each patient. Secondarily, 3D-printed models are also beneficial training tools for surgical residents, with simulation practice of authentic anatomical forms. Training has the potential for greater surgical competence and confidence, and consequently, better patient care. As orthopedic surgery progresses, the utilization of digital technologies and 3D printing is a commitment to increasing the quality of care, with the technology having the promise to deliver improved surgical outcomes. The rapid adoption of digital health technology during the COVID-19 pandemic further amplified the influence of technology on orthopedic practice, providing opportunities for successful deployment of innovations like 3D printing. The revolution in rules and the reimbursement system at that point in time enabled faster incorporation of these technologies, remapping the destiny of orthopedic surgery. As explained in various studies, not only have computer tools facilitated remote management of the patient but also offered valuable aid in operating rooms through better planning and preparation capabilities (Ast et al., 2020). Besides, comparative studies revealed that while both open and endoscopic procedures have positive results, using advanced manufacturing techniques like 3D printing has the potential to tailor procedures and promote successful use in complicated situations (Bini et al., 2020). Thus, future orthopedic surgery will become increasingly incorporated with digital and 3D printing technologies, which will result in improved care delivery and patient satisfaction (Figure 1.14).

1.5.2. Use in Dental Applications

The integration of 3D printing technologies in dentistry is a milestone achievement in biomedical engineering. Through this new approach, dentists can design highly customized dental appliances like crowns, bridges, and orthodontic aligners according to the unique anatomical needs of individual patients. With the use of patient-specific anatomical data, dental practitioners are able to produce models that not only optimize fit and comfort but also aesthetic outcomes. With the development of such technologies, it becomes increasingly feasible to create complex structures, for instance, dental implants and tissue engineering scaffoldings, rendering conventional dentistry irrelevant while making treatment protocols more effective (Chia et al., 2015). The possibility of rapid prototyping of dental products also has far-reaching implications for patient care, particularly in treatment plan implementation. Personalization is not merely limited to end products, as 3D printing makes it possible to produce pre-surgical visualization models that can aid practitioners in expecting and preparing for difficult cases. Through enhanced communication among patients and experts, printed models offer a tangible illustration of available treatments, leading to informed discussions and concrete treatment decisions. In essence, the development of additive manufacturing technologies is not merely technological innovation; it is a paradigm shift in how dental healthcare providers interact with their patients throughout treatment (Ali et al., 2019). Despite the promising advances, the extensive incorporation of 3D printing technology in dentistry has its downsides. Difficulty in material properties, printer ability, and regulatory requirements are obstacles that must be overcome prior to the application of these technologies in day-to-day practice. The field is witnessing ongoing research and research activity to overcome these limitations, like exploring a vast array of biomaterials that can mimic biologically behaving structures and materials. As such technological issues are addressed, the potential for 3D printing to revolutionize dental solutions—from surgical guides to fully functional implants—is increasing, which holds out the possibility of a new age in customized dental care and treatment (Chia et al., 2015) (Figure 1.15).

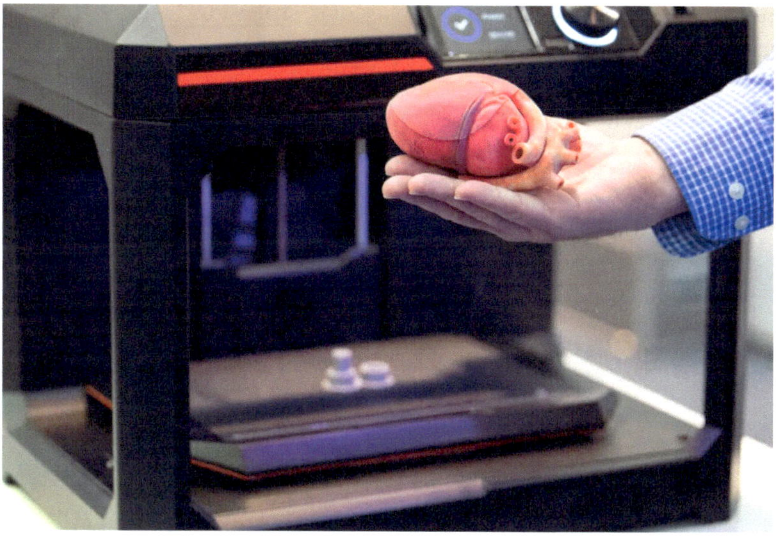

Figure 1.15. Customization extends beyond just the final products, as 3D printing allows for the generation of pre-surgical visualization models that can help practitioners anticipate and adapt to unique case challenges.

Source: https://www.thomasnet.com/insights/_next/image/?url=https%3A%2F%2Fthomasmkt.wpengine.com%2Fwp-content%2Fuploads%2F2023%2F10%2F3d-printed-heart.jpg&w=3840&q=75.

1.5.3. Advancements in Cardiovascular Treatments

The cardiovascular treatment scenario has undergone a revolutionary shift, particularly with the integration of state-of-the-art technologies such as 3D printing. Previously, generic devices and implants were traditionally used, which with high probability tended to cause problems due to mismatched anatomical and patient-specific requirements. The evolution of 3D printing technology has revolutionized the production of patient-specific cardiovascular devices, including stents and heart valves. This technology allows for an exact replica of a patient's anatomy, enhancing surgical accuracy and potentially patient outcomes. The ability to produce custom implants translates not only to a more precise fit but to reduced recovery time as well, aligning with the increasing trend toward personalized medicine based on customized treatment protocols. In addition, innovations in cardiovascular treatments over the last several years extend far beyond implant customization. 3D printing has enabled one to create complex anatomical models that are actually useful for preoperative planning and training. Such models can facilitate surgeons to see and manually manipulate a patient's specific cardiovascular structure, leading to improved surgical procedures and less intraoperative difficulties.

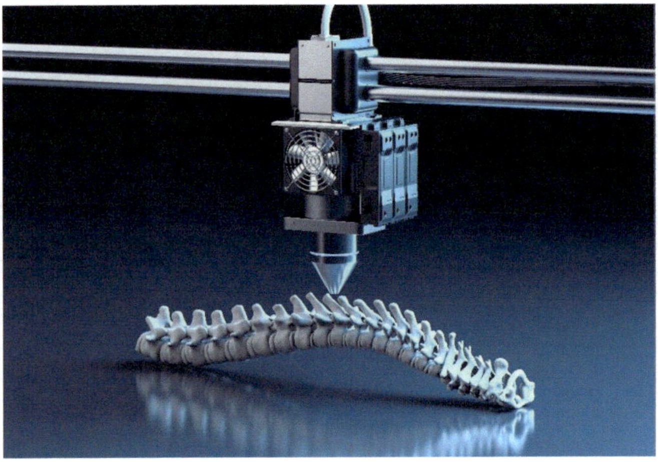

Figure 1.16. 3D printing has enabled the creation of complex anatomical models that are invaluable for pre-surgical planning and education.

Source: https://www.futurebridge.com/wp-content/uploads/2024/05/3D-Anatomical-model.jpg.

The integration of 3D printing technologies within learning environments also enhances the training of health professionals, best preparing them for real-world procedures. As has been noted, the continued advancement in pervasive health monitoring technologies fits with growing demand for these kinds of technologies, promising to open up to an ever more efficient and effective healthcare system dedicated to effective patient management and outcomes (Perez et al., 2015). Additionally, 3D printing is beginning to become an important factor in the development of bioengineered tissues and organs for cardiovascular applications. Promising studies have led to the development of vascular grafts and heart tissues replicating natural biological properties, bypassing donor organ deficits, and issues in artificial implants. The studies continue to reveal the potential of tissue engineering techniques, with emphasis on scaffold constructs for regeneration and body integration. The positive prospect of such advancements marks a paradigm change in cardiovascular therapies wherein engineered treatments would function in concordance with native tissues, ultimately aiming to offer enhanced functionality and longevity of cardiovascular implants. Such advancements justify the necessity of merging engineering concepts with medical knowledge, dictating the future of cardiovascular care on both efficiency and sustainability lines (Kalaskar et al., 2017) (Figure 1.16).

1.6. CONCLUSION

In short, integration of 3D printing within biomedical engineering is a paradigmatic shift in the development and delivery of medical solutions. Through 3D printing, prosthetics and implants can be tailored to fit the individual patient's needs, boosting results and quality of life. The capability to print scaffolds with more than one polymer and biopolymer facilitates the precise replication of complex anatomical structures, a method supported by advanced software using patient-specific data. According to recent studies, the 3D bioplotting approach offers the possibility of incorporating cells during scaffold construction, paving the way for novel organ printing techniques. This innovation not only makes production easier but also solves the problems entailed in tissue engineering, thereby elevating the quality of care in healthcare centers (Carvalho et al., 2004). Moreover, the ever-changing research and technology in 3D printing in biomedical engineering hold a promising future with enhanced functions and applications. Paradigm shift to personalized medicine is seen as 3D printing allows customization of medical devices and treatment strategies according to patient profiles. With the ability to create complex geometries and adjust material properties, it has stimulated research on novel biomaterials that can enhance biocompatibility and bioactivity. With educational institutions now incorporating hands-on experiences through 3D manufacturing into their learning programs, students are enabled to create innovative solutions addressing current challenges in medicine. Not only do these experiences deepen their knowledge of theoretical principles, but they also equip them with capabilities suited for a career in an emerging field where collaboration across disciplines is essential (Nagurka et al., 2015). The impact of 3D printing on biomedical engineering is more than mere technological advances; they are the proper reaction to new healthcare realties. Since it is now possible to prototype and print rapidly in medicine, practitioners in the field can respond and address new needs, such as those that arise with world health crises. Furthermore, the more favorable and supportive regulatory frameworks promote such innovations to prosper, the larger the application of 3D printing in medical settings is likely to expand. Researchers and professionals must thus remain vigilant and proactive in current debate on the ethical and practical consequences emerging from such technology. By establishing a culture of collaboration and creativity, the biomed community can actually invoke the best of 3D printing, in the end making it a more positive experience for patients and advancing medical science.

1.6.1. Summary of Key Points Discussed

The integration of 3D printing in biomedical engineering has ushered in a new dawn of innovation, particularly concerning the design and manufacturing of medical devices and prosthetics. One of the significant challenges addressed is that of developing low-cost molding inserts used in particulate injection molding (PIM) applications. Traditional machining methods have come into the spotlight, with scientists walking the path towards the creation of hybrid methods that combine additive and subtractive processes. The study showed that while conventional methods produce superior surface finish quality, the rapid evolution of additive manufacturing is accompanied by significant cost reduction, thereby making quality manufacturing services more accessible to health professionals (Ewart et al., 2019).

The hybrid method guarantees the delicate handling of complex geometries, appropriate for the specific needs of medical applications where customization is of utmost value. Another significant point of 3D printing in biomedical engineering is how to overcome inherent limitations when it comes to traditional additive manufacturing methods, particularly speed and geometric constraint. Research on volumetric additive fabrication has responded by providing solutions for these problems by presenting a new paradigm that involves the use of holographic patterning to enable the production of complex geometries in seconds. With the help of this advanced technique, it is possible to reduce how complex photopolymer structures are fabricated to a minimum, significantly reducing the cost and time involved in fabricating components to be employed in biomedical applications.

By virtue of bestowing light pattern qualities and fabrication of low-absorbing resins, the results demonstrate great promise in creating complex geometries at record-breaking speeds, making way for the next generation of biomedical devices (Browar et al., 2017). Last but not least, the evolution of 3D printing technologies indicates the mutual coupling between engineering innovation and biomedical application. Efforts to enhance function in 3D-printed parts often turn on overcoming surface quality and strength issues. The aforementioned studies indicate both benefits and drawbacks of various fabrication methods, illuminating the path to future improvement and optimization. By having a profound understanding of the challenges both new and old ways present, researchers can establish best practices that will produce top-notch results in medical device production. All these breakthroughs testify to the revolutionary potential of 3D printing in making it easier to address essential requirements within the healthcare industry, pushing personalized medicine, and improving patient outcomes.

1.6.2. The Potential Impact of 3D Printing on the Future of Healthcare

The integration of 3D printing in the medical sector represents a paradigm shift in the creation and design of medical devices, implants, and prosthetics. Personalization is the core of this revolution, which allows for precision-based design of customized medical products to meet the needs of individual patients. Traditional manufacturing techniques have a tendency to restrict such adaptations in terms of time, cost, and complexity. However, 3D printing enables rapid production of tailored solutions, minimizing distress to patients and maximizing treatment efficacy. For instance, biocompatible material may be employed in the creation of bespoke implants, assisting in easier integration into the human body. With advancements in healthcare, the capability to create personalized solutions through 3D technologies is both a challenge and an opportunity that requires continuous research and development for efficacy and safety in clinical settings. Further investigation into what 3D printing can do shows that it is also capable of improving drug delivery systems. By utilizing additive manufacturing techniques, researchers are developing complex geometries for drug drugs that maximize bioavailability as well as targeted delivery within the body. For example, 3D-printed drug delivery devices can be programmed to release drugs in pre-specified sequences, thus improving therapeutic benefits and minimizing side effects. This personalized approach not only improves patient compliance but also allows physicians to customize treatment regimens based on patients' individual outcomes. The combination of 3D printing and pharmacy would lead to revolutionary innovation in the way medicine is prescribed and dispensed, paving the way for a more individualized experience of healthcare that goes beyond the limitations of the past. Furthermore, 3D printing holds enormous scope in regenerative medicine, particularly in tissue and organ engineering. With developments still in progress, the field is getting closer to the possibility of creating fully viable bio-printed organs to be transplanted, which can also plug the global gap in organ donors. Technologies including bio-responsive hydrogels and organic thin film electronic devices, presented by Oliver et al. (2009), are at the center of such innovation. Such materials can facilitate the development of structures that mimic the biological microenvironment, allowing cell growth and improving functionality. Further, the research on low-cost molding inserts, as studied by Ewart et al. (2019), is a crucial steppingstone toward mass production methods in tissue scaffold fabrication. This development also marks the extensive impact of 3D printing on the future of medicine, announcing a shift toward sustainable and innovative approaches in addressing medical requirements.

1.6.3. Call to Action for Further Research and Development in the Field

The leading edge of biomedical engineering is experiencing revolutionary advances with 3D printing technology, yet the promise of this technology remains in stasis until there is ongoing research and development. Specifically, while current uses, such as pre-surgical models and patient-specific implants, have proven to be highly successful, the technology needs to be further studied to transcend inherent technological limitations. Challenges such as the biocompatibility of materials, the resolution of printed structures, and the complexity of vascularization within engineered tissues have to be seriously explored. By aggressively searching for focused research to address these challenges, researchers can open new realms of 3D printing technology in regenerative medicine and move toward fully functional, implantable organs and tissues that can revolutionize patient care and patient-specific healthcare solutions (Chia et al., 2015). Moreover, the integration of novel printing techniques and new materials is a requirement for 3D printing advancement in the field of medicine. Materials like photopolymerizable hydrogels can mimic native-like tissue properties, which is a prerequisite for creating conditions to activate biological activity within engineered constructs. Examining techniques, such as microfluidic manufacturing and biomass engineering, could lead to the development of more sophisticated scaffolds that do not only support cell growth but also provide the necessary mechanical properties for various tissues. For instance, as visualized in current work, the manufacturing of multilayered hollow microfibers allows for the reconstruction of complex tissue structure, hence tissue engineering a far more mature discipline. An interdisciplinarity effort to further expand these methods will propel advancements in developing functionalized biomimetic tissues applicable for therapeutic purposes (Bolderson et al., 2017). Lastly, to ensure an all-around advancement of 3D printing technology in biomedical engineering, interdisciplinarity collaboration is imperative. The interdisciplinarity collaboration among engineers, biologists, and clinicians will facilitate interdisciplinarity perspectives and include the existing knowledge base across disciplines. These collaborations may also facilitate the transition from bench-side experimentation to clinical application, thereby making 3D-printed solutions more applicable in clinical settings. As research explores the complete potential of 3D printing, an active call for investment in the area becomes ever more critical. An investment in such a direction can drive innovative solutions that not only provide solutions to the needs of today but also predict future needs in the healthcare sector and ultimately lead to revolutionary medical practice and patient care. By constantly laying emphasis on research and development, the potential of 3D printing in biomedical engineering can be completely utilized.

REFERENCES

1. Abbaszadeh, Z., D'Oria, V., Dalla Cort, A., et al. (2018). MicroRNAs delivery into human cells grown on 3D-printed PLA scaffolds coated with a novel fluorescent PAMAM dendrimer for biomedical applications. https://core.ac.uk/download/188824005.pdf (accessed on 14th October 2025).
2. Abhijit Kumar, Ghosh, B., Mallik, M., Das, S., Ghosh, S., Banerjee, S., Pal, S., et al. (2023). Advancing biomedical frontiers: Unveiling the potential of 3D bioprinting in organ regeneration. https://core.ac.uk/download/603897473.pdf (accessed on 14th October 2025).
3. Ali, M. M., Otte, J. N., Rai, R., et al. (2019). A product life cycle ontology for additive manufacturing. https://core.ac.uk/download/186332015.pdf (accessed on 14th October 2025).
4. Almeida, L. E., Dashtimoghadam, E., Fahimipour, F., et al. (2017). A current overview of materials and strategies for potential use in maxillofacial tissue regeneration. https://core.ac.uk/download/213072267.pdf (accessed on 14th October 2025).
5. Andreu Perez, J., Ip, H., Leff, D., et al. (2015). From wearable sensors to smart implants–Towards pervasive and personalized healthcare.
6. Ast, M. P., Bini, S. A., Chung, C. C., et al. (2020). Digital orthopedics: A glimpse into the future in the midst of a pandemic. https://core.ac.uk/download/323308683.pdf (accessed on 14th October 2025).
7. Bini, S. A., Jäger, M., Maslaris, A., et al. (2020). Equivalent mid-term results of open vs endoscopic gluteal tendon tear repair using suture anchors in forty-five patients. https://core.ac.uk/download/323073887.pdf (accessed on 14th October 2025).
8. Bolderson, J., Cusack, M., Dalby, M. J., et al. (2017). Continuous fabrication and assembly of spatial cell-laden fibers for a tissue-like construct via a photolithographic-based microfluidic chip. https://core.ac.uk/download/77601453.pdf (accessed on 14th October 2025).
9. Branch, C. (2015). *3D Printing in Healthcare*. https://core.ac.uk/download/48617394.pdf (accessed on 14th October 2025).
10. Browar, A. E. M., Fang, N. X., Henriksson, J., et al. (2017). One-step volumetric additive manufacturing of complex polymer structures. https://core.ac.uk/download/323063262.pdf (accessed on 14th October 2025).
11. Carvalho, C., Landers, R., & Mülhaupt, R. (2004). Soft and hard implant fabrication using 3D-Bioplotting™. https://core.ac.uk/download/287648471.pdf (accessed on 14th October 2025).

12. Chia, H. N., & Wu, B. M. (2015). Recent advances in 3D printing of biomaterials. https://core.ac.uk/download/323078409.pdf (accessed on 14th October 2025).

13. Cho, H., Jammalamadaka, U., & Tappa, K. (2018). Nanogels for pharmaceutical and biomedical applications and their fabrication using 3D printing technologies. https://core.ac.uk/download/212859248.pdf (accessed on 14th October 2025).

14. Chunmin, M., Wen, D., Chen, G., Xu, H., Lei, H., Xia, L., Song, L., et al. (2016). A multi-robot cooperation framework for sewing personalized stent grafts. http://arxiv.org/abs/1711.03195 (accessed on 14th October 2025).

15. Dautenhahn, K., Novanda, O., Robins, B., et al. (2017). The iterative development of the humanoid robot Kaspar: An assistive robot for children with autism. https://core.ac.uk/download/287727381.pdf (accessed on 14th October 2025).

16. Day, S. J., & Riley, S. P. (2018). Utilizing 3D printing techniques when providing unique assistive devices: A case report. https://core.ac.uk/download/132205880.pdf (accessed on 14th October 2025).

17. De Beule, M., Deckers, J. P., Forward, M., et al. (2019). A validated computational framework to evaluate the stiffness of 3D printed ankle foot orthoses. https://core.ac.uk/download/237010383.pdf (accessed on 14th October 2025).

18. Dehghanghadikolaei, A., Emamian, S. S., Fotovvati, B., et al. (2019). The potential of additive manufacturing in the smart factory industrial 4.0: A review. https://core.ac.uk/download/231748826.pdf (accessed on 14th October 2025).

19. Ewart, P. (2019). A comparison of processing techniques for producing prototype injection molding inserts. https://core.ac.uk/download/322841895.pdf (accessed on 14th October 2025).

20. Farahi, E., Gibbons, G. J., Lv, Y., Purnell, P., & Williams, R. (2010). 3D printing of cement composites. https://core.ac.uk/download/44217.pdf (accessed on 14th October 2025).

21. Hu, Y., Huang, B., Lee, S. L., et al. (2017). A multi-robot cooperation framework for sewing personalized stent grafts. https://core.ac.uk/download/132200785.pdf (accessed on 14th October 2025).

22. Jung, T. K. (2016). Micro computed tomography based finite element models of calcium phosphate scaffolds for bone tissue engineering. https://core.ac.uk/download/81578125.pdf (accessed on 14th October 2025).

23. Kalaskar, D., Leong, J., & Provaggi, E. (2017). Applications of 3D printing in the management of severe spinal conditions. https://core.ac.uk/download/79531622.pdf (accessed on 14th October 2025).
24. Macwan, I., Patra, P., Shinde, D., et al. (2018). 3D printed hyaluronic acid hydrogels using free form fabrication technique for tissue engineering. https://core.ac.uk/download/156902195.pdf (accessed on 14th October 2025).
25. Miura, B., Wagner, A., & Wu, P. (2017). Phosphate contaminant detection in water through a paper-based microfluidic device. https://core.ac.uk/download/127619787.pdf (accessed on 14th October 2025).
26. N/A. (2016). *The Boston University Photonics Center Annual Report 2015–2016.* https://open.bu.edu/bitstream/2144/29754/1/Photonics-Center-Annual-Report-2016-final.pdf (accessed on 14th October 2025).
27. Nagurka, M. L., & Slightam, J. E. (2015). Machine design experiments using gears to foster discovery learning. https://core.ac.uk/download/213088465.pdf (accessed on 14th October 2025).
28. Oliver, R., Tillotson, J., & Toomey, A. (2009). Bioengineered textiles and nonwovens–The convergence of bio-miniaturization and electroactive conductive polymers for assistive healthcare, portable power and design-led wearable technology. https://core.ac.uk/download/9587153.pdf (accessed on 14th October 2025).
29. Phelps, C. L. (2004). *Advances in Teaching & Learning Day Abstracts 2005.* https://core.ac.uk/download/46714715.pdf (accessed on 14th October 2025).
30. Rosa, A., & Salaris, F. (2019). Construction of 3D *in vitro* models by bioprinting human pluripotent stem cells: Challenges and opportunities. https://core.ac.uk/download/231747057.pdf (accessed on 14th October 2025).
31. Santello, M., & Valero-Cuevas, F. J. (2017). On neuromechanical approaches for the study of biological grasp and manipulation. http://arxiv.org/abs/1710.08557 (accessed on 14th October 2025).

CHAPTER 2

FUNDAMENTALS OF ADDITIVE MANUFACTURING TECHNOLOGIES

Contents

INTRODUCTION

Additive manufacturing (AM), or 3D printing, is a disruptive production technology that enables the creation of complex and customized parts in many industries, particularly biomedical engineering. AM creates the potential for accurate design freedom, enabling the quick production of customized prosthetics and implants with enhanced performance in individualized medicine. The application of AM in healthcare is an important development since it more than halves production time and material loss relative to conventional manufacturing processes. Additionally, its use in the Industry 4.0 environment highlights its relevance in modern manufacturing practices, promoting innovation through decentered production approaches and smart manufacturing systems that can address the specific demands of biomedical applications, ultimately optimizing the overall effectiveness of medical device design and manufacturing (Dehghanghadikolaei et al., 2019). The versatility of AM technologies is also used in producing customized tools and instruments, such as surgical guides and molds for other medical procedures. Research has demonstrated that AM can effectively produce these components with precise accuracy, fulfilling specific anatomical needs and improving the outcomes of surgical interventions. A study of the different AM technologies, such as fused deposition modeling and selective laser sintering, demonstrates how the processes are able to create soft and hard tissue scaffolds, thereby contributing towards the progress of tissue engineering. By enabling the production of complex geometries that mimic natural tissue architectures, AM has the ability to transform how healthcare professionals tackle patient treatment and rehabilitation, paving the way for more effective and targeted therapeutic strategies previously inaccessible (Ewart et al., 2019). Furthermore, the inclusion of AM technologies in biomedical science raises vital questions regarding cost-effectiveness and accessibility. With the advancement of the technology, more applications in the production of inexpensive inserts and molds for uses like particulate injection molding are being found. Mutual use of the additive and subtractive processes demarcates the way hybrid systems can cross material property and design complexity hurdles. Through providing sustainable solutions to issues such as surface finish and structural integrity, these strategies emphasize the multi-aspect benefits of AM in accessibility for lower-scale practitioners and institutions. As the environment of biomedical engineering continues to change, understanding these integrative strategies will be vital in realizing AMs full potential, ultimately leading to improved patient care and innovation in medical technology (Dehghanghadikolaei et al., 2019).

Definition and Overview of Additive Manufacturing

Additive manufacturing (AM), also known as 3D printing, is a new technique for the build of components and products by successive addition of materials in layers in sequence according to digital models. The new technology branches out widely from traditional subtractive manufacturing, where material is removed from a solid block in an effort to achieve the desired shape. The versatility of AM spans across different materials like plastics, metals, and ceramics, and thus has applications in all industries. In biomedical engineering, most significantly,

AM can provide for the fabrication of customized implants and prosthetics that can be manufactured to match the patient's anatomy uniquely, thus resulting in enhanced efficiency of medical treatment and patient outcome. Furthermore, the ability to produce intricate geometries that would be difficult to produce using conventional manufacturing methods displays AMs great potential in designing intricate medical devices and biological scaffolds. The advancement of additive manufacturing technologies has been significantly influenced by the application of lasers. Laser is a critical equipment in various AM processes, such as selective laser sintering (SLS) and selective laser melting (SLM), where the laser melts powdered material with great accuracy. Precision is necessary in biomedical uses, where the geometric accuracy of devices and implants can heavily impact their functionality and compatibility with biological structures. With continuous research, the integration of state-of-the-art laser technology into AM keeps on converting into increased processing speed and properties of materials, hence enhancing the overall reliability and quality of manufactured biomedical products.

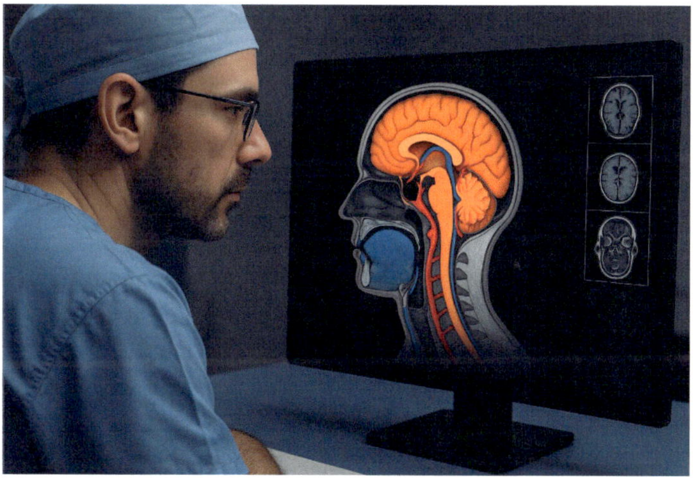

Figure 2.1. 3D printing has enabled the creation of complex anatomical models that are invaluable for pre-surgical planning and education.

Source: https://pareidolia.in/wp-content/uploads/2025/04/ChatGPT-Image-Apr-22-2025-11_43_35-AM.png.

Meanwhile, the economic implications of adopting AM, particularly in high-risk fields such as healthcare, continue to attract attention, driving its overall adoption and prospects for growth in the industry (Pinkerton et al., 2015). Despite the promising developments, numerous impediments still remain that hinder the application of additive manufacturing on a larger scale in biomedical engineering. Issues with regulations, material limitations, and the need for rigorous quality control processes are some of the foremost impediments. Regulators need to confirm that AM devices are extremely safe and effective, and it may slow down the innovation process. In addition, the economic benefits of AM, while considerable, come with the disadvantages of the high initial investment in sophisticated technology and hardware. The future of additive manufacturing looks promising, as studies indicate an ongoing refinement of techniques to enable increasingly complicated applications in the biomedical industry. While AM is not likely to completely overwhelm all manufacturing sectors, it is clear that it guarantees new possibilities that are capable of enhancing the performance of existing technologies (Figure 2.1).

Historical Development of Additive Manufacturing Technologies

The development of additive manufacturing (AM) technologies dates back to the 1980s, which was a revolution in manufacturing and engineering. The initial processes such as stereolithography (SLA) were employed in generating prototypes in a short span of time, allowing for designers to revise their designs at a pace unchallenged by others. This revolutionized the very nature of how products were designed and brought to market and stimulated a move away from traditional subtractive manufacturing techniques. Over the years, a number of AM technologies have been created, including selective laser sintering (SLS) and fused deposition modeling (FDM), which provide specific benefits in terms of material versatility and rate of build. As a consequence, AM uses expanded by leaps and bounds, resulting in its adoption in aerospace and automobile industries that require accuracy and customization. This historical sequence of events finally paved the way for AMs strong entry into biomedical engineering with complexity and customization as its thrust. By the early 2000s, advancements in material science and engineering further added to the capability and versatility of AM technologies, particularly in the field of biomedicine. Since there was increasing focus on patient-specific therapy, scientists began to investigate the potential of AM in manufacturing complex anatomical structure and personalized medical devices. For instance, the application of biocompatible materials in 3D printing has created interest in producing prosthetics and implants to serve the special needs of patients. More significantly, the potential for producing intricate geometries not achievable with conventional methods has become an essential feature for enhancing the performance of biomedical devices. Thus, additive manufacturing started to receive acclamation for accelerating the arrival of personalized medicine, proving its utility beyond traditional applications in manufacturing. This is a mark that indicates the manner in which AM has revolutionized the healthcare sector, fulfilling efficiency and personalization in healthcare. As the history of the evolution of AM technologies was unfolding, their use in the biomedical sector became increasingly more complex and multidirectional. Much research works indicated using a combination of additive and subtractive manufacturing methods to simplify the manufacturing processes, especially for the creation of advanced biomedical devices. For example, the simultaneous use of both methods in crafting molding inserts used in the injection molding process indicates the possibility of better designs and reduced production costs. This hybrid process allows for cleaner surface finishes and minimizes defects usually encountered with traditional manufacturing. With concerted research and development, the future of AM in biomedical engineering is bright with innovations that are constantly rewriting the way medical devices are conceived and made. These innovations not only improve functionality but also abide by the sustainability concept by minimizing wastage of resources and allowing localized production (Dehghanghadikolaei et al., 2019; Ewart et al., 2019).

Importance of Additive Manufacturing in Biomedical Engineering

The applicability of additive manufacturing (AM) to biomedical engineering is highlighted by its ability to provide highly customized medical devices that accommodate specific patient needs. Traditional production techniques impose complexity and size restrictions, which hamper the fabrication of complex geometries required in the biomedicine field. AM technologies, such as 3D printing, give engineers the potential to produce personalized implants and prosthetics tailored for anatomical needs, thereby enhancing functioning and comfort for the patient. For instance, the use of AM can generate complex geometries, e.g., scaffolds applicable for tissue engineering purposes, which can stimulate cellular growth and integration within the human body. The technology represents a shift from mass production to personalized medicine, which implies that AM is essential to the evolution of biomedical engineering, accommodating unique patient anatomy and improving surgical outcomes. Additionally, the integration of hybrid manufacturing systems with additive and subtractive processes becomes a revolutionary aspect of AM in biomedical applications. These hybrid systems capitalize on the strengths of both production approaches, allowing for effective production of intricate medical devices with fewer limitations inherent in either approach individually. With the ability to produce previously unachievable complex geometries, hybrid machines are a significant milestone in the ability to create parts of improved material properties and greater performance. Furthermore, additive and subtractive process interaction is the driver of innovation in the form of transcending technical barriers such as effective process design and resource allocation. With additional developments in such hybrid systems emerging, the biomedical engineering sector gets more important with a potential of bringing in a new era of enhanced device performance and manufacturing efficiency (Arrate et al., 2018). When used in pharmaceuticals, additive manufacturing can revolutionize drug delivery systems and dosage form design. The development of 3D-printed drugs, like the first FDA-approved 3D-printed drug, proves the capability of AM technology to personalize drug formulations and simplify release profiles to meet the unique patient needs. This versatility can support the design of complex geometries in oral tablets, which can enhance the bioavailability of active pharmaceutical ingredients with innovative designs that ensure better drug absorption. Moreover, as the technologies advance in AM, they begin to offer new possibilities in the field of pharmaceutical application, such as incorporating multiple active ingredients and tailoring dosage forms to specific therapeutic objectives. This growing interest in AM within the pharmaceutical industry reflects both the potential for change and the regulatory challenges that must be surmounted if it is to realize its maximum potential within healthcare (Goyanes et al., 2016) (Figure 2.2).

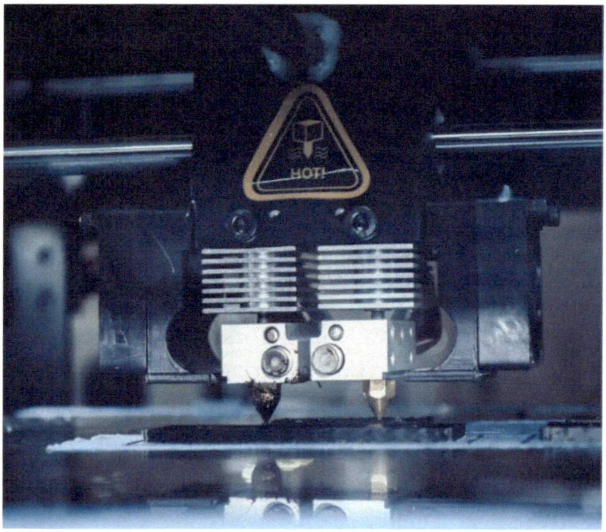

Figure 2.2. Traditional manufacturing methods often impose limitations related to complexity and size, hindering the creation of intricate designs required in the field of biomedicine.

Source: https://elimold.com/wp-content/uploads/2025/06/sls-3d-printing-service1-1024x877.webp.

2.1. TYPES OF ADDITIVE MANUFACTURING TECHNOLOGIES

Additive manufacturing (AM) methods encompass a wide range of techniques through which three-dimensional objects are created in a layer-by-layer fashion. Among the most widely utilized methods is Fused Deposition Modeling (FDM), where thermoplastic substances are melted and sprayed out of a heated nozzle to produce complex structures. This technique finds widespread application in biomedical engineering for creating scaffolds employed during tissue regeneration. FDM allows precision in mechanical properties and porosity, which are key parameters in scaffold performance. This is crucial since the scaffolds should mimic the natural extracellular matrix for cell adhesion and proliferation. The ability to customize the makeup of the material with biocompatible polymers increases even further the potential of FDM for the development of applications in tissue engineering, thus providing a groundbreaking instrument for researchers' intent on innovating in the biomedical area. Stereolithography (SLA), which via light polymerizes liquid resin into solid structures, is another dominant technology among the additive manufacturing process. This technique is particularly renowned for having high resolution and the capability of forming delicate details that other methods are unable to. In biomedical engineering, SLA is widely used to produce dental and orthopedic implants that require precise fit and operation. The capability of SLA to produce intricate internal geometry makes it highly useful in the production of porous structures mimicking the mechanical response of bone tissue. Furthermore, advances in material science have introduced bio-resorbable resins that degrade slowly in the body, providing a pathway for temporary scaffolding in regenerative medicine. Collectively, they signal SLAs pioneering potential for enhancing patient outcomes with patient-specific medical devices and implants. Selective Laser Sintering (SLS) is also a promising additive manufacturing technique that uses a high-powered laser beam to melt powdered material into solid structure. It is the flexibility of SLS that distinguishes it, as it can be used with a variety of materials, from polymers to metals, and thus can be utilized for both the creation of soft tissue scaffolds and load-bearing orthopedic implants. The most important advantage of SLS is that it can create parts with internal lattices and intricate geometries, which cannot easily be achieved through traditional manufacturing methods. This characteristic is extremely significant in biomedical devices, where mechanical properties and structural integrity are of major interest. Recent advances have also opened up the SLS opportunity for fabricating Ionomeric polymer-metal composites (IPMC) actuators, which have been promising in biomedical devices due to their high displacements and rapid responses. The convergence of innovative design and material technology positions SLS in a pivotal role in the field of biomedical additive manufacturing (Lipson et al., 2005).

2.1.1. Fused Deposition Modeling (FDM)

Fused deposition modeling (FDM) is one of the leading companies in the additive manufacturing industry and more generally in the biomedical engineering industry. Based on layer-by-layer deposition, FDM transforms thermoplastic material into durable structures by precisely extruding it out of a heated nozzle. FDM has been extremely helpful in creating bespoke medical devices and prostheses to fit the patient's anatomy. Its comparably low cost and ready availability make FDM a serious option for both research and clinical applications, allowing for quick prototyping of complex geometries prevalent in medical therapy. The ability to use biocompatible polymers also enhances its potential in the development of implants and scaffolds that comply with high-level regulatory standards of biomedical applications while ensuring effectiveness and patient safety. The growth of FDM technology has been influenced to a great extent by advances in engineering and architecture. A variety of polymers, including poly(lactic acid) (PLA), acrylonitrile butadiene styrene (ABS), and more complex composite materials, are being exploited to improve mechanical properties and biocompatibility. More recent studies indicate that the introduction of fiber reinforcement into FDM processes can deliver improved structural integrity, which is of paramount concern for load-carrying applications in biomedical devices. The incorporation of advanced materials not only broadens the applications of FDM but also the potential for customization offered by the technology. As per new reviews, the advances portray the dramatic improvement taken in the past five years, demonstrating the adaptability of FDM in the construction of implants and tissue scaffolds mimicking the complexity of human anatomy (Chia et al., 2015). While it has advantages, FDM technology is also faced with a number of challenges requiring more R&D. Dimensional accuracy, surface finish, and layer adhesion remain significant limitations that can impact the functionality of biomedical devices. For instance, achieving the exact resolutions typically required for the complex tissue engineering tasks may be a significant challenge. Furthermore, the thermal and mechanical properties of FDM-printed products may not always meet the stringent requirements for specific biomedical applications. Breaking these confines will be essential in facilitating the ready adoption and common implementation of FDM in regenerative medicine. Continuous innovation and exploration in the additive society will ultimately result in methods to bypass these limitations, and this can unveil revolutionary developments in customized and regenerative medicine (Hansen et al., 2017) (Figure 2.3).

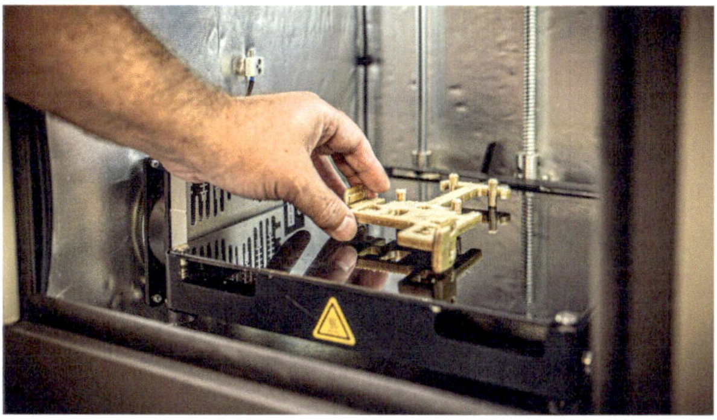

Figure 2.3. Fused deposition modeling (FDM) has emerged as a key player in the landscape of additive manufacturing, particularly within the field of biomedical engineering.

Source: https://media.licdn.com/dms/image/v2/D4E12AQEndKKiws6UGA/article-cover_image-shrink_720_1280/B4EZZJbNtNHYAI-/0/1744988594011?e=2147483647&v=beta&t=Nb6XIr3XFROGrhHVbSWqjjJEnZS5_-DAAlbsgTltk0U.

2.1.2. Stereolithography (SLA)

Stereolithography (SLA) is one of the first additive manufacturing technologies to have received special reference in the field of biomedical engineering. Invented during the 1980s, SLA uses the process of curing ultraviolet (UV) light on photopolymer resins, layer by layer, to produce three-dimensional objects. It is a remarkable process for producing prototypes with extremely fine details and accuracy, which is crucial in biomedical applications such as customized prosthetics and anatomical models. The precision of SLA allows for precise designs to meet specific patient needs, which facilitates innovation in personalized medicine. Moreover, the ability to create complicated geometries and polishing surface finishes in SLA prints makes it a desirable choice for highly biocompatible and aesthetically demanding medical devices, which fulfills growing demands for cost-efficient and effective solutions for the health care sector. With advancement in the field of biomedical, economic factors of implementing SLA technology become increasingly relevant. Initial investment in SLA equipment and materials could be extremely expensive; however, long-term benefits repay this expense in terms of enabling rapid prototyping and reducing material waste. Traditional manufacturing methods involve a long-time cycle and higher cost due to material machining and wastage. On the other hand, SLAs layer-by-layer method minimizes wastage of material and allows for quick iteration of designs, thus smoothing out the process of development. According to recent research, the increasing application of SLA in the biomedical field could lead to deep market transformation, benefiting manufacturers by allowing them to meet regulations and customize products effectively. By expanding the production capabilities, SLA not only promotes innovation in the healthcare setting but also emerges as a prime mover in the economic development of additive manufacturing technology (Pinkerton et al., 2015). In the coming years, the future of SLA in biomedical engineering appears promising, particularly with advancements in material science and technology. Recent work is tackling the creation of improved properties for SLA materials, including the development of bioresorbable and biocompatible photopolymers with direct contact with human tissues. Multi-material advancements also offer the promise of creating intricate structures with varying mechanical properties required to create functional tissue scaffolds and other medical devices. The integration of Industry 4.0 ideas, such as automation and data processing, will also further enhance the reliability and effectiveness of SLA processes (Jena et al., 2024). Through the overcoming of existing barriers, such as material limitation and energy consumption, the adaptation and development of SLA technology can potentially result in revolutionary uses in regenerative medication and advanced surgical practices, ultimately towards an effective healthcare delivery system (Figure 2.4).

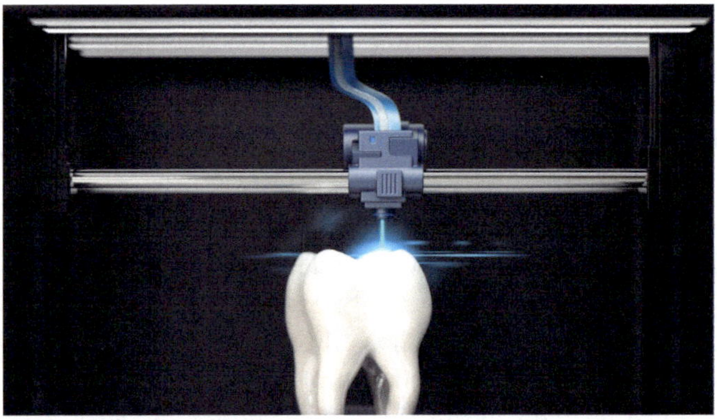

Figure 2.4. Stereolithography (SLA) is one of the pioneering technologies in the field of additive manufacturing, particularly notable for its application in biomedical engineering.

Source: https://cdn.hswstatic.com/gif/Stereolithography-process-steps.jpg.

2.1.3. Selective Laser Sintering (SLS)

Selective laser sintering (SLS) has been one of the principal technologies in the realm of additive manufacturing, particularly in biomedical engineering. The method involves the use of high-energy lasers to selectively sinter powdered materials to form intricate geometries and structures rapidly. This capability plays a crucial role in the production of patient-specific implants, prosthetics, and scaffolds, which can be tailored with high accuracy to match anatomical features. SLS stands out for its ability to print with multiple materials like polymers, ceramics, and metals, and this makes it flexible for various applications. Not only does this enhance the degree of customizations for biomedical devices, but it also serves a critical role in making treatments more efficient, paving the way for future innovations in personalized medicine and regenerative therapies, according to recent improvements in 3D Printing technologies (Chia et al., 2015). The integration of SLS with biomedical engineering has facilitated the production of complex scaffolds for tissue engineering, which are central to regenerative medicine.

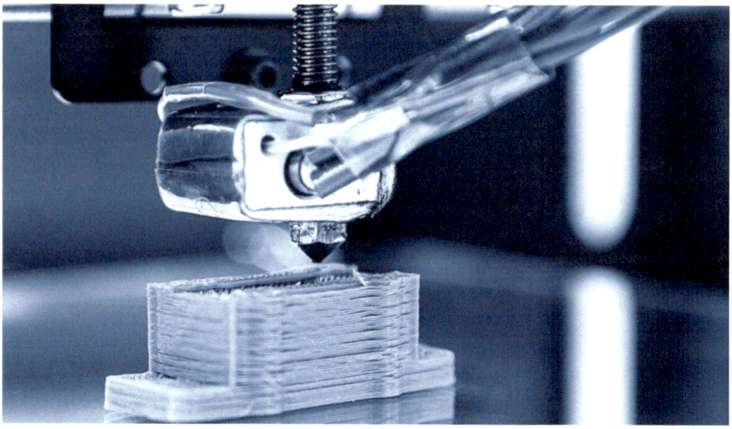

Figure 2.5. Selective laser sintering (SLS) has emerged as a pivotal technology within the landscape of additive manufacturing, particularly in biomedical engineering.

Source: https://media.licdn.com/dms/image/v2/D5612AQGatKoZhjJszg/article-cover_image-shrink_720_1280/article-cover_image-shrink_720_1280/0/1729684806250?e=2147483647&v=beta&t=m7mRNIJHCbzZelxHOnmGn93CtZZEKddj-3wDMKhZ-zA.

Scaffolds are in essence templates that direct the growth of cells and tissue formation and are required for uses ranging from bone repair to vascular grafts. Since SLS can be used to create complex structures with very high precision, it meets one of the primary needs of tissue engineering—the development of scaffolds with microarchitectures similar to those of natural tissue. This technology facilitates the objective of improving biocompatibility and fostering cell adhesion and growth, thus enhancing the probability of successful tissue integration and function. Although very promising, SLS technology poses challenges of material limitation and processing parameter challenges to be overcome, and there is a requirement for ongoing research for enhanced outcome and enhanced utilization (Chia et al., 2015). The future of SLS in biomedical engineering holds promise, but future widespread use depends on the defeat of significant obstacles. Opportunities lie in continued material science and laser development; whereby improved properties and capabilities can be obtained in devices produced by SLS. Increased investment in the technology is also on the rise, particularly as recognition of its worth is growing in all sectors of industry, including the medical sector. SLS's efficiency in reducing waste and streamlining manufacturing is keeping up with the growing requirement for sustainability, further cementing its position in today's manufacturing environment. However, it continues to be vital to continue examining the economic viability and scalability of SLS solutions so that they may effectively address the biomedical industry requirements, as seen in recent studies on additive manufacturing's paradigm shift (Figure 2.5).

2.2. MATERIALS USED IN ADDITIVE MANUFACTURING

Material selection is a primary importance in additive manufacturing (AM), particularly in biomedical engineering, where functionality and biocompatibility are also of prime concern. Metals, ceramics, and polymers constitute the three main material systems applied in AM processes, and each of them has various benefits for various applications. For instance, biocompatible polymers like polycaprolactone and polylactic acid are commonly employed to fabricate tissue engineering scaffolds due to their favorable mechanical properties and tailored degradation profiles. In contrast, metals such as titanium and cobalt–chromium alloys are employed to fabricate durable implants that are capable of withstanding significant mechanical loads. The inbuilt versatility in such materials enables innovations in patient-specific implants (PSI) that are customized to individual anatomical necessities and demands of mechanical performance, thereby ensuring the overall efficacy of treatments in biomedical applications. In addition, integrating advanced materials in AM processes has enabled realizations of design complexity and functionality that were heretofore impossible. As explained in current research, the reverse engineering and design functionality have revolutionized the development of medical devices. Using AM technologies, it is possible to produce intricate geometries not achievable with traditional manufacturing methods, thereby generating additional therapeutic potential. For example, algorithms can be employed to design a cranial PSI to optimize its shape by simulating stress and strain patterns for varying load conditions and thus ensuring the stability of the implants while minimizing failure. This new style not only maximizes the mechanical performance of the implants but also the interface with adjacent tissues, and this highlights the paramount importance of material selection in order to achieve successful patient outcomes (Díaz et al., 2017). Additionally, developments in AM technology have stimulated innovative pathways towards more sustainable production methods for biomedical devices. Through enabling additive rather than subtractive production, waste generation is minimized—a critical aspect of manufacturing sustainability. The newfound trend for the utilization of recycled parts and advanced composites in AM processes complements the biomedical sector's goals on sustainability. Furthermore, Industry 4.0 concepts facilitate the achievement of intelligent manufacturing systems that improve material usage and efficiency in terms of production, with profound influences on overall costs and environmental footprints. With developing additive manufacturing, it becomes necessary to explore how the advances in new materials and technologies impact sustainability, flexibility in design, and efficiency in biomedical engineering, with focus on the profound transformation that needs to be experienced in this industry (Dehghanghadikolaei et al., 2019) (Figure 2.6).

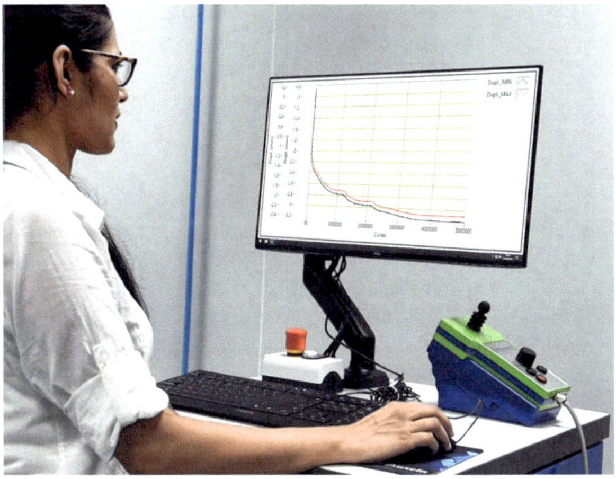

Figure 2.6. The versatility inherent in these materials allows for innovations in patient-specific implants (PSI) that cater to individual anatomical requirements and mechanical performance needs, thereby enhancing the overall efficacy of treatments in biomedical applications.

Source: https://www.vibronicslab.com/wp-content/uploads/2020/05/Simmulator.jpg.

2.2.1. Biocompatible Polymers

Biomedical engineering has made huge strides with the advent of biocompatible polymers in additive manufacturing technologies. Biocompatible polymers are central to the development of medical devices, implants, and tissue engineering scaffolds. Their intrinsic properties, such as biocompatibility, mechanical stiffness, and tailorability, make them great candidates for numerous biomedical applications. Moreover, the ability of these polymers to be altered in their physical properties and chemical structure makes it possible to tailor interactions between biological tissue and the material, including tissue that promotes integration and functionality. As additive manufacturing techniques change, the use of such polymers also continues to advance to create developments in personalized medicine and regenerative therapy that are key to addressing individual patient requirements in clinical practice. Additive manufacturing has enabled the creation of complex structures with morphology resembling that of human tissues by using biocompatible polymers. Other methods such as 3D printing have enabled printing patient-specific scaffolds and implants required for tissue regeneration.

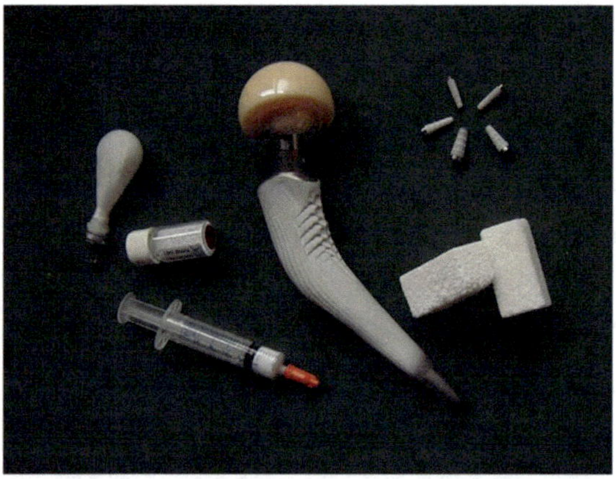

Figure 2.7. Biocompatible polymers serve a crucial role in the development of medical devices, implants, and scaffolds designed for tissue engineering.

Source: https://images-provider.frontiersin.org/api/ipx/w=1200&f=png/https://www.frontiersin.org/files/Articles/169485/fbioe-03-00202-HTML/image_m/fbioe-03-00202-g001.jpg.

The use of these advanced manufacturing techniques allows for controlled material deposition, resulting in new geometries that promote cell growth and adhesion, which are essential in tissue engineering. Biocompatible polymers possess favorable degradation rates, matching the development of tissues, thereby creating a dynamic scaffold for cellular development. As research further develops, the identification of new polymer-additive combinations, including bioactive molecules, will further enhance the efficacy of these constructs for medical applications (Chia et al., 2015). The development of porous scaffolds from biocompatible polymers represents a significant potential to propel tissue engineering applications. Scaffolds need to be precisely designed in order to maintain appropriate cell migration, delivery of nutrients, and waste removal, all of which are critical for tissue repair and growth. Using the support of additive manufacturing technologies, scaffolds with predetermined porosity and mechanical properties for various tissues can be designed by engineers—a feat that traditional manufacturing methods have not yet achieved. Cellular material research, particularly through the employment of solid freeform fabrication processes, emphasizes the use of geometric modeling and the potential of layered structures for cell function (Concheri et al., 2018). As advancements in scaffold design continue, the creation of advanced regenerative capacity will put biocompatible polymers at the forefront of biomedical engineering innovations (Figure 2.7).

2.2.2. Metals and Alloys for Biomedical Applications

Application of metals and alloys in biomedical engineering has gained momentum due to their excellent mechanical properties, biocompatibility, and corrosion resistance. The material chosen is titanium alloys, stainless steel, and cobalt–chromium alloys, which are used widely in medical devices, implants, and prosthetic devices. The titanium alloys, especially Ti-6Al-4V, have gained popularity for orthopedic and dental implants due to its good strength-to-weight ratio and bone tissue compatibility. Aside from this, advances in technology during additive manufacturing have made it easier to produce very complex geometries beneficial to enhanced clinical performance. With advancing manufacturing procedures, it becomes increasingly feasible to tailor implants for fit to patient anatomy individually, based on the growing trend towards personalized medicine and improving the performance of implants in bio-medical contexts. The intricate relationship between the metal and alloy microstructure and resultant properties is of deep significance in the field of biomedical applications. Additive manufacturing technologies, such as selective laser melting and electron beam melting, offer precise control over cooling rates and thermal gradients during solidification. Additive manufacturing processes have profound impacts on microstructural characteristics, such as dendritic arm spacing and grain morphology, which ultimately decide mechanical performance and biocompatibility. Microstructure evolution must be understood in order to optimize these additive processes, as it will allow for the prediction of material behavior under physiological conditions. Recent studies indicate that parameter modifications can produce significant differences in the mechanical properties, underlining the need for extensive investigation of the microstructural effect of additive processing on metals and alloys used in biomedical applications, as exemplified by studies of Ti-6Al-4V and its application in implants (Meng et al., 2019). At the heart of the topic concerning metals and alloys for medical applications is sustainability and reduced waste through additive manufacturing technologies. Subtract manufacturing techniques, however, are apt to involve a great deal of wastage of materials, whereas AM is cost-effective by employing the minimum amount of material necessary in order to produce parts.

This does the double good of not merely saving money but also adhering to recent sustainability initiatives in medicine. Furthermore, on-demand part manufacturing cancels out the logistics and storage capacity problems, and the manufacturing process becomes even more streamlined.

The integration of additive manufacturing within the biomedical industry not only streamlines the manufacturing process but also allows for the development of new materials and designs and, in turn, contributes to enhanced patient outcomes with the acceptance of the environmental problems associated with manufacturing (Dehghanghadikolaei et al., 2019). As the industry evolves to meet these advances, the future for biomedical metal and alloy application is bright prospect for future innovation and sustainability (Figure 2.8).

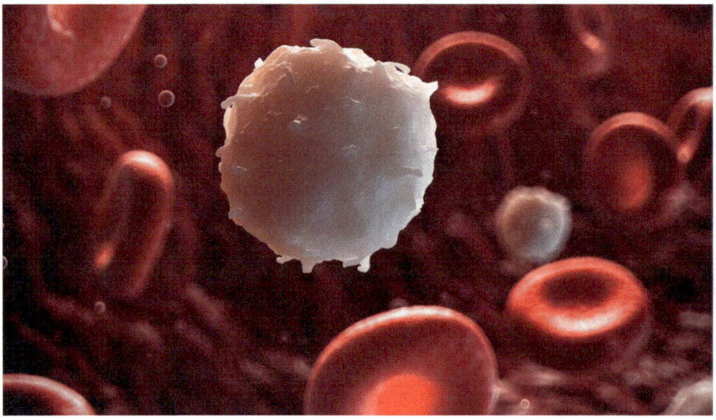

Figure 2.8. Understanding microstructure evolution is essential for optimizing these additive processes, as it facilitates the prediction of material behavior under physiological conditions.

Source: https://static.horiba.com/fileadmin/Horiba/_processed_/5/c/csm_shutterstock_133426889_b4fa283c57.jpg.

2.2.3. Ceramics and Composite Materials

The use of ceramics and composite materials in additive manufacturing has transformed the biomedical engineering field, offering excellent progress in the manufacture of implants and prosthetics. The materials exhibit interesting properties, such as biocompatibility and strength, which are advantageous when used within the human body. Ceramics are special because they possess useful properties such as low thermal conductivity and high hardness that make them very suitable for load-bearing applications. Moreover, their microstructurability allows complex shapes to be formed that can mimic the intricate structure of biological tissue. This is in accordance with the objectives of additive manufacturing, where one can easily attain complex design, thereby eliminating the limitations placed by traditional manufacturing technologies. The synergy between additive manufacturing and ceramics has the potential for groundbreaking solutions to meet the demanding requirements of biomedical applications. Composite materials have also attracted significant attention in additive manufacturing due to the fact that they can be customized with their properties and better performing features. By combining different materials, such as ceramics and polymers or metals, researchers are able to engineer composites that exhibit increased strength, toughness, and stiffness at reduced weight. These are greatly sought after in biomedical applications where implants not only need to withstand physiological stresses but also should be able to reside peacefully alongside adjacent biological tissues. The use of additive manufacturing technologies offers the ability to control precisely the distribution of constituent materials, enabling the synthesis of functionally graded materials with the ability to optimize artificial device interaction with biological systems. The use of bioactive ceramics in composites also offers a better osseointegration, allowing for more favorable outcomes for healing following surgical intervention (Farahi et al., 2010). Thus, the research of ceramic composites within additive manufacturing is a crucial field for biomedical engineering advancement. As technology further advances the field, the implications of additive manufacturing technologies on ceramics and composites are increasingly clear. The application of such advanced materials under the Industry 4.0 environment highlights the union between the new manufacturing methods and the need for sustainable production. The shift towards decentralized manufacturing methods is also in accordance with the approaches of waste reduction, supporting improved resource and material utilization, which is particularly applicable to the biomedical sector (Dehghanghadikolaei et al., 2019). The capability of rapid prototyping of patient-specific implants tailored to accommodate certain anatomy of a single patient not only enhances the success of surgery but also a tremendous step towards personalized medicine. With growing research, the future of additive manufacturing with ceramics and composites is likely to redefine the game in biomedical engineering, allowing innovations that spur faster patient care and the broader effect of medical intervention.

2.3. APPLICATIONS IN BIOMEDICAL ENGINEERING

The integration of additive manufacturing technology into biomedical engineering has initiated significant developments, particularly in scaffold design and production for tissue engineering. Using solid freeform fabrication techniques, porous structures with geometries that are similar to the natural extracellular matrix of tissues can be produced. This is vital in facilitating cell attachment and growth because the architecture of scaffolds dictates cellular behavior and tissue formation. The tunability offered by these technologies allows scaffolds with tailored porosity and mechanical properties to be created to specifically suit the needs of various kinds of tissue. These developments matter as they make it possible to enhance the regenerative capability of engineered tissues so that they can integrate more favorably when implanted. As noted by current studies, cellular material geometric modeling explains how the structure of scaffolds can be optimized, addressing some of tissue engineering's most significant challenges, and paving the way for customized medicine (Concheri et al., 2018). In actuators and soft robotics, additive techniques have evolved into a revolutionary instrument to fabricate flexible and lightweight devices. An especially relevant example is the Ionomeric Polymer-Metal Composite (IPMC) actuators, which have been recognized for their capability of creating large displacements through low voltage inputs. Freeform fabrication of these actuators allows for designers to test out unconventional geometries that promise to improve movement and performance, thus expanding their applicability in biomedical devices. For instance, by making significant strides in freeform fabrication, researchers are able to create IPMC actuators that have integrated functionalities when coupled with other devices that are manufactured. This may be utilized for the creation of more sophisticated biomedical devices that respond dynamically to physiological stimuli and lead to improved patient outcomes (Lipson et al., 2005). Moreover, the impact of additive manufacturing is also experienced in the field of personalized implants and prosthetics, where patient-specific models can improve performance and compatibility significantly. The ability to produce complex, tailored devices through additive manufacturing technologies ensures that each product accurately fits the anatomical and functional specifications of individual patients. As an example, 3D printing technologies enable the fabrication of orthopedic implants specifically conforming to the unique geometry of a patient's bone structure, therefore enhancing healing and reducing the likelihood of complications. The technology continues to advance with further potential for the design of multi-material implants with varying mechanical properties in a single device. This technology is a paradigm shift in biomedical device design and development, and it guides a future of patient-specific health care solutions that promise to enhance the quality of life of patients (Concheri et al., 2018; Lipson et al., 2005).

2.3.1. Custom Prosthetics and Implants

With the development of additive manufacturing technologies, it became feasible to produce personalized prosthetics and implants, which brought a significant revolution to the care of patients in biomedical engineering. 3D printing makes it possible to create strongly individualized medical devices that are precisely developed for compliance with the patient's anatomical and functional needs, enhancing the accuracy and efficiency of treatment. One of the primary advantages of employing this technology is the reduction of operation time and improved patient outcomes, as evidence has shown that individually designed 3D-printed implants can potentially lead to optimal anatomical fit and function. By allowing patient-specific anatomical information to be integrated, additively manufactured prosthetics can easily minimize complications normally associated with traditional manufacturing methods. Thus, this ongoing integration of 3D printing in medicine works to highlight a paradigm shift towards personalized medicine, and the importance of the technology in modern healthcare (Annemans et al., 2016). Additionally, design and material selection at the time of 3D printing are important aspects in determining the success and longevity of custom prosthetics and implants. For instance, in temporomandibular joint replacement (TMJR) patients, stock versus custom prosthetic system choice can make a tremendous difference in outcome. Research has indicated that custom prostheses not only allow for better anatomical reconstruction but also enhanced range of motion, which is essential for joint function (Centeno et al., 2018). Furthermore, the application of materials that have high performance and are capable of imitating the physical characteristics of natural tissue enhances the body's integration of the implants and reduces the possibility of rejection and increases long-term success. As additive manufacturing technologies progress, focus will be key on achieving optimized material performance as well as biocompatibility in the creation of future prosthetic products. Generally, the union of additive manufacturing technologies with custom prosthetics and implants is a revolutionizing development in the biomedical engineering field. Potential for improved surgical outcomes, individualized solutions, and complication reduction characterizes the benefits of integrating customized designs into practice. Also important is additional research to further elucidate the cost-effectiveness of these interventions as compared to traditional methods, as healthcare systems strive towards sustainable practice. As seen from the advancement in manufacturing methods and the application of new materials, the future of custom-made implants and prosthetics will be more durable and functional in orientation, therefore improving the quality of life for millions of patients worldwide (Annemans et al., 2016) (Figure 2.9).

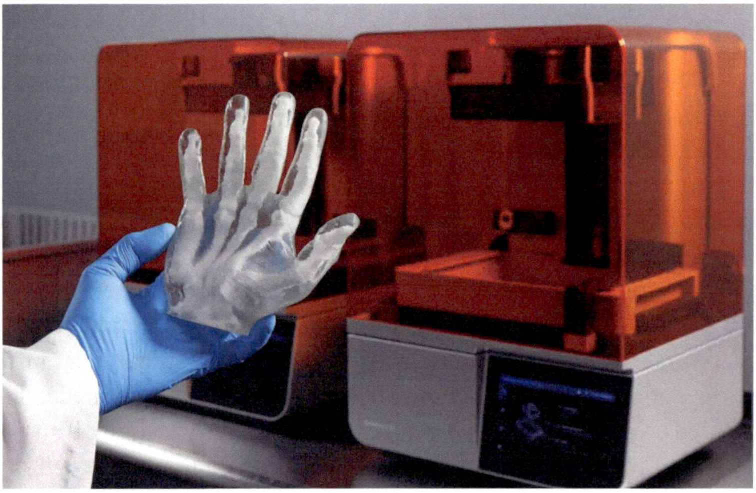

Figure 2.9. 3D printing enables the creation of highly individualized medical devices tailored to the anatomical and functional needs of patients, enhancing the accuracy and efficacy of treatment.

Source: https://formlabs.com/_next/image/?url=https%3A%2F%2Fformlabs-media.formlabs.com%2Ffiler_public_thumbnails%2Ffiler_public%2Ffd%2F46%2Ffd465dbb-99de-4899-99a3-33985c7424cb%2Fformlabs-biocompatible-resins-a-comprehensive-guide-to-choosing-the-right-material.jpg__1354x0_q85_subsampling-2.jpg&w=3840&q=75.

2.3.2. Tissue Engineering and Regenerative Medicine

The advances in Tissue Engineering and Regenerative Medicine have become integral to addressing the growing demands for effective therapy in regenerative health. Of central focus in these advances are the abilities of additive manufacturing technologies wherein complex biological structures that can replicate the function of native tissues are within reach. Since the development of the field, the terminology and definitions related to biofabrication have expanded and required more precision regarding the methodologies involved. Understanding biofabrication concepts—towards approaches like bioprinting and bioassembly—can significantly enhance the design and functionality of engineered tissue. This openness enables researchers and practitioners to ascertain the appropriate strategies to bridge the laboratory-clinical gap properly, thereby propelling the field forward (Blunk et al., 2016). The most advanced application of additive manufacturing techniques is the use of 3D printing, which has greatly accelerated the development of customized biomedical devices and scaffolds. By taking patient-specific anatomical data into account, 3D printing allows clinicians to create personalized implants and scaffolds to suit particular patient needs. While initial applications focused on surgical models and tooling, the real strength of 3D printing has already been employed to produce personalized scaffolds for tissue engineering, diagnostic platforms, and drug delivery devices. Yet complex tissue regeneration as a capability remains a challenge that has to overcome significant technological barriers. Developing, for example, scaffolds that can sustain the intricate microarchitecture of tissues in vascular and nervous systems, for example, requires sustained innovation in materials and printing technologies (Chia et al., 2015). Furthermore, the discipline of Tissue Engineering is characterized by the convergence of the life sciences and advanced manufacturing technologies, and this has spurred inquiry into the application of hybrid methods of fabrication. Current research investigates the combination of stem cells and personalized 3D scaffolds, with a view toward encouraging a more individualized strategy to regenerative medicine. This union of technology and biology offers not just better outcomes in tissue regeneration but also addresses a number of ethical problems in the procurement and transplantation of tissues. Moreover, continuous studies also hope to break barriers such as material biocompatibility and scaffold functionality so that successful integration into the human body is possible. As these obstacles are removed through innovative techniques developed within the additive manufacturing space, the possibility of successfully regrowing sophisticated tissue and organs becomes increasingly a reality, opening the door to revolutionary health interventions (Blunk et al., 2016).

2.3.3. Surgical Planning and Simulation Models

The confluence of additive manufacturing processes with surgical planning and simulation models has revolutionized the biomedical engineering paradigm. With patient-specific anatomical models, surgeons can now visualize intricate anatomy and modulate their approach based on individual anatomical variations. Such individualization not only supports increased precision in surgery but also aids in pre-predicting related complications, thereby improving patient outcomes. Advances in three-dimensional printing technology have made it possible to produce low-cost, patient-specific medical implants and, particularly in spinal surgery, this is very useful. The ability to produce highly detailed models of patients' anatomy means not only improved planning of surgery but also reassures patients about what is to be done, resulting in greater confidence in their surgical teams (Kalaskar et al., 2017). Also, the additive manufacturing (AM) and X-ray computed tomography (XCT) synergy has played a central role to enhancing surgical simulations. XCT provides useful data regarding the three-dimensional anatomy of anatomical structures, which can be employed to produce real surgical models using AM.

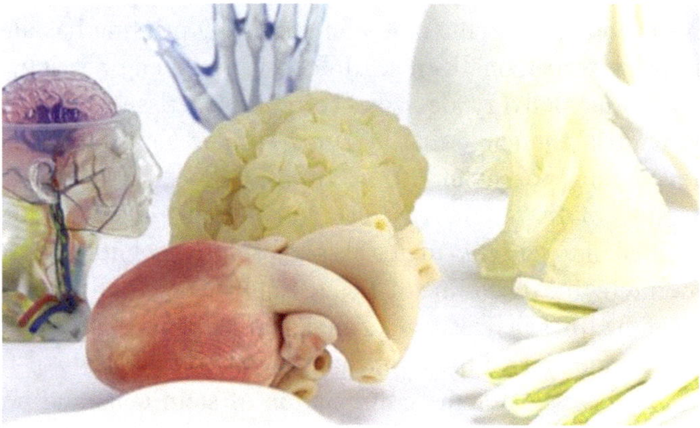

Figure 2.10. By creating patient-specific anatomical models, surgeons can visualize complex structures and tailor their approach based on unique anatomical variations.

Source: https://www.3dnatives.com/en/wp-content/uploads/sites/2/2020/11/surgery_cover-600x353.jpg.

They complement each other to promote a transition from rudimentary medical modeling to the production of personalized guides and implants, enhancing the accuracy of surgery. With the support of these technologies, physicians are able to simulate various types of surgical cases and thus prepare for unexpected complexities in each case. Increased utilization of XCT and AM technologies may establish new gold standards in surgical models and implant manufacturing as well as decrease further the gap between preoperative planning and intraoperative realities (Appleby et al., 2017). Although their translational potential is high, the universal adoption of the new technologies is not problem-free. The greatest barrier remains the extraordinary cost associated with XCT imaging as well as additive manufacturing processes. The initial investment cost of the technology and training, coupled with the need for lengthy clinical trials to prove efficacy of the methods, can deter them from being adopted in standard surgical procedures. Besides, the requirement for regulatory approval when manufacturing customized implants can complicate the achievement of timeliness in their use in real-life scenarios. These challenges will have to be overcome in maximizing the benefits of surgical planning and simulation models, eventually driving the functionality of customized medicine in biomedical engineering (Appleby et al., 2017; Kalaskar et al., 2017) (Figure 2.10).

2.4. ADVANTAGES OF ADDITIVE MANUFACTURING IN HEALTHCARE

Additive manufacturing (AM) has a number of advantages to the healthcare sector, particularly in the fabrication of medical equipment and prosthetics. Traditional manufacturing methods have limits in terms of the design complexity due to the fabrication constraints. AM, on the other hand, allows the generation of complex geometry that can be tailored for a specific patient. This ability is essential in areas like prosthetics and orthotics, where customized devices can increase functionality as well as comfort for patients. Further, AM allows quick prototyping, allowing healthcare professionals to go through several iterations of designs rapidly and test them without long lead times, thus speeding up the innovation process in medical uses. As such, additive manufacturing not only enhances patient-specific solutions but also enhances a more agile development culture within the space of biomedical engineering. Another advantage of AM within healthcare is the provision of material efficiency and reduced waste. Traditional subtractive manufacturing methods leave a tremendous amount of wasted material in their wake as raw material is cut away to create desired shapes. Simultaneously, AM builds items layer by layer, which means that there is considerably less waste and improved material utilization. This sustainability aspect is an advantage of the utmost significance to the growing emphasis in the medical field on sustainability, because producers and hospitals would like to lessen their ecological footprint. Besides, the application of biocompatible materials in AM makes implants and devices not just custom-fitted for patients but also meet regulatory standards for safety and effectiveness. Such dual focus on environmental sustainability and medical efficacy makes additive manufacturing an important technology for the future of healthcare. Finally, additive manufacturing has changed the learning environment within biomedical engineering by providing new ways of training future health practitioners. The ability to produce models for training that precisely imitate human anatomy enables the use of immersive learning spaces in which students and practitioners can practice surgical procedures or explore complex anatomical routes. Using AM allows institutions to create affordable, custom-made training material that exposes medical practitioners to hands-on experience with patient-specific cases without the ethical considerations and cost factors associated with employing traditional methods of training. The addition of AM in the field of education not only enhances learners' competence but also prepares them to embrace a dynamically shifting landscape in healthcare where personalized treatment plans become increasingly relevant. The marriage of technology and education thus empowers the next generation of healthcare professionals to optimally utilize the potential of additive manufacturing in their practice.

2.4.1. Customization and Personalization of Medical Devices

Additive manufacturing (AM) has revolutionized the field of biomedical engineering, particularly the aspect of customization and personalization of medical devices. This technology offers engineers and clinicians the possibility of creating highly specialized components that are tailored to the anatomy of unique patients, hence more efficient treatment. Design freedom offers the possibility of creating complex geometries using traditional manufacturing capabilities, thereby enhancing the functionality and comfort of medical devices. On top of that, Industry 4.0 through the connectivity of intelligent manufacturing systems enhances further AMs capability that enables fast prototyping and decentralized production more adaptable to patient individualized needs (Dehghanghadikolaei et al., 2019). Thus, customization through additive manufacturing not only meets personalized medicine needs but also enables future economic and environmental drivers in modern healthcare. In the particular instance of cranioplasty and prosthetic implants, AM has demonstrated its ability to deliver very bespoke solutions for enhancing patient outcomes. Advanced methodologies, including design for additive manufacturing and reverse engineering, have been instrumental in developing hybrid structures tailored for complex anatomical details (Ida et al., 2021). For instance, cranioplasty entails precise fitments in order to restore cranial integrity—a procedure aided significantly by the customization feature offered by AM. These customized medical devices not only enhance aesthetic results but also functional recovery, pointing toward the trend in patient-centric healthcare solutions. Moreover, these innovations highlight how AM enables medical devices to be tailored according to specific needs, thereby resulting in more efficient and effective clinical procedures. The convergence of technology and customization in additive manufacturing points to the promising innovations of the future in biomedical devices. With material science advancements and design practices currently undertaken, it is anticipated that the effectiveness of customized medical devices will continue to increase. For example, the inclusion of machine learning and data analysis in the design would yet enhance device customization, making them more responsive to patient-specific data. In addition, with sustainability increasingly becoming an imperative in healthcare, the ability of AM to reduce waste and optimize resource utilization will be the key determinant of biomedical engineering in the future. Lastly, personalization and customization of medical devices using additive manufacturing is a revolutionary strategy that embraces individuality while, at the same time, pursuing broader solutions to healthcare problems (Dehghanghadikolaei et al., 2019; Ida et al., 2021).

2.4.2. Reduction of Waste and Cost Efficiency

The integration of additive manufacturing (AM) technologies within biomedical engineering is a landmark change toward reducing wastage and enhancing cost-effectiveness. Traditional manufacturing methods usually succumb to massive wastage of resources through subtractive processes, which eliminate surplus raw material. By comparison, AM builds parts layer by layer with just the amount of material necessary to produce complex designs. This additive approach minimizes scrap and excess material, towards a greener manufacturing context. Secondly, the precision made possible by AM allows the creation of intricate and customized medical devices, which have the possibility to achieve improved patient outcomes while reducing the cost of overproduction and material waste. As more industries become incorporated with AM, the possibility of massive economic gains with accompanying environmental benefits becomes clear, further establishing the technology's place in a sustainable healthcare future (Dehghanghadikolaei et al., 2019). In addition, additive manufacturing cost-effectiveness extends beyond direct material savings to other savings in the area of production time and labor. The traditional manufacturing processes use giant tooling and setup processes that are both time and financially costly. On the other hand, AM allows rapid production and prototyping and the capacity to create quicker iterations and modifications to medical designs based on individual patient specifications. For instance, personalized implant design can be designed much more rapidly through the utilization of AM technologies, thereby reducing lead time from design to clinical application. This acceleration not only creates a reduction in warehousing and inventory expenses but also facilitates increased treatment of patients, thus resulting in improved efficiency in health. These advances demonstrate AMs capacity for optimizing procedures within biomedical engineering—resulting in the reduction of waste and lower total production (Ewart et al., 2019). Moreover, the ability to combine additive and subtractive manufacturing processes creates a sophisticated method for maximizing production efficiency in the biomedical sector. As demonstrated by examining molding inserts for the particulate injection molding (PIM) process, a hybrid system with both methods can address specific manufacturing challenges while being cost-effective. By leveraging the power of each method, manufacturers are able to optimize surface finishes and intricate geometrical details essential to biomedical applications. This fusion process not only prevents material loss and enhances product quality but also significantly reduces upfront tooling costs during prototyping and production runs. Thus, the combined application of additive and subtractive approaches shows how technology can strategically be applied to maximize cost-effectiveness while minimizing waste and further establish additive production as the basis of sustainable practice in biomedical engineering (Ewart et al., 2019) (Figure 2.11).

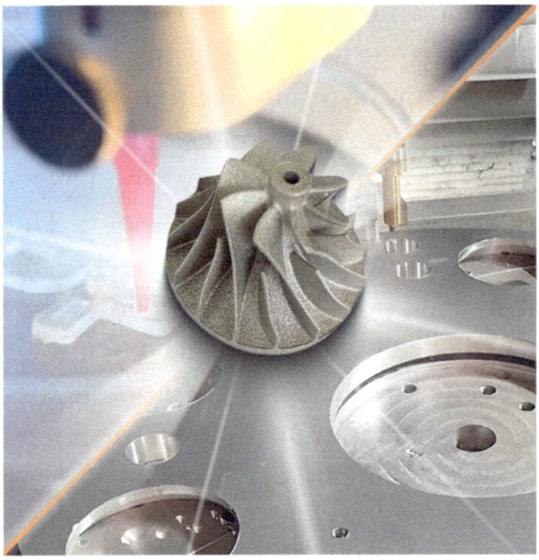

Figure 2.11. Traditional manufacturing methods often succumb to significant material waste due to subtractive processes that cut away excess raw materials.

Source: https://firstmold.com/wp-content/uploads/2024/05/additive-manufacturing-and-subtractive-manufacturing-featured-image.webp.

2.4.3. Speed of Production and Prototyping

The rapid pace of production and prototyping facilitated by additive manufacturing (AM) is arguably its most significant advantage throughout the discipline of biomedical engineering. AM technologies, particularly 3D printing, allow for the speedy construction of intricate and customized parts that meet precisely the specific needs of patients as well as of professionals. Because traditional manufacturing methods can be associated with significant setup time and rigorous design specifications, the flexural nature of AM allows for rapid iteration and optimization of models. Such responsiveness during the design phase not only shortens the development cycle but also enables the manufacture of customized medical devices ranging from prosthetics to intricate surgical devices. Thus, the integration of AM technologies into biomedical engineering constitutes a paradigm shift in production speed and innovation efficiency, enabling quicker reaction to clinical requirements and eventually better patient care outcomes (Dehghanghadikolaei et al., 2019). Moreover, prototyping in biomedical engineering is significantly advantageous with respect to the ability to manufacture iterations extremely quickly.

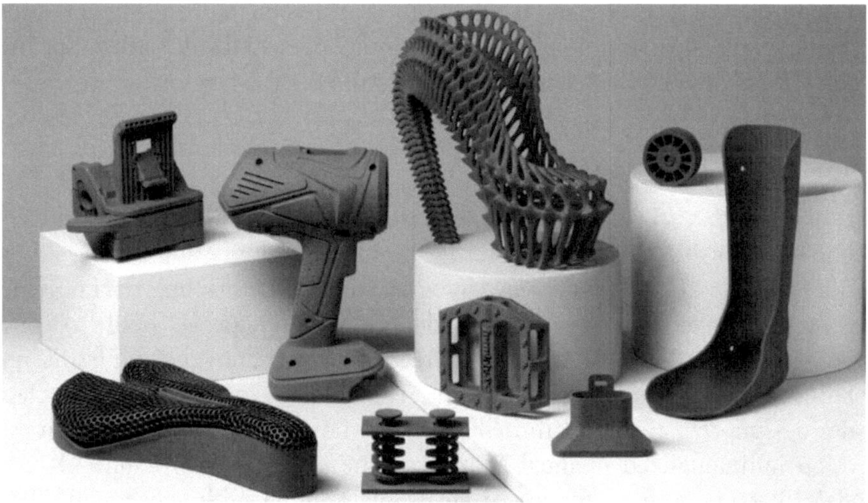

Figure 2.12. AM techniques, particularly 3D printing, facilitate the swift creation of complex and customized components that meet the specific needs of patients and practitioners alike.

Source: https://www.3dnatives.com/en/wp-content/uploads/sites/2/2024/04/RP-Parts-1-1280x720.jpg.

With AM, engineers can create prototypes very close to the final product with the significant reduction in long lead times typical manufacturing processes have. Not only are product testing and validation faster, but there is less material waste through enabling precise fine-tuning during the prototyping phase to be made. For instance, during medical implant design, prototypes are readily created to test fit, function, and compatibility with biological structures. Such rapid prototyping has proved priceless in medical uses where timely solutions are issues of life and death. Through speeding up the amount of prototypes that can be made, AM facilitates an iterative and rapid-response design process so that biomedical engineers can innovate effectively and maximize the potency of their solutions (Ewart et al., 2019). In the broader industry 4.0 context, additive manufacturing speed in production and prototyping embodies a convergence of digital advanced technologies with smart manufacturing systems. This does not only ensure maximum workflow efficiency but also shapes the face of production by embracing distributed manufacturing paradigms. Thus, AM technologies enable the decentralization of manufacturing for localized production of customized biomedical devices, with likely reduced costs and greater access within healthcare systems. As the industry becomes more advanced, the potential for hyper-personalized medicine approaches becoming a reality, demonstrating that manufacturing speed and prototyping in additive manufacturing is not just efficiency but a paradigm of becoming more personalized, patient-specific health (Dehghanghadikolaei et al., 2019) (Figure 2.12).

2.5. CONCLUSION

The end of this chapter on the fundamentals of additive manufacturing technologies in biomedical engineering highlights the revolutionizing nature of these new technologies. The integration of 3D printing technologies has revolutionized the biomedical device manufacturing field to offer customizability, efficiency, and design freedom without match from traditional techniques. For instance, technological advancements in 3D printing, such as in the design of patient-specific AFOs, show how crucial it is to design and develop individualized medical solutions. The verification of finite element models that measure stiffness and stress distribution with success indicates how crucial proper manufacturing is for better patient outcomes. With the utilization of these skills, the discipline of biomedical engineering can address unique healthcare issues, moving towards individualized medicine that respects individual patient needs and biomechanics, paving the way for future advancements. The use of additive manufacturing also has connotations extending beyond mere fabrication; it covers the whole cycle of biomedical device development, from initial concept design to actual practice. As demonstrated in research on ionomeric polymer-metal composite (IPMC) actuators, such as new geometries through freeform fabrication, can enable biomedical applications to be more functional. The study of IPMC indicates that such materials, when artificially molded through advanced manufacturing techniques, can lead to significant performance gains. Their integration into devices is a testament to the capability to create more complex functionalities in a smaller package. Such advancements bode towards a shift to even more advanced biomedical devices that are not only more effective but also more harmonized with the dynamically evolving environment of medical technology. Cumulatively, such advancements foster an even deeper investigation into the potential of additive manufacturing as a means of revolutionizing healthcare delivery. In encapsulating this analysis, it becomes clear that the biomedical engineering of the future is quite naturally harmonized with the evolution of additive manufacturing technologies. These technologies not only promise to upgrade existing medical devices but also to motivate the creation of never-before-seen solutions for special patient requirements. The research into how to incorporate advanced polymers and personalized medical devices is part of a broad trend towards more flexible and responsive healthcare solutions. As scientists continue to advance these technologies, future investigations will need to try to address their cost-effectiveness as well as possible scalability of manufacture. This future drive suggests that with additive manufacture progressing further, it will inevitably play an influential part in making the future of biomedical engineering, with the end goal of improving patient care and outcomes within increasingly personalized healthcare systems.

2.5.1. Summary of Key Points

Additive manufacturing technologies, particularly in the biomedical field, have breakthrough capabilities that are commensurate with the demand for customized medical solutions. The primary area to consider is that of developing personalized prosthetics and implants with customized designs suited to the individual patient anatomies. Not only does this personalization provide for greater comfort and fit of the devices but potentially also clinical performance. By employing technologies such as 3D printing, medical specialists are in a position to develop personalized implants, thus better addressing individual patient needs than might be achieved with traditional manufacturing. The implications of this shift are profound, as they herald a movement toward patient-oriented healthcare and additive manufacturing as a leading tool in the delivery of improved therapeutic solutions. The other fundamental aspect of additive manufacturing in biomedicine concerns the impact it exerts on material selection and mechanical behavior. Research indicates that infill direction and deposition patterns play decisive roles in influencing the strength and fracture resistance of products fabricated through 3D-printed PLA. Interestingly, PLA research showed that infill orientation changes do not have a material effect on overall strength or fracture toughness, indicating some level of manufacturing process design tolerance. Moreover, the ability to model mechanical behavior of 3D-printed materials without complex non-linear models can make the engineering design process easier. These findings underscore the importance of material property understanding in biomedical uses, ultimately ensuring consistency and effectiveness of medical devices produced through additive manufacturing (Anderson et al., 2017). Last, the wider business impacts of additive manufacturing technology become ever more visible as it disrupts conventional operating paradigms within the health sector. Research identifies that additive manufacturing not only enhances manufacturing but also demands a reframing of business models for organizations involved in biomedical engineering. Companies need to change to value proposition and customer dynamics shifts driven by the power of 3D printing technology. The conversion calls for an increased integrated perspective, looking at how creative manufacturing techniques engage with evolving customer needs. Such forthcoming research is on the verge of penetrating deeper into these crossroads so as to realize the full capabilities of additive manufacturing in the context of biomedical engineering (Asnafi et al., 2018).

2.5.2. The Impact of Additive Manufacturing on Future Biomedical Engineering

The advent of additive manufacturing (AM) has revolutionized the field of biomedical engineering, with unprecedented flexibility for medical device and implant design and manufacture. Unlike traditional manufacturing processes, in which intricate geometry often restricts the process, AM allows for the creation of extremely complex and tailored structures. This capability comes very useful while designing custom prosthetics that fit a specific patient anatomy, hence making them functional and comfortable. With the introduction of Industry 4.0, the integration of smart technology further maximizes the application of AM in medicine, making processes even more efficient and enabling design changes in real-time based on patient-specific needs, and lastly making a contribution to improved clinical outcomes (Dehghanghadikolaei et al., 2019). The revolutionary impact of such technology is likely to not only reshape the accessibility of products but also accuracy in meeting the diverse demands of physicians and patients. Moreover, the economic contribution of additive manufacturing in biomedical engineering is significant. Traditionally, medical device production is characterized by a high rate of material loss and extended lead times due to the need for multiple manufacturing processes. In contrast, AM processes prioritize efficiency through layer-by-layer fabrication, reducing the usage of material. This capability becomes a necessity when reflecting on the fast-evolving need for healthcare products, as AM can facilitate quick prototyping of tools that can be adjusted and optimized prior to mass production. In addition, the technology facilitates local production, which significantly saves shipping time and costs, apart from fulfilling its function in sustainability programs through minimizing carbon footprints associated with logistics (Dehghanghadikolaei et al., 2019). Accordingly, the future of biomedical engineering is increasingly intertwined with the economic benefits and efficiencies introduced by additive manufacturing technologies. AM's future advancement will continue to extend its range of applications in biomedical engineering, particularly concerning biocompatible materials and tissue engineering. The ability to print living cells and biomaterials sets the stage for developing regenerative medicine products, including organ printing and wound healing. Hybrid methodologies, which combine additive and subtractive processes, were found to maximize production of intricate tissue scaffolds and resolve processing issues associated with traditional processing methods, according to a recent study. Breakthroughs in material science enable metals, polymers, and bioactive agents to be combined and enable the formation of multifunctional devices that actively interact with biological systems. With further advances in research, prospects for AM use in the biomedical sector appear limitless, with a potential future for customized, functional, and sustainable medical devices matched closely to patient needs and healthcare demands.

2.5.3. Final Thoughts on the Evolution of the Field

The speedy evolution of additive manufacturing (AM) technologies has drastically transformed the area of biomedical engineering. This transformation has granted designers and engineers greater liberty in fabricating complex components tailored to the specific needs of medical devices. The foundation of this transformation is the capacity of AM in enabling rapid prototyping, an element which allows for swift repetition of designs and accelerates collaboration among multi-disciplinary teams. Its inclusion in the framework of Industry 4.0 has further enhanced its impact, promoting efficiency, waste reduction, and material conservation. The technologically driven renaissance also presents an opportunity to tackle issues of sustainability, hence balancing the field of biomedicine with greater environmental ends. The ability of AM to revolutionize traditional ways of making and improve patient recovery is what ultimately makes it a turning point agent in the future of biomedical engineering (Dehghanghadikolaei et al., 2019). In light of the specific advancements witnessed in AM technologies, appreciation should be given to the way such innovations have led to the growing personalization of medical implants and devices. The ability to design patient-specific solutions, including orthopedic and dental prosthetics, encourages not only increased compatibility but also increased efficiency in healing and rehabilitation. Development and research into many materials, including biocompatible polymers and metal alloys, are based on knowledge of the interaction between these substances and biological systems. A multi-processing method of manufacturing that combines additive and subtractive processes is proof of the innovative strategies being used to counter challenges that are native in the biomedical industry. For instance, the use of low-cost molding inserts reflects the potential of hybrid manufacturing techniques to fight surface finish and part removal defect issues, finally ending up in more advanced and functional finished goods in the application of biomedical (Ewart et al., 2019). Given the trajectory that AM technologies have followed in biomedical engineering, the future looks rosy for increased developments. Given that scientists continue to explore the intersection of AM with other emerging technologies, the potential for developing new materials and methodologies is unlimited. This trend of further exploration for efficiency, coupled with an unabiding passion for sustainability, will likely drive even greater infusion of smart manufacturing principles into biomedical processes. With the technology coming of age, the amalgamation of different sciences—materials science to mechanical engineering to biology—will lead to new applications previously impossible. Thus, embracing the development process of AM technologies not only places their relevance in the current time into context but also highlights their role in shaping the destiny of biomedical engineering as a tool towards improved patient-focused solutions and, by extension, the destiny of health care as a whole (Dehghanghadikolaei et al., 2019).

REFERENCES

1. Anderson, I., de Ciurana, J., Fernandez-Vicente, M., Hamad, W. Y., Lanzotti, A., Susmel, L., Susmel, M., et al. (2017). Additively manufactured PLA under static loading: Strength/cracking behaviour vs. deposition angle. https://core.ac.uk/download/144881174.pdf (accessed on 14th October 2025).
2. Annemans, L., Gemmel, P., Tack, P., et al. (2016). 3D-printing techniques in a medical setting: A systematic literature review. https://core.ac.uk/download/84043719.pdf (accessed on 14th October 2025).
3. Appleby, A., Azari, B., Bache, B., Bernhard, J., Berry, D., et al. (2017). X-ray computed tomography and additive manufacturing in medicine: A review. https://core.ac.uk/download/132846284.pdf (accessed on 14th October 2025).
4. Arrizubieta Arrate, J. I., Cortina Burón, M., Lamikiz Mentxaka, A., et al. (2018). Latest developments in industrial hybrid machine tools that combine additive and subtractive operations. https://core.ac.uk/download/187772345.pdf (accessed on 14th October 2025).
5. Asnafi, N., Oberg, C., & Shams, T. (2018). Additive manufacturing and business models: Current knowledge and missing perspectives. https://core.ac.uk/download/222841326.pdf (accessed on 14th October 2025).
6. Ast, M. P., Bini, S. A., Chung, C. C., et al. (2020). Digital orthopedics: A glimpse into the future in the midst of a pandemic. https://core.ac.uk/download/323308683.pdf (accessed on 14th October 2025).
7. Blunk, T., Boland, T., Burdick, J. A., et al. (2016). Bio fabrication: Reappraising the definition of an evolving field. https://core.ac.uk/download/77034391.pdf (accessed on 14th October 2025).
8. Centeno Báez, G., González Pérez, L. M., González-Pérez-Somarriba, B., et al. (2018). On the analysis of the contact conditions in temporomandibular joint prostheses. https://core.ac.uk/download/225123757.pdf (accessed on 14th October 2025).
9. Chia, H. N., & Wu, B. M. (2015). Recent advances in 3D printing of biomaterials. https://core.ac.uk/download/323078409.pdf (accessed on 14th October 2025).
10. Concheri, G., Meneghello, R., Rosso, S., et al. (2018). Geometric modeling of cellular materials for additive manufacturing in biomedical field: A review. https://core.ac.uk/download/154326170.pdf (accessed on 14th October 2025).

11. De Beule, M., Deckers, J. P., Forward, M., et al. (2019). A validated computational framework to evaluate the stiffness of 3D printed ankle foot orthoses. https://core.ac.uk/download/237010383.pdf (accessed on 14th October 2025).
12. Dehghanghadikolaei, A., Emamian, S. S., Fotovvati, B., et al. (2019). The potential of additive manufacturing in the smart factory industrial 4.0: A review. https://core.ac.uk/download/231748826.pdf (accessed on 14th October 2025).
13. Díaz, J., González-Estrada, O. A., & López, C. (2017). Biomechanical analysis of a cranial patient specific implant on the interface with the bone using the finite element method. http://arxiv.org/abs/1709.06632 (accessed on 14th October 2025).
14. Ewart, P. (2019). A comparison of processing techniques for producing prototype injection molding inserts. https://core.ac.uk/download/322841895.pdf (accessed on 14th October 2025).
15. Farahi, E., Gibbons, G. J., Lv, Y., Purnell, P., & Williams, R. (2010). 3D printing of cement composites. https://core.ac.uk/download/44217.pdf (accessed on 14th October 2025).
16. Goyanes, A., Goyanes, A., Goyanes, A., Goyanes, A., Melocchi, A., Maier, A. K., Buanz, A. B., et al. (2016). Emergence of 3D printed dosage forms: Opportunities and challenges. https://core.ac.uk/download/42138948.pdf (accessed on 14th October 2025).
17. Hansen, H. N., Hofstätter, T., Pedersen, D. B., et al. (2017). State-of-the-art of fiber-reinforced polymers in additive manufacturing technologies. https://core.ac.uk/download/84005855.pdf (accessed on 14th October 2025).
18. Ida, P. (2021). *Integrated Methodologies and Technologies for the Design of Advanced Biomedical Devices*. https://core.ac.uk/download/574199143.pdf (accessed on 14th October 2025).
19. Jena, M. C., Mishra, S. K., & Moharana, H. S. (2024). Application of 3D printing across various fields to enhance sustainable manufacturing. https://core.ac.uk/download/635776175.pdf (accessed on 14th October 2025).
20. Kalaskar, D., Leong, J., & Provaggi, E. (2017). Applications of 3D printing in the management of severe spinal conditions. https://core.ac.uk/download/79531622.pdf (accessed on 14th October 2025).
21. Ledbetter, F., Morgan, K., Prater, T., et al. (2025). A portfolio of fabrication and recycling technology development for the International Space Station. https://core.ac.uk/download/pdf/161998639.pdf (accessed on 14th October 2025).

22. Ledbetter, F., Morgan, K., Prater, T., et al. (2025). In-space manufacturing at NASA Marshall Space Flight Center: A portfolio of fabrication and recycling technology development for the International Space Station. https://core.ac.uk/download/pdf/161998643.pdf (accessed on 14th October 2025).
23. Lipson, H., & Malone, E. (2005). Freeform fabrication of ionomeric polymer-metal composite actuators. https://core.ac.uk/download/287648532.pdf (accessed on 14th October 2025).
24. Meng, L., Wu, L., Zhang, J., et al. (2019). Phase field simulation of dendritic microstructure in additively manufactured titanium alloy. https://core.ac.uk/download/227054203.pdf (accessed on 14th October 2025).
25. Pinkerton, A. J. (2015). *Lasers in Additive Manufacturing*. https://core.ac.uk/download/42415986.pdf (accessed on 14th October 2025).

CHAPTER 3

MATERIALS FOR BIOMEDICAL 3D PRINTING

Contents

INTRODUCTION

The invention of 3D printing technology has revolutionized numerous fields, particularly in the field of biomedicine, where it offers new solutions to long-existing issues in tissue engineering and regenerative medicine. The possibility of creating patient-specific scaffolds and implants has gained significant attention, highlighting the necessity of developing appropriate materials that can meet the sophisticated biological requirements for those applications.

This union of technology and materials science enables new possibilities, making it possible to generate constructs that not only mimic the mechanical and biological behaviors of human tissues but also support cellular behavior required for healing and regeneration. Consequently, the research on diversified materials like polymers and biopolymers is important to drive this emerging science forward and face severe healthcare issues such as organ deficiency and the need for better drug testing facilities. It has been identified through studies that organ deficiency for transplantation has made frank appeals for new solutions, particularly in the form of developing artificial human tissue. This requirement becomes increasingly important as traditional organ transplant waiting lists continue to escalate, placing many patients in life-threatening situations. Furthermore, the drug market is plagued by lengthy human trial phases, provoking a search for alternative testing arenas mimicking *in-vivo* environments. 3D printing technologies allow the fabrication of tissue-like structures, both addressing organ deficiencies and enhancing drug development processes. Current trends in the techniques, whether laser or laser-free, demonstrate various spatial resolutions and print speeds, which are indicative of this technology heading towards rapid development and application in the clinical sector (Bakhshinejad et al., 2015). With the developing 3D printing technology, there has been a need to create new materials and processes that can intermingle cells seamlessly, thereby enhancing the efficacy of biofabrication. The development of technologies such as 3D Bioplotting™ illustrates the potential for working with various polymers and biopolymers in the development of patient-specific scaffolds for organ printing. With the utilization of personal computer tomography scans of patients, scientists can create biodegradable patient-specific scaffolds with superior *in-vitro* and initial *in-vivo* results. These advances not only make the possibilities of enhanced organ regeneration approaches available but also teach us about how to better optimize scaffolding materials for a variety of biomedical applications (Carvalho et al., 2004). With continued development, interaction between material scientists, engineers, and clinicians will be essential in translating laboratory advances into effective therapeutic interventions.

Importance of Materials in 3D Printing

The role of materials in 3D printing cannot be overemphasized, especially in biomedical applications. Proper selection of materials determines the structural integrity and biocompatibility of the printed structures. For instance, studies on biopolymers and hydrogels have added to the material list used to generate scaffolds that allow cellular growth. Specifically, techniques such as 3D Bioplotting allow a variety of polymers, including collagen and chitosan, to be employed in scaffolding constructs that are not just supportive but also facilitate cell proliferation and viability (Carvalho et al., 2004). Since the patients all have unique anatomical requirements, individual patient-derived scaffolds can be constructed based on individual patient information, illustrating the requirement for elastic materials to maximize personalized treatment and medicine outcomes. Materials used in 3D printing also have a fundamental function in improving the productivity and versatility of the manufacturing process. Additive manufacturing offers the capability to produce intricate designs with significantly reduced material loss, which is concurrent with sustainability goals in manufacturing (Dehghanghadikolaei et al., 2019). This is especially significant in the biomedical field, where precision of component generation is critical to procedures such as organ printing.

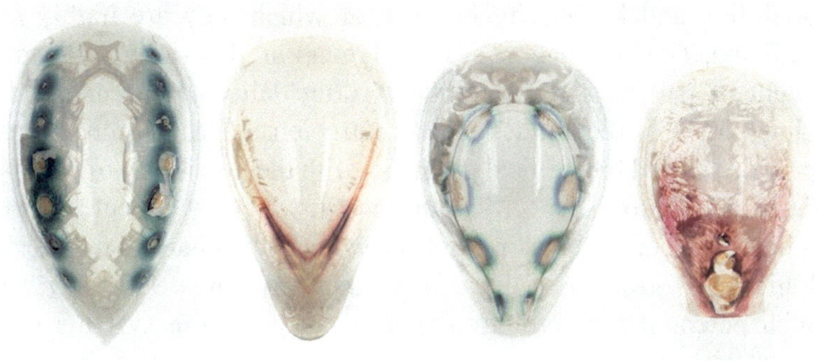

Figure 3.1. The significance of materials in 3D printing cannot be overstated, particularly in the context of biomedical applications.

Source: https://news.mit.edu/sites/default/files/styles/news_article__image_gallery/public/images/202001/MIT-3D-Bioprinting_0.jpg?itok=9Y6_DqMc.

Technological advancements in eco-friendly materials are not just critical for economic efficiency but also contribute to the overall environmental impact of 3D printing technologies. To have the ability to employ biodegradable materials when making models and prototypes highlights the importance of material selection since it provides opportunities for green practices that enable sustainability within the healthcare industry. Lastly, the future of biomedical 3D printing rests in ongoing research and material development for the response to different biomedical applications. As the technology itself evolves, the materials being researched range from advanced thermoplastics to emerging biocompatible composites. Adding 3D printings to broader industry trends, such as Industry 4.0, emphasizes the need for breakthrough material solutions enabling rapid prototyping and distributed manufacturing (Dehghanghadikolaei et al., 2019). The potential of these materials to revolutionize the character of patient care—by facilitating custom-made solutions to enhance healing and recovery—bears testimony to their increasing relevance. In the long term, the continued discovery of new materials will not only refine existing applications but also introduce revolutionary breakthroughs in the area of biomedical engineering (Figure 3.1).

3.1. TYPES OF MATERIALS USED IN BIOMEDICAL 3D PRINTING

Biopolymers are one of the most promising categories of materials used in biomedical 3D printing due to their unique properties and environmental friendliness. These bio-based materials exhibit features such as biocompatibility, biodegradability, and bioactivity because of which they are highly safe for use in medicine. The application of biopolymers in 3D printing allows for the development of patient-specific implants, drug delivery systems, and tissue engineering scaffolds. Techniques such as extrusion and laser printing have been used to produce varied biomedical products, with the possibility of personalized applications tailored to the specific requirements of every patient. Advances in blending biopolymers with nanoparticles have further enhanced the mechanical and biological performance of these 3D-printed structures. This new approach holds much potential for revolutionizing advanced health systems in such a way that materials can be properly integrated into the human body and deliver functionality and sustainability (Hossain, 2023). Another vitally important category of material gaining more attention in biomedical 3D printing includes nanogels. These are materials that incorporate nanoscale structures, which are created by connecting micelles within aqueous solutions, and have the ability to enclose different therapeutic payloads. The multi-functionality of the nanogels makes them ideal prospects for drug delivery, with applications extending into tissue engineering and surgical tools. The advancements in 3D printing technology have opened new avenues for the specific, tailor-made, and efficient production of nanogels that are at the core of personalized medicine. As researchers go on to develop such materials, the potential to prepare tailored nanogel formulations through 3D printing is a major step towards improving targeted drug delivery. Such a shift in the process of nanogel production enhances their application potential as a solution for various biomedical applications, opening the door towards improvements in patient care and treatment efficacy (Cho et al., 2018). The exploration of composite materials in biomedical 3D printing integrates the advantages of various materials, thus optimizing their overall performance. Biopolymers are often combined with metals or ceramics to upgrade mechanical properties as well as biological performance. For instance, metal-enriched biopolymers can provide structural integrity in load-bearing applications such as orthopedic implants and maintain the required biocompatibility. In addition, composites may be engineered with precise bioactive properties to support cellular adhesion and growth, essential for tissue engineering applications. As researchers continue to investigate more of the interactions between different material phases, optimization of composite materials will contribute to pushing patient-specific treatments in biomedical 3D printing forward. Lastly, this innovative approach highlights the potential of interdisciplinarity in producing highly complex materials that meet the diversity of issues facing modern healthcare (Hossain, 2023).

3.1.1. Polymers

Polymers are a groundbreaking material in the field of biomedical engineering, particularly with 3D printing technology. Engineers are able to employ various polymeric materials to create scaffolds that replicate the complex microarchitectures found in living tissues. The scaffolds serve as templates for cell adhesion and development, thus leading to tissue development and healing. Particularly, biological polymers like gelatin, alginate, and hyaluronic acid have gained special attention due to their extracellular matrix (ECM) mimicking properties and biocompatibility. The application of these polymers for 3D printing allows for the possibility of having customizable properties, which are designed to meet particular medical applications, thereby providing both mechanical strength and biological activity. Overcoming the particular challenge presented in tissue engineering requires a nuanced understanding of polymer properties and behavior within biological environments, and it is a vital platform for regenerative medicine innovation. Chemically cross-linked polymers are a significant step forward in the production of 3D-printed scaffolds. It enhances the mechanical strength of hydrogel constructs, typically compromised in non-cross-linked materials, suitable for biomedical applications. For instance, gelatin, alginate, and hyaluronic acid scaffolds can be cross-linked chemically using calcium chloride to produce a stable scaffold that is more resistant to physiological conditions than traditional hydrogels. Such advances are necessary for developing scaffolds that can be employed for tissue engineering in applications from liver regeneration to eye implantation. It brings into focus the importance of polymer chemistry in the determination of the properties and performance of 3D-printed materials within the clinical context, hence providing a pathway for successful tissue integration and function (Macwan et al., 2018). Advances in recent 3D printing technologies have also increased the potential areas of application for polymers in biomedical applications. The ability to fabricate patient-specific scaffolds and devices has transformed the science of personalized medicine with the promise of individualized treatment strategies that more effectively address anatomical differences on a patient-to-patient basis. As highlighted in recent literature, 3D printing not only facilitates the creation of bespoke implants and scaffolds but also incorporation with cellular material to bring the field further toward the regeneration of complex tissues. However, reproducibility and scalability of 3D-printed constructs, especially those that mimic complex tissue architectures such as liver or cardiac tissue, remain challenges. These will be overcome through further research into material properties as well as printing technologies in an effort to achieve maximum efficacy and safety for clinical applications (Chia et al., 2015). With ongoing incremental advances, polymers will continue to open new paths in the interface of medicine and technology, ultimately revolutionizing treatment modalities within the biomedical community (Figure 3.2).

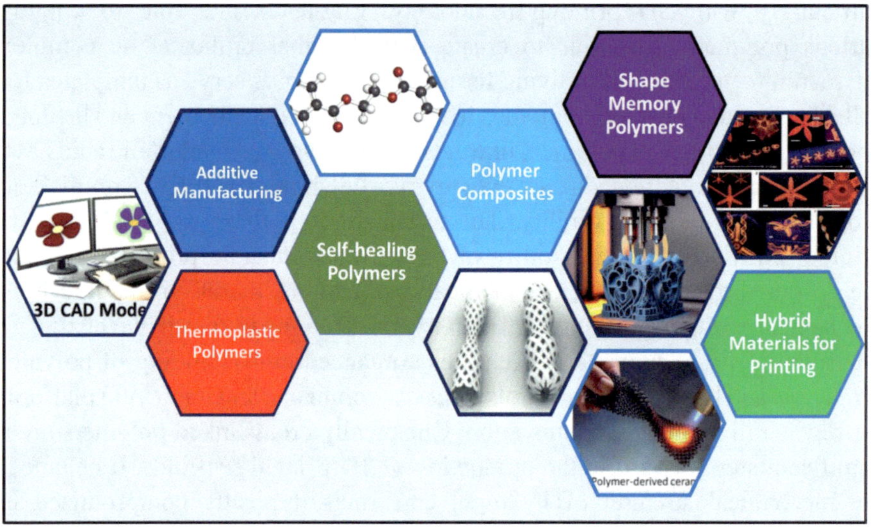

Figure 3.2. Polymers play a transformative role in the field of biomedical engineering, particularly in 3D printing applications.

Source: https://pub.mdpi-res.com/molecules/molecules-29-00319/article_deploy/html/images/molecules-29-00319-ag.png?1704931573.

3.1.2. Metals

In the area of biomedical 3D printing, metals are found to be essential materials due to their unique mechanical characteristics and biocompatibility. Stainless steel and titanium are commonly applied in the fabrication of implants and prosthetics due to their hardness, toughness, and resistance to physiological conditions. The property of metal to be precisely molded and designed with additive manufacture is of particular significance for the development of complex geometries that may be individually customized to fit individual patient needs. Not only does such versatility enhance the operational efficacy of biomedical devices but also patient outcomes through minimizing the danger of complications due to improperly fitting implants. Thus, the use of metals in biomedical 3D printing is a giant leap towards personalized medicine, highlighting the groundbreaking nature of new materials for medical applications. To that, the advances of additive manufacturing (AM) technologies are complemented with the uses of metals in biomedical 3D printing. These technologies, in the form of additive manufacture of metal components layer by layer, enable the synthesis of complicated shapes that in theory cannot be produced by traditional manufacturing methods. For instance, AM enables the production of porous metal structures that can stimulate osseointegration, which is yet another step towards developing even more functional orthopedic implants (Dehghanghadikolaei et al., 2019).

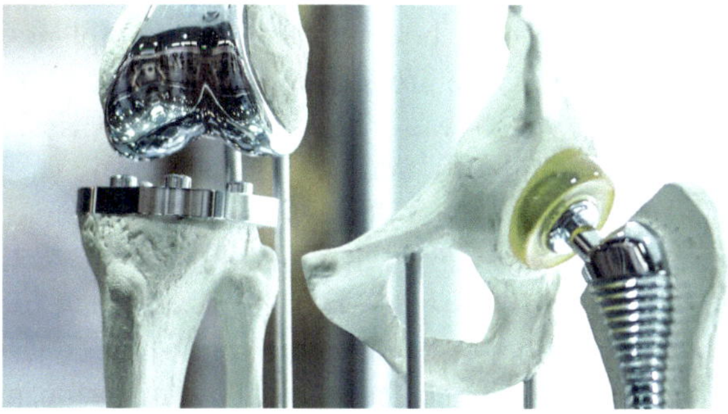

Figure 3.3. Metals, such as titanium and stainless steel, are frequently utilized in creating implants and prosthetics due to their strength, durability, and ability to withstand physiological conditions.

Source: https://images.theconversation.com/files/275791/original/file-20190521-23835-38tcg8.jpg?ixlib=rb-4.1.0&rect=0%2C614%2C2856%2C1428&q=45&auto=format&w=1356&h=668&fit=crop.

The increased design freedom associated with AM not only enables innovation in implant design but also promotes sustainability via material conservation, as wastage is minimized. These are areas of technological overlap that highlight the deep potential that metals have for advancing existing biomedical use, ultimately leading to better treatment and improved healthcare provision. Besides traditional metallic applications, research into new metal-based alloys has opened up avenues for enhanced functionality within biomedical devices 3D-printed. Alloy developments, such as adding bioactive coatings and modifications to improve corrosion resistance, have significant implications for the longevity and performance of implants. Moreover, utilization of advanced production techniques allows for the control of metal characteristics during printing to guarantee the formation of devices able to adapt to the biological environment in which they are inserted. These advances have some resonance with the growing emphasis on personalized medicine, in which patient-specific needs lead the character of the advancing implants. Thus, while the field of biomedical engineering continues to expand, metals are sure to be part of the key in charting the future of biomedical engineering and improving the quality of patient care in various modes of therapy (Figure 3.3).

3.1.3. Ceramics

Ceramics have emerged as a critical material in biomedical 3D printing, largely due to the fact that they are bioinert and mechanically stable. They provide the possibility of a favorable environment for osseointegration, and consequently, they can be used in bone scaffolds and implantable devices. Based on conventional methods, the production of ceramic components relied on traditional approaches, which were known to restrict design freedom. However, with the evolution of additive manufacturing technologies, particularly in processes such as stereolithography and powder bed fusion, it is feasible to create complex geometries that enhance the interaction between ceramic implants and biological tissues. With the enablement of customized design and porosity optimization, researchers are capable of creating scaffolds that not only facilitate cell attachment but also allow diffusion pathways for nutrients, hence enabling tissue regeneration and healing processes. Aside from that, the incorporation of ceramics within 3D printing is highly compatible with the overall trends of Industry 4.0, which include the integration of intelligent manufacturing with smart materials. Ceramics blended with other polymers and biopolymers can enhance significantly the mechanical strength of the resulting hybrid materials. This versatility allows for the production of custom-made implants precisely designed for individual patients' requirements based on precise imaging data. The potential for real-time prototyping made possible through additive manufacturing techniques not only helps the efficient production process but also assists in greater customization of biomedical implants. As companies increasingly turn towards sustainable practices, ceramics also demonstrate favorable characteristics, such as biocompatibility and the ability to minimize waste, helping to solidify their role within the future of biomedical 3D printing (Dehghanghadikolaei et al., 2019). Aside from their mechanical and biological advantages, the chemical resistance and thermal stability of ceramics also qualify them for use in various biomedical environments. For instance, bioactive ceramics such as bio-glasses and calcium phosphate ceramics can actively participate in biological processes, promoting interfacial bonding to surrounding tissue and bone healing. The ceramics are also identified to function as drug delivery systems due to their porosity with controlled release profiles. Moreover, with research taking place, developments in ceramic formulations and processing methods are creating avenues for more efficient manufacturing of premium-quality medical devices. The integration of ceramics onto 3D printing platforms is therefore a fundamental aspect of the engineering of future biomedical applications, since current research continues to prove the promising results of a number of *in vitro* and *in vivo* tests that have now been conducted using these new materials (Carvalho et al., 2004) (Figure 3.4).

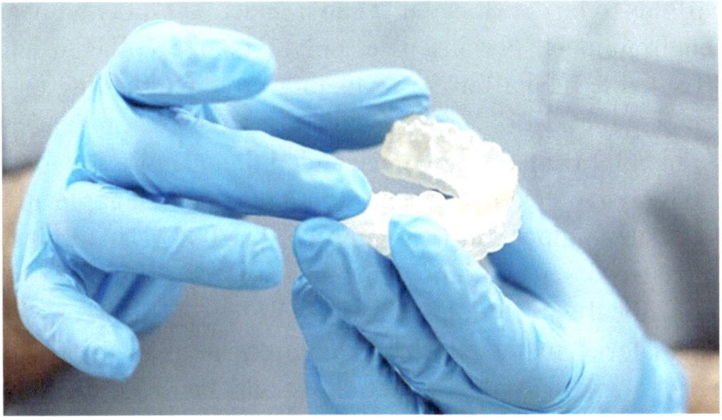

Figure 3.4. Ceramics have emerged as a crucial material in the realm of biomedical 3D printing, primarily due to their bioinert properties and structural integrity.

Source: https://cheersonic-liquid.com/wp-content/uploads/2022/03/Ceramic-3D-printing-is-a-step-forward-for-dental-products-Cheersonic.jpg.

3.2. PROPERTIES OF IDEAL 3D PRINTING MATERIALS

The ideal 3D printing materials' properties form the backbone of successful utilization of biomedical constructs. They ought to be biocompatible in order not to react when they come into contact with living tissue. Moreover, they must possess appropriate mechanical strengths such as strength and elasticity similar to the natural tissue that will be replaced or supported. This type of biomimicry is essential to the point that printed structures will be capable of withstanding physiological loads and operations in the long term. The materials must also demonstrate printability, i.e., be comfortable to deal with during the printing process without deteriorating. This may include maintaining viscosity, flow characteristics, as well as thermal stability under various conditions. Full comprehension of such material properties allows scientists to better optimize implant and device design and performance, tailored to some specific biomedical application, significantly enhancing regenerative medicine (Chia et al., 2015). Another property that needs to be perfect for materials used in 3D printing is the ability to incorporate bioactive agents or cells during the printing process. This compatibility is key to the development of scaffolds that not only provide structural support but also stimulate cellular activity, stimulation of which results in the regeneration of tissue. New materials, such as biodegradable polymers and hydrogels, have also made this possible, allowing complex scaffolds to be developed that can interact favorably with surrounding biological environments. For instance, polymers like collagen and chitosan can serve as suitable media for encapsulating protein signaling or stem cells, thereby enhancing the scaffolds functionality. Based on research advancements, technologies like 3D Bioplotting have enabled the use of a broad spectrum of polymers and biopolymers, thereby expanding the range of application in organ printing and tissue engineering (Carvalho et al., 2004). This trait mirrors the necessity of material science innovation in terms of facilitating increasingly advanced biomedical applications. Last but not least, fast processing rate and simplicity of material manufacturing remain essential in the biomedical 3D printing environment. The ideal materials should facilitate rapid prototyping in a bid to fulfill the urgent needs of patient-specific solution treatment. Development of processes that facilitate quick redesign and material change can significantly reduce the time from idea to clinical application. Furthermore, advancements in multi-material printing technologies allow hybrid structures to be built with a variety of various material qualities, leading to performance improvement and tissue compatibility. Blending material technology with high-technology printing procedures is critical in order to bypass drawbacks presently experienced in custom implants and prosthetic manufacturing. Focused research effort on multi-material strategies can push the field forward, providing tailored solutions that maximize patient advantage in regenerative treatments and surgical interventions (Chia et al., 2015).

3.2.1. Biocompatibility

The concept of biocompatibility is most crucial in biomedical 3D printing as it addresses the compatibility of materials being used in medical implants and devices with the biological system. Biocompatibility not only depends on the ability of a material to perform its assigned function without inducing a reaction that one would not desire but also on how it can interact peacefully with the human body. In the case of 3D-printed devices, this involves that the selected material must support cellular functions and promote tissue regeneration and minimize inflammatory responses. The materials science achievements have provided the development of a variety of polymers, including photo-initiator-modified and crosslinking agent-modified polymers, which support tailorability of mechanical properties and degradation rates required for specific biomedical application. Studies have established that some material blends for 3D-printed biomedical devices also affect their biocompatibility to a large extent.

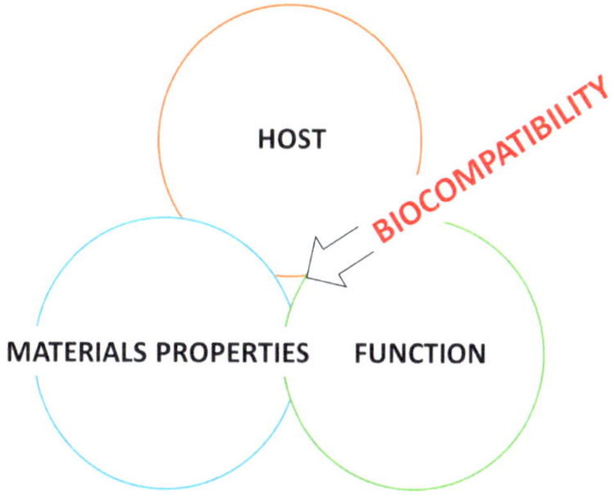

Figure 3.5. Biocompatibility is defined not only by a materials ability to perform its intended function without eliciting an adverse reaction but also by its potential to integrate seamlessly with the human body.

Source: https://pub.mdpi-res.com/materials/materials-16-06881/article_deploy/html/images/materials-16-06881-g001.png?1698324301.

For example, combining hydrogels like PEGDA blended with alginate or PVA has been proven to exhibit good mechanical properties suitable for use in medicine. As in new research, it has been noted that these materials, when exposed to various crosslinking procedures like UV exposure or *in-situ* reticulation, also exhibit varying mechanical strengths and elasticity suitable for the use of prosthetics. A systematic investigation of such comparisons establishes that higher concentrations of PVA can enhance Young's Modulus, thereby enhancing load-carrying properties. Such enhancements underpin the notion that the selection of material is a direct function of achievable mechanical properties, which in turn influence the longevity and functional success of devices in a biological setting (Cristóvão et al., 2018). Moreover, the evolving nature of 3D printing technologies poses a tipping point for personalized medicine in that it has the ability to offer customizing of devices based on patient-specific anatomies. The ability to produce complex geometries that mimic the infrastructure of native tissues offers opportunities for application in tissue engineering and regenerative medicine. However, the challenge remains to maintain biocompatibility while achieving intricate geometrical structures and microstructural characteristics that support cellular processes. With rising interest in personalized scaffolds and implants, overcoming the material functionality and biocompatibility technological limitations becomes a need of utmost importance. This problem, in conjunction with pushing continued research on novel materials and printing techniques, also prompts a multidisciplinary approach to develop the field, with aspects from material science, biology, and medical engineering being incorporated into it (Chia et al., 2015) (Figure 3.5).

3.2.2. Mechanical Strength

The concept of mechanical strength is of utmost significance for the case of materials used in biomedical 3D printing. In contrast to conventional manufacturing techniques, 3D printing enables the creation of geometries that are highly complex and are often tailored to the specific anatomy of a patient. Personalization has the effect of improving the functionality of biomedical devices, but it also means the materials must exhibit proper mechanical behavior. Mechanical strength, encompassing tensile strength, compressive strength, and fatigue resistance, determines the ability of such materials to withstand physiological stresses without failure. With continued technological development in 3D printing, the selection of materials with necessary mechanical strength for specific biomedical applications—e.g., bone or cartilage substitutes—becomes increasingly vital. Such material characteristics need to be known to guarantee the longevity and effectiveness of implants and scaffolds in tissue engineering. Within three-dimensional printed structures, coordination of mechanical strength and manufacturing processes is what defines biomedical application fate. Additive manufacturing techniques such as Fused Deposition Modeling (FDM) and Selective Laser Sintering (SLS) possess distinct capabilities and limitations in relation to mechanical strength. For example, the layering process employed in FDM can be prone to developing anisotropy where mechanical properties are directionally dependent. Conversely, SLS can be more mechanically strong with a homogeneous powder particle fusion. Brittleness present in certain materials, like titanium alloys utilized in Particulate Injection Molding (PIM) trial runs, necessitates material choice and processing adjustment to be taken into serious account. These changes are required to reverse surface finish defects and part removal, ultimately leading to the production of robust biomedical devices that can endure dynamic physiological conditions

(Ewart et al., 2019). Progress in material science is also driving innovations that enhance the mechanical performance of 3D-printed biomedical devices. Innovation has focused more and more on combining traditional polymers with bioactive compounds to enhance the mechanical and biological compatibility of scaffolds. For example, the incorporation of composite materials that include bioactive glass or ceramics may increase mechanical strength while ensuring osteoconductivity for bone scaffolds. Not only do such advancements aim to replicate the mechanical integrity of native tissue but also the biological necessities needed for successful integration and healing. As highlighted by current research into materials and technologies, the congruence of utmost mechanical strength and biocompatibility is a problem still fueling development and innovation in biomedical 3D printing (Chia et al., 2015). This congruence between mechanical properties and bio-functionality is of utmost importance for the future success of personalized regenerative medicine initiatives (Figure 3.6).

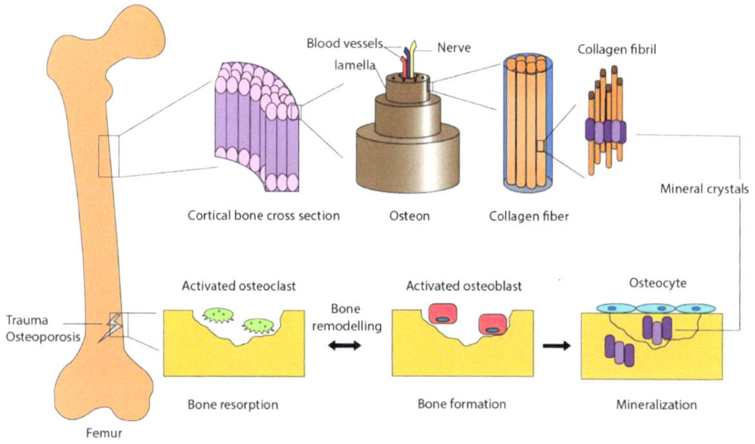

Figure 3.6. Utilizing composite materials that integrate bioactive glass, or ceramics can augment the mechanical properties while enabling osteoconductivity in bone scaffolds.

Source: https://www.mdpi.com/jcs/jcs-05-00259/article_deploy/html/images/jcs-05-00259-g001.png.

3.2.3. Printability

One of the main characteristics of biomedical 3D printing is the concept of printability as a material's capability to be properly processed and formed into complex structures through additive manufacturing technologies. For materials that are to be used in applications such as drug-eluting implants, printability entails the mechanical properties and printing flow behavior of the polymer, biocompatibility, as well as long-term stability after processing. Advanced materials like the thermo-responsive supramolecular polyurethane show appreciable advantage to achieving ideal printability. The ability of the material to self-assemble depending on hydrogen bonding and π-π stacking interactions enables the material to create a processable structure at comparatively low temperatures, retaining the functional properties required for biological application.

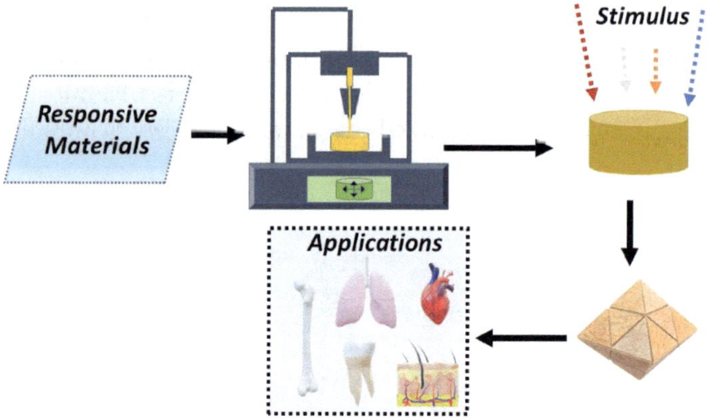

Figure 3.7. Innovative materials, like the thermo-responsive supramolecular polyurethane, demonstrate significant advantages in achieving ideal printability.

Source: https://www.mdpi.com/pharmaceutics/pharmaceutics-15-02743/article_deploy/html/images/pharmaceutics-15-02743-g001.png.

These functionalities are essential for ensuring successful layer bonding and creating intricate geometries for fulfilling the demands of some medical applications, without degrading material integrity upon printing (Clark et al., 2020). Another facet of printability is the formulation of inks that can display stability and performance upon going through printing technologies like inkjet technology. Novel findings on biodegradable polyurethane polymers derived from sugar indicate a hopeful trajectory in this direction. These polymers not only contribute the rheological properties necessary for printability but also contribute to a better understanding of how different formulations can contribute to the resolution and geometrical complexity of printed objects. Stabilizing gold nanoparticles in these inks is novel and has broad implications in making possible advanced biomedical sensors and showcasing the synergy between printing technology and material formulation. These developments reveal the ways in which factors such as polymer stability, print resolution, and functional additive incorporation potential can significantly contribute to the overall functionality and printability of biomedical applications (Vel et al., 2019). Innovation in materials to enhance printability also plays a key role in achieving tailored patient-specific solutions in the biomedical field. Precise calibration of materials allows for tailoring of mechanical properties and degradation rates to meet the need of different applications, from orthopedic implants to drug delivery systems. Continued work on improving printability will surely yield materials that allow for better bioactivity and cell growth promotion, which are essential to successful integration in biological systems. As proven in studies on 3D printed drug-eluting implants, the possibility of drug release profiles being controlled through polymer composition emphasizes the importance of printability to achieve functional results. Further research into printability in biomedical materials is therefore needed to fully unlock the potential of 3D printing technologies in the healthcare sector (Clark et al., 2020) (Figure 3.7).

3.3. COMMON POLYMER MATERIALS

In biomedical 3D printing, the choice of polymer material plays an important role in the success of most applications such as implants, scaffolds, and drug delivery devices. Polymers are becoming increasingly popular due to their beneficial properties such as biocompatibility, ease of processing, and versatility. Some of the most popular polymers are poly(lactic acid) (PLA), polycaprolactone (PCL), and poly(ethylene glycol) (PEG), each with different properties suited for various biomedical applications. For instance, PLA is renowned to be biodegradable and utilized in frequent use in temporary implants, while PCL is prized for its degradation rate as slow and suitable for use on a long-term basis in tissue scaffolding. The availability to tailor these materials makes them more practical and is targeted at the aim of creating patient-specific solutions, emphasizing the significance of continuous research in polymer processing techniques and chemistry in biomedical 3D printing (Chia et al., 2015). The integration of several processing techniques allows for new advances in biomedical device creation. For instance, techniques such as fused deposition modeling (FDM) and stereolithography (SLA) are capable of accelerating the manufacturing capacity for sophisticated designs required in biomedical applications. FDM based on thermoplastic polymer usage presents a low-cost and inexpensive technique for the fabrication of bioactive scaffolds, while SLA presents high precision in creating complex geometry structures with high smoothness of surface finish. Scientists have explored hybrid methods that combine additive and subtractive operations to advance the production of components needed for applications like particulate injection molding (PIM) with handling of delicate materials. Overcoming challenges related to surface finish and structural integrity through such advanced technologies will enhance the performance and reliability of 3D-printed biomedicals significantly (Ewart et al., 2019). Despite the prospective characteristics of polymers in biomedical 3D printing, there are many limitations that need to be resolved in order to enable their regular application. One of the principals among them is the mechanical behavior of printed materials, especially for load-bearing functions such as orthopedic implants. A majority of the used polymers in biomedical functions have insufficient mechanical properties relative to bone and therefore require reinforcement or blending with stronger materials. In addition, their biocompatibility with living tissues is of the utmost significance; most crucial is that they should not result in adverse immune reactions. Enhancing drug delivery efficiency and ensuring sustained release factors has been the focus of research by modifying polymer structures. Overcoming these technological limitations will not only further enhance the efficiency of biomedical devices but also make them more integratable within clinics, resulting in more personalized and efficient care (Chia et al., 2015).

3.3.1. Polycaprolactone (PCL)

In biomedical 3D printing, Polycaprolactone or PCL has emerged as a key material due to its biocompatibility and ability to biodegrade. PCL is a renewable polyester that has favorable mechanical properties, which make it suitable for several applications ranging from tissue engineering scaffolding to enabling long-term drug delivery and slow tissue regeneration. Its low rate of degradation makes it a valuable tool in regenerative medicine. The printability of PCL by using traditional 3D printing technologies such as Fused Deposition Modeling (FDM) has made it more applicable in manufacturing complex structures that are tailored to meet patient-specific anatomical requirements. As the demand for personalized medicine rises globally, PCL's malleability renders it a valuable asset in the production of custom-made implants and devices that can be seamlessly absorbed into the human body, creating avenues for innovative therapeutic strategies in medicine (Chia et al., 2015). The applications of PCL are not limited to scaffolding. It is possible to mix this with other compounds or change its composition to make it stronger, hence a potential hybrid material for tissue engineering. Recent developments have proved that the addition of inorganic elements to PCL improves mechanical strength markedly and encourages cell growth and adhesion. All these alterations allow for the creation of bespoke scaffolds that are capable of mimicking the extracellular matrix (ECM) in tissues, which is essential for cell growth as well as overall tissue functionality. PCLs biocompatibility also allows one to introduce growth factors and antibacterial agents into the scaffolds, hence enabling faster healing phenomena as well as reducing infection possibilities upon implantation (Abalymov et al., 2020). While scientists keep discovering and actualizing the potential of PCL, its role in 3D printing also keeps growing, addressing some of the issues in biomedical application. Ultimately, the applicability of PCL in biomedical 3D printing hinges on its ability to keep up with the demands of a continually evolving field. The integration of new manufacturing technologies with materials like PCL is a paradigm shift in the designing and manufacturing of medical devices and tissue engineering scaffolds. By facilitating the creation of intricate geometries tailored to a specific patient, PCL not only enhances the efficacy of biomedical implants but also facilitates the attainment of the ultimate goal of precision medicine. Ongoing research on modifying PCL composites and deciphering their effects with biological systems will naturally create new applications, pushing development towards improved clinical performance. As new materials are investigated, PCL is a cornerstone of biomedical 3D printing, demonstrating its fundamental worth towards creating functional and customized medical devices (Abalymov et al., 2020; Chia et al., 2015) (Figure 3.8).

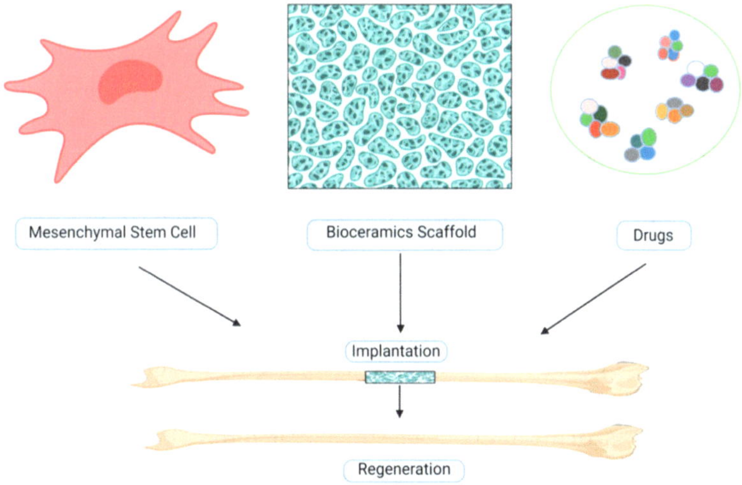

Figure 3.8. PCLs compatibility with bioactive molecules enables the incorporation of growth factors and antibacterial agents within the scaffolds, thereby facilitating enhanced healing processes and reducing the risk of infection post-implantation.

Source: https://pub.mdpi-res.com/biomimetics/biomimetics-09-00230/article_deploy/html/images/biomimetics-09-00230-g001.png?1713176291.

3.3.2. Polylactic Acid (PLA)

Polylactic acid or PLA is one of the most sought-after biopolymers for 3D printing, particularly biomedical applications, due to its biodegradability and biocompatibility. PLA is produced from renewable resources such as cornstarch, which apart from enhancing its sustainability, renders it an environmentally friendly material in materials science. This biopolymer is especially noteworthy based on the fact that it is capable of replicating the mechanical properties of biological tissues precisely and thus is an appropriate candidate for scaffold fabrication in tissue engineering. Scaffold development from PLA allows for successful creation of structures capable of supporting cell growth and extracellular matrix (ECM) deposition necessary for successful tissue repair and regeneration. Moreover, the modularity of PLAs molecular weight and composition can endow with targeted mechanical and degradation properties appropriate for personal biomedical applications. PLA application in 3D printing is not only confined to structural support but also entails complex functionality that is critical for therapeutic discovery. Altered PLA-based scaffolds have been demonstrated by existing research to be designed to fit drug delivery systems for localized controlled delivery of therapy agents. This technology offers an enhancement of the scaffolds overall performance in treating numerous diseases by ensuring that growth factors or antibacterial agents can be directly applied at the point of injury. Hence, PLA scaffolds are not mere passive containers but become active participants in the healing process. Foraying in this field of research opens the window of possibility for hybrid materials where PLA is mixed with bioactive agents, further augmenting the potential of the scaffold to facilitate cell growth and tissue integration. This multidisciplinary endeavor is a new direction in biomedical engineering. It is also worth mentioning that ongoing developments in additive manufacturing technologies on PLA are redefining the fabrication aspect on an ongoing basis. The latest developments have utilized the application of PLA fiber-reinforced composites to enhance mechanical properties, surpassing the traditional limitations against the inherent brittleness of neat PLA. The resultant improvement allows for the production of strong yet flexible structures resisting physiological stresses. The use of additives, including carbon fiber or glass fiber, proves the versatility of PLA as an application in advanced biomedical fields. This growing body of work also highlights the necessity for print parameter and material formulation optimization to enable optimal properties tailored to specific clinical demands. As the landscape of biomedical 3D printing advances, PLA continues to spearhead the effort, reinforcing its credentials time and again for its flexibility and potential to enhance patient treatment and care practices, as reported by Abalymov et al. (2020) and Hansen et al. (2017) (Figure 3.9).

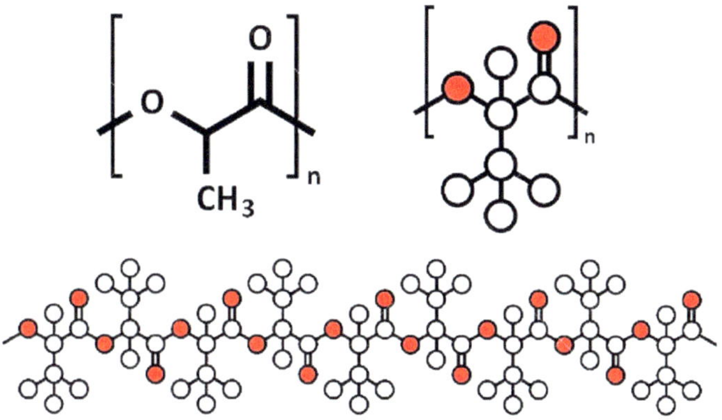

Figure 3.9. Polylactic acid (PLA) has emerged as a favored biopolymer in the realm of 3D printing, particularly for biomedical applications, due to its biocompatibility and biodegradability.

Source: https://media.springernature.com/lw1200/springer-static/image/art%3A10.1007%2Fs00170-022-10795-y/MediaObjects/170_2022_10795_Fig1_HTML.png.

3.3.3. Thermoplastic Elastomers (TPE)

Thermoplastic elastomers (TPE) are a class of materials with the characteristics of thermoplastics and elastomers and thus the best materials for biomedical applications, particularly for 3D printing. Their unique properties of flexibility, toughness, and processability are important in the fabrication of intricate structures with the ability to mimic biological tissues. TPEs may be engineered with a wide range of mechanical properties, as long as the final solutions are shaped to meet personalized biomedical applications, such as drug delivery devices, soft implants, and tissue engineering scaffolds. The ability to print TPEs contributes to their appeal in biomedicine as, in being printed, they can be utilized to design devices that require customized dimensions and geometry without compromising the biocompatibility — a secret of medical devices to be utilized for quite a period of time within the human body. The flexibility of TPEs encompasses their mixing with functional additives that enhance their performance in specific applications. With the addition of conductive nanofillers, researchers can design piezoresistive sensors to monitor the physical condition of infrastructure *in situ*, aside from their use in biomedical applications. Such addition demonstrates TPE's potential in transforming products like organ-on-chip technologies, whose correct environmental factors are critical. TPE's ability to be formed into films, coatings, and complex geometries makes them viable in intelligent biomedical devices that respond adaptively to the physiological environment of the body. Further, the profound effect of polymer processing and design on the final properties of TPE composites underscores their utility in future biomedical engineering applications, particularly as the medical field increasingly turns to targeted and individualized therapies (Costa et al., 2021). For organ-on-chip platforms, TPEs offer important advances through cost-effective and broadly applicable solutions for microfluidics applications. These systems promise to revolutionize the drug discovery process and personalized medicine by the accurate recapitulation of human physiology in a test tube. TPE materials enable rapid microfabrication processes, which are critical in the scale-up of organ-on-chip technology.

TPEs also permit the creation of functional microtissues and blood perfusion networks without the burdensome tubing and pumping, thus simplifying experimental designs. Scalable organ-on-disc technologies created via the application of TPEs demonstrate their use in overcoming the fabrication constraints traditionally associated with microphysiological systems to make them affordably and on a large scale (Schneider et al., 2022). In conclusion, the multifaceted use of TPEs in biomedical 3D printing supports their basic role as pioneers in next-generation healthcare technologies and applications (Figure 3.10).

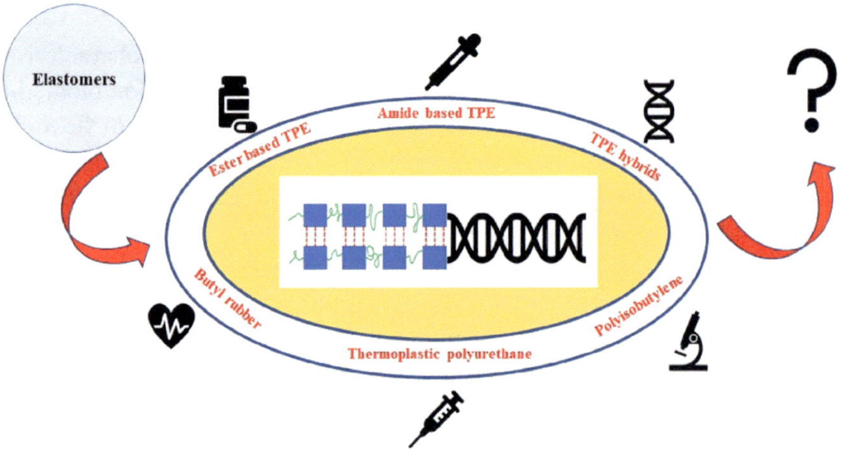

Figure 3.10. Thermoplastic elastomers (TPE) represent a class of materials that blend the characteristics of thermoplastics and elastomers, making them ideal candidates for biomedical applications, particularly in 3D printing.

Source: https://www.tandfonline.com/action/showGraphicalAbstractImage?doi=10.1080%2F10601325.2021.1922086&id=lmsa_a_1922086_uf0001_c.jpg.

3.4. METAL MATERIALS IN BIOMEDICAL APPLICATIONS

The application of metal materials to biomedical devices has revolutionized the 3D printing technology, particularly in fabricating complex structures necessary for medical implants and devices. Titanium and titanium alloys are chosen due to compatibility with biological systems, mechanical properties, and corrosion resistance, hence appropriate for load-bearing orthopedic implants. In addition, cobalt–chromium alloys and stainless steel are both widely used in various surgical instruments and dental implants due to their resistance and strength in the physiological environment. Incorporation of these metal components maximizes implant durability and reliability as well as potentially reducing post-surgery complications, thereby significantly enhancing patient outcome. The multidisciplinary 3D printing technologies enable the possibility of personalizing these materials, thereby enabling the production of patient-specific anatomy models and devices that are specifically designed to fulfill certain medical specifications, a critical step towards personalized medicine (Chia et al., 2015). Moreover, additive manufacturing technologies have also expanded the potential for introducing metal materials in biomedical devices. Techniques such as selective laser sintering and electron beam melting have realized revolutionary leaps in accuracy and complexity that can be achieved in metallic structures. The methods facilitate the creation of porous scaffolds that not only replicate the mechanical behavior of natural bone but also increase greater biological integration because of the elevated surface area for cell attachment as well as nutrient delivery. The structures are uniquely applied in tissue engineering applications. Furthermore, the novel material processing and design minimization technologies are overcoming some of the inherent limitations for metallic implants, such as stress shielding and wear of the device over time. As such, the novel dynamics of metal materials in 3D printing are, therefore, inducing novel avenues of research and application in regenerative medicine (Dehghanghadikolaei et al., 2019). With the development of technology in biomedical 3D printing, there is still a great need to address the challenge of metal materials. The primary challenge is the need for improved material properties to enhance tissue integration and functional performance within the body. In recent studies, the focus is on the design of bioactive metallic materials that can enhance osseointegration while maintaining the mechanical integrity for load-bearing applications. Furthermore, the environmental and economic impacts of metal production are being brought under greater scrutiny, resulting in advances in green manufacturing processes. By implementing the dimensions of Industry 4.0, wherein efficiency and waste minimization are paramount, the future of metal materials in healthcare use could not just provide useful patient products but also prioritize environmental stewardship. In such a changing environment, sustained innovation in metal 3D printing technologies is key to realizing their potential in customized healthcare (Chia et al., 2015) (Figure 3.11).

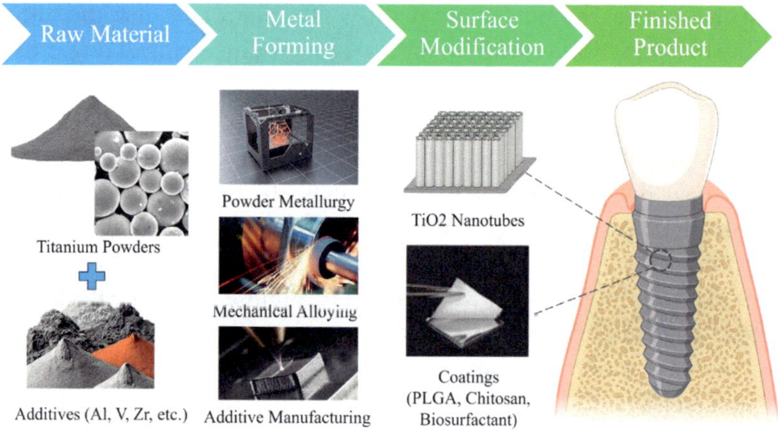

Figure 3.11. Metals such as titanium and its alloys are favored due to their biocompatibility, mechanical strength, and corrosion resistance, making them ideal candidates for load-bearing orthopedic implants.

Source: https://pub.mdpi-res.com/materials/materials-16-06860/article_deploy/html/images/materials-16-06860-g002.png?1698312011.

3.4.1. Titanium Alloys

Titanium alloys are increasingly valued for their superior attributes in biomedical engineering, particularly in 3D printing technology. The alloys are characterized by excellent strength-to-weight ratios and better resistance to corrosion, proposing them as ideal implants and prosthetics. This worth is further boosted by their compatibility with biology, allowing lesser side effects within the human body. Titanium's ability to form stable surfaces within biological systems in addition to its mechanical properties makes it possible to produce complex geometries and inner shapes required for individualized medical solutions. As there is an ever-growing demand for personal medical devices, titanium alloys using 3D printing are one way of producing personal implants that meet individual patients' needs, resulting in better surgical outcomes and patient satisfaction. The convergence of 3D printing technology and titanium alloys is a paradigm-shifting new path for traditional manufacturing methods in the biomedical sector. Additive manufacturing is a process that makes it possible to produce patient-specific models and implants, which cannot be produced using traditional methods. Owing to the complexity of human anatomy, porous structures and complex internal geometries can be produced with physiological requirements specific to patients, which by itself is an advancement. Additionally, additive manufacturing, as one of the Fourth Industrial Revolution, embodies the spirit of operational sustainability and effectiveness in terms of minimizing wastage of materials while compressing the production timeline. The combination of titanium alloys with 3D printing maximizes design possibility together with adherence to the imperatives of these modern times of rapid prototyping and bespoke therapeutic intervention, which take the lead in driving innovation along with healthcare provision (Dehghanghadikolaei et al., 2019). Moreover, continuous research and development of titanium alloys and processing routes through 3D printing are providing avenues for future advancements in biomedical applications. Material science advancement has met the challenge of enhancing the mechanical properties of titanium alloys and exploring their production efficiencies. Introduction of many alloying elements allows tailoring mechanical properties to suit the requirements of specific biomedical applications, such as orthopedic implants for various tensile strength and ductility needs. Moreover, ongoing work on surface treatments and coatings of titanium alloys holds the potential for improved osseointegration and overall biological behavior after implantation. As the biomedical industry more and more applies 3D printing as its foundation of progress, titanium alloys are destined to play a progressively vital function in the development of future medical devices and treatments methods, thereby addressing the complex challenges of modern medicine (Cho et al., 2018).

3.4.2. Stainless Steel

In the arena of biomedical 3D printing, stainless steel is a particularly intriguing material due to its favorable characteristics that make it most suited for use in surgical implants and medical devices. Commended for its better biocompatibility, stainless steel showcases the capacity to inhibit adverse reactions when in contact with biological tissues. Moreover, its mechanical properties and corrosion resistance are essential in attaining the durability and reliability of implants in dynamic biological environments. The successful integration of stainless-steel parts determines the success of tissue engineering and regenerative medicine therapy overall. Stainless steel is being used more and more by researchers in 3D printing to fabricate intricate geometries that respond to patient-specific use, ultimately more personalizing medical procedures. Novel applications of stainless steel in the development of biomedical devices are among the key drivers of healthcare technology advancement. The capability to fabricate complex geometries that have the ability to replicate the multi-faceted nature of biological tissues is one of the key advantages of using stainless steel in additive manufacturing. As reported in recent studies, stainless steel has been incorporated into numerous biomedical applications, such as orthopedic implants and dental appliances, in which precision of the mechanical properties is imperative for functionality. Furthermore, advancements in processing techniques have facilitated easier production of stainless-steel components with enhanced surface quality, which are critical to improve osseointegration and reduce the risk of infection. This varied application of stainless steel reflects its core role in the evolution of the potential of biomedical 3D printing technology. Nevertheless, without all its benefits, the application of stainless steel to biomedical 3D printing is also confronted by setbacks. The intricacy in the printing process, including the selection of appropriate parameters for the energy input and layer adhesion, is observed to affect predominantly the material performance and mechanical strength. Furthermore, post-processing techniques, as researched in the fabrication of cavities for metal alloys like titanium, highlight the need for careful attention to surface quality and structural soundness. Research on the optimal manner in which additive and subtractive processes are combined illustrates the ability to overcome such difficulties. With continued evolution of the discipline, it will be essential to address these issues to obtain the maximum benefit of stainless steel in biomedical applications, to make the prototype-to-ready-to-use-device process effective and reliable (Ewart et al., 2019) (Figure 3.12).

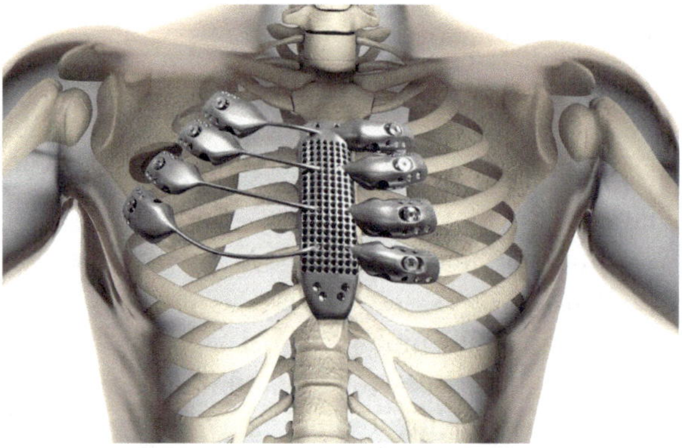

Figure 3.12. In the realm of biomedical 3D printing, stainless steel has emerged as a noteworthy material due to its advantageous properties, making it particularly suitable for surgical implants and medical devices.

Source: https://habrastorage.org/getpro/habr/upload_files/748/440/097/748440097b5fff77e94cb7c0168c0121.png.

3.4.3. Cobalt–Chromium Alloys

The cobalt–chromium alloys are increasingly recognized as a primary factor in biomedical 3D printing, particularly in the manufacture of orthopedic implants and dental appliances. Cobalt–chromium alloys possess an excellent combination of mechanical properties including great strength, wear resistance, and corrosion resistance, which are of utmost importance for those materials applied under load-bearing situations inside the human body. The ability of cobalt–chromium alloys to adapt allows them to be susceptible to being manufactured using various additive manufacturing technologies, hence ability to manufacture structures with complex geometries that are challenging using traditional machining processes (Attar et al., 2018). This concurs with the evolution of additive manufacturing technologies to enable cellular material design with desired functional attributes, particularly scaffolds for tissue engineering (Concheri et al., 2018). Hence, cobalt–chromium alloys are good targets for innovation in individualized medicine, where implants can be precisely fitted to enhance patient performance. The use of cobalt–chromium alloys in biomedical 3D printing also addresses required issues of biocompatibility. In their use in implants, the alloys will not only have to satisfy requirements for mechanical performance but also have to be well compatible with living tissues in order to inhibit immune responses. Recent studies have identified successful approaches in surface modification of cobalt–chromium implants for improving their biocompatibility. For instance, techniques of introducing self-assembled monolayers (SAMs) can enhance the surface properties to reduce post-implant complications (Ask et al., 2014). Such treatments can facilitate the attachment of biomolecules that improve cellular interactions, with the ultimate goal of better integration with surrounding tissues. As scientists continue to explore these shifts, the potential of cobalt–chromium alloys to sustain function biologically yet retain mechanical strength is an exciting frontier in biomaterials technology. From the perspective of additive manufacturing, the level of structural complexity attainable with cobalt–chromium alloys is a clear sign of the direction of healthcare to come. The fabrication of porous scaffolds, for instance, avails itself of the specific capability of these alloys to improve bone in-growth and tissue regeneration. Geometrical flexibility offered by 3D printing facilitates the fabrication of scaffolds with tailor-made porosity and mechanical properties to duplicate those of alternating bone structures, allowing for improved biological performance (Concheri et al., 2018). Besides, studies still strive to refine the printing method to maximize the surface quality and mechanical strength of cobalt–chromium parts. Ultimately, the combination of sophisticated fabrication techniques and the biocompatibility of cobalt–chromium alloys enhance the likelihood of developing implants and scaffolds that not only perform but also respond to the biological environment they inhabit. This dual capacity underscores their revolutionary impact on modern biomedical engineering (Figure 3.13).

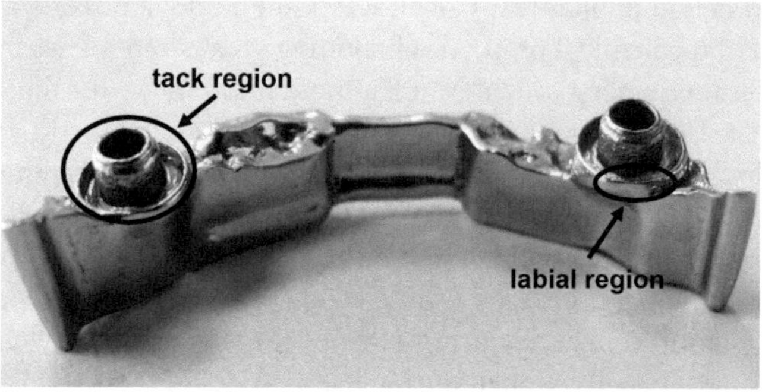

Figure 3.13. Cobalt–chromium alloys are increasingly recognized for their significant role in the field of biomedical 3D printing, particularly in the manufacture of orthopedic implants and dental applications.

Source: https://www.mdpi.com/materials/materials-13-05390/article_deploy/html/images/materials-13-05390-g001.png.

3.5. CERAMIC MATERIALS FOR 3D PRINTING

The incorporation of ceramic materials into 3D printing technology has, in a large manner, revolutionized the aspect of biomedical applications, particularly in tissue engineering and regenerative medicine. Ceramics are noted for their mechanical properties, biocompatibility, and bioactivity, hence ideal for various biomedical devices, including implants and scaffolds. Unlike traditional production techniques, 3D printing allows for the personalization of ceramic structures to the unique anatomical requirements of specific patients. This capability is crucial for the creation of patient-specific implants that can facilitate better biointegration with biological tissue and facilitate healing processes. The transition from simple printing for pre-surgical models to the design of complex biocompatible constructs is a demonstration of the utility of ceramics in facilitating personalized medicine, and this highlights the necessity of overcoming existing technological limitations in print resolution and material properties prior to clinical use becoming common practice (Chia et al., 2015). Furthermore, progress in the field of additive manufacturing has opened avenues for the study of several ceramic materials for enhancing the mechanical and biological properties of printed components. Specifically, the use of bioactive ceramics, such as calcium phosphate ceramics, has been promising due to their ability to stimulate bone regeneration. The flexibility of these materials allows for the incorporation of other bioactive agents within the ceramic matrix, allowing for the development of drug delivery systems incorporated into 3D-printed scaffolds. Besides their structural benefits, these composite materials may respond to physiological signals, releasing therapeutic agents in a controlled manner, thereby enhancing their efficacy in regenerative applications. But the specific mechanical properties and biocompatibility of these novel ceramic compositions must be studied comprehensively for confirming their suitability for application in clinics (Farahi et al., 2010). In order to use the full potential of ceramics in biomedical 3D printing, the problem regarding the process of printing itself must be addressed. The use of the ceramic materials has a tendency to pose issues in achieving intricate designs and high precision due to their brittle nature and difficulty in layer-wise deposition. Remedies such as modifying the polymer-ceramic composite concentrations and optimizing the print parameters are being explored in order to mitigate these challenges. For instance, research has indicated that the incorporation of additives is used to improve the flow properties of ceramic pastes to achieve higher print resolutions and mechanical strengths. Furthermore, post-processing operations like sintering and soaking in hydration media assist in realizing improved mechanical properties and avoiding the layered appearance typical of 3D-printed geometries. To address these technology hurdles is essential to drive the field of biomedical 3D printing into fruition to produce dainty, functional, and bio-compatible ceramic implants (Chia et al., 2015).

3.5.1. Hydroxyapatite

The advent of hydroxyapatite as a key material in biomedical 3D printing has revolutionized the scope of regenerative medicine to a great extent. Hydroxyapatite, which is the natural mineral form of calcium apatite, best replicates the mineral structure of bone tissue. It is a suitable candidate for bone tissue engineering applications owing to its osteoconductivity and biocompatibility, improving the integration of implants with adjacent bone tissue, hence enabling natural healing mechanisms. Latest breakthroughs in 3D printing technology allow for the precise manufacturing of hydroxyapatite scaffolds that may be tailored to fit unique patient anatomies and thus revolutionize surgical processes. Based on various research, the applications of such tailored scaffolds are extended beyond simple scaffolding to even complex architectures that have the potential to sustain regrowth of complex tissue architectures required for maximum outcomes in regenerative medicine (Chia et al., 2015). Apart from its advantageous biological properties, the versatility of hydroxyapatite in 3D printing methods also establishes it as crucial in biomedical engineering.

Stereolithography, Selective Laser Sintering, and Fused Deposition Modeling are among various printing methods applied in creating hydroxyapatite-based constructs that mimic the natural bone's mechanical and biological properties. Such constructs not only enhance the scaffold properties but also allow the delivery and incorporation of growth factors and stem cells necessary for tissue development. Incorporation of hydroxyapatite into composite scaffolds, which could be combined with polymers and other biomaterials, has been reported to enhance both the functionality and the durability of the printed constructs and thus bypass some of the pitfalls observed in traditional grafting procedures. These innovations are part of a trend towards personalized regenerative therapies using 3D printing technology for better clinical outcomes (Almeida et al., 2017). Besides, the therapeutic capability of hydroxyapatite to heal complex tissue deficiencies places it at the forefront of biomaterials used in contemporary surgeries. The traditional method of dealing with maxillofacial defects, which typically relies on autografts or allografts, is challenged with donor site morbidity and restricted accessibility. Hydroxyapatite scaffolds, especially those that are produced with advanced 3D printing technology, are a satisfactory option through their ability to present a template that can sustain cellular proliferation and differentiation *in vivo*. More recent research highlights the efficacy of hydroxyapatite for both hard and soft tissue regeneration, showing its capability for incorporation and functional integration within the craniofacial and other regions. This potential is significant for future treatment regimes for diseases such as temporomandibular joint disorders and bone fractures, hence paving the way for further research in the field of biomedical 3D printing (Chia et al., 2015) (Figure 3.14).

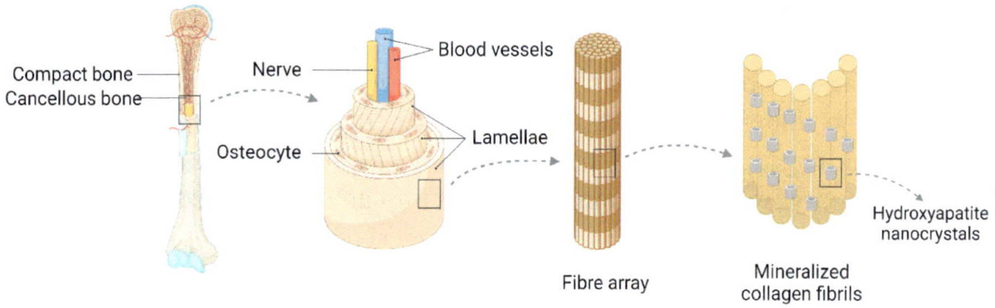

Figure 3.14. Hydroxyapatite, a naturally occurring mineral form of calcium apatite, closely resembles the mineral component of bone, making it an ideal candidate for applications involving bone tissue engineering.

Source: https://pub.mdpi-res.com/ijms/ijms-24-12492/article_deploy/html/images/ijms-24-12492-g001.png?1691318983.

3.5.2. Bioglass

The invention of Bioglass as an innovative biomaterial signifies its key contribution to biomedical 3D printing. It was discovered in the 1960s, but today Bioglass has been famous for its bioactivity that allows it to bond with surrounding bone tissue and stimulate natural mechanisms of healing. Such a characteristic is crucial while manufacturing scaffolds used in tissue regeneration in medical devices for applications in orthopedics and dentistry. Unlike traditional materials, Bioglass can participate in dynamic biological interaction and promote osteoconductivity and hydroxyapatite formation, the primary bone mineral matrix.

As a result, Bioglass scaffolds are ideal candidates for 3D printing technology, with the potential to manufacture patient-specific implants that offer sophisticated mimicking of bone morphology, eventually leading to enhanced integration and functionality in the body. Application of Bioglass in 3D printing technology offers high potential for the personalization of scaffolds according to the specific needs of individual patients. The versatility of 3D printing allows the rational design of porous structures that can facilitate cell invasion and nutrient supply, both being crucial for successful tissue engineering. Moreover, Bioglass can be doped with various dopants, e.g., metal ions, which can enhance its bioactivity and antimicrobial properties. These technologies have the promise to overcome shortcomings of traditional graft materials that are often faced with integration and biocompatibility challenges.

Continued research, the marriage of Bioglass with advanced 3D printing technologies has the promise of revolutionizing regenerative medicine to deliver tailored solutions to complicated human anatomical restorations. Recent research recognizes the role of Bioglass in scaffolds development for a number of applications, including maxillofacial defect repair. Such an ability to create biodegradable and customized scaffolds is characteristic of the interdisciplinarity of contemporary material science. This is especially valid taking into account the growing requirement for new developments in tissue engineering with the involvement of cooperation between clinicians and bioengineers in order to improve the effectiveness of treatments. Substantial *in vitro* and *in vivo* tests have established the effectiveness of Bioglass in cartilage and bone regeneration, thereby pointing towards its use as a new material basis in biomedical applications. As various reports have confirmed (Almeida et al., 2017), the uses of Bioglass are not merely for structural support but also as a healing catalyst and tissue integrator—a cornerstone in the future of biomedical 3D printing (Figure 3.15).

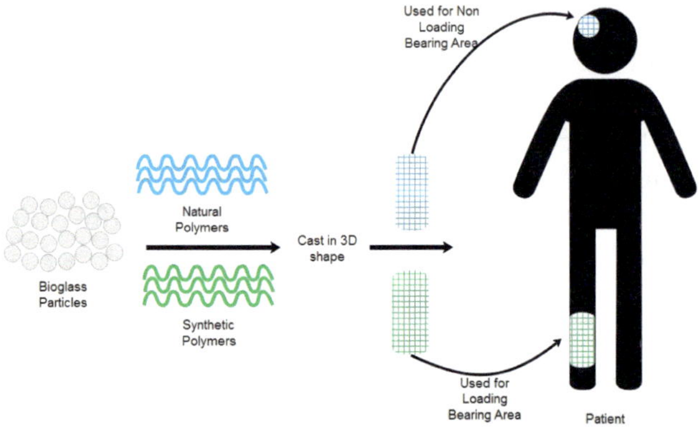

Figure 3.15. Bioglass scaffolds are ideal candidates in the realm of 3D printing, enabling the fabrication of patient-specific implants that closely mimic natural bone structures, ultimately enhancing integration and functionality within the body.

Source: https://www.tandfonline.com/action/showGraphicalAbstractImage?doi=10.1080%2F00914037.2023.2186864&id=gpom_a_2186864_uf0001_c.jpg.

3.5.3. Alumina

Alumina or aluminum oxide is one of the key materials in biomedical 3D printing with primary uses being the high biocompatibility and mechanical properties. Having good strength and durability makes it suitable for a broad scope of applications, particularly bone and dental implants. Incorporating alumina into structures printed by 3D printing provides the ability to produce intricate structures that mimic the architecture of natural bone, hence improved osseointegration. The use of 3D printing technology combined with alumina also facilitates the creation of porous scaffolds that can aid in cellular growth, thereby increasing the overall efficiency of the implant. This versatility is one of the main aspects in modern biomedical engineering since it broadens the application of conventional materials used in human health. In addition to its mechanical properties, alumina has chemical stability and wear resistance, which are important for long-term biomedical applications. Being a material processed in conjunction with advanced 3D printing technologies, alumina can be engineered to produce specific microstructural configurations that are crucial to the material's overall functionality. For instance, the inclusion of nanoscale features in alumina composites enhances its mechanical strength and biocompatibility. Recent studies have indicated that the combination of alumina with other biocompatible substances can yield composites that not only resist crack advancement but also offer better integration with the surrounding tissues. These advancements underscore the potential of alumina-based materials in revolutionizing the manufacturing of reliable and durable implants, addressing the growing demand for customized medical solutions. The use of alumina in 3D printing is synchronized with the newest research avenue in the production of nanocomposites for medical applications. Previous research on micro-nano composites has shown that the addition of alumina enhances the characteristics of polymer matrices significantly, resulting in tougher and more durable structures for implants. Furthermore, 3D printing's ability to create layered architectures provides control over porosity and interconnectivity of the scaffold, which is required for cell proliferation and nutrient transport. These advances in 3D printed material with alumina are an important step towards the creation of implants whose longevity approaches that of the patients themselves, dramatically expanding the reach of biomedical manufacturing (Farahi et al., 2010; Torrecillas et al., 2009). As research continues to evolve, exploring the synergy of alumina and emerging printing technologies promises even greater breakthroughs in this intriguing field.

3.6. CHALLENGES IN MATERIAL SELECTION

Selecting proper materials for biomedical 3D printing is plagued by many challenges that greatly impact the safety and efficacy of the resulting devices. The greatest challenge among them is achieving the required biocompatibility, which will ensure that the materials do not cause unwanted immune responses upon implantation into the human body. Several materials such as metals, ceramics, and polymers exhibit various types of responses in biological systems, thus making it highly significant to find out about interactions with body tissues. Advancements in material science are purely necessary; however, the complexity of conditions in the human bodies such as pH variation and mechanical stress provides an additional level of challenge. Besides, with the expansion of biomedical uses to cover tissue engineering scaffolds as well as organ models, the selection of material must also cover novel mechanical properties typical of natural tissues, thus representing a challenge in multiple dimensions to researchers in 3D printing (Chia et al., 2015). Another significant challenge is presented by the technology limitations of current 3D printing technologies. The ability of various methods, such as Fused Deposition Modeling and Stereolithography, often dictates the type of materials that can be successfully employed, which can limit material design innovation. For instance, certain materials may require elevated temperatures incompatible with the heat-sensitive biological components to be added into the printed structures. This is compounded by the need to obtain precision when creating complex geometries, critical when mimicking biological tissue fine architectures. As additive manufacturing technologies continue to advance, it becomes increasingly necessary to overcome such limitations in terms of material capabilities and performance in order to effectively exploit the potential of 3D printing in biomedicine (Dehghanghadikolaei et al., 2019). Moreover, economic and regulatory aspects associated with material selection in biomedical 3D printing also present immense challenges. Development of new biomaterials is likely to be extremely expensive, both in terms of research and development, and possess a rigid regulatory requirement from health authorities. Approvals of new materials can be lengthy and expensive, thus hindering development in the field. Moreover, the material sustainability of additive manufacturing remains an issue; environmental impact of raw material procurement and biomedical waste treatment pose significant material considerations. These financial and regulatory restraints might limit researchers' alternatives, pushing them toward proven materials that will not entirely meet the innovative challenges of modern biomedical engineering (Chia et al., 2015; Dchghanghadikolaei et al., 2019).

3.6.1. Regulatory Considerations

The advent of 3D printing technology in the biomedical domain has necessitated a complete analysis of regulatory factors to ensure the safety and efficacy of materials produced. With the development of industry, the challenge for regulatory organizations is to reengineer systems to accommodate the unique properties of 3D-printed biomaterials. Such factors are crucial, as they have significant implications for patient health and safety. The regulatory landscape is complex, with different stakeholders including manufacturers, clinicians, and regulators. This is further compounded by the diversity of materials utilized in 3D printing, whose biocompatibility, mechanical performance, and regulatory status also differ largely. Compliance with the existing regulations and driving innovation in the technology is thus essential in order to advance biomedical 3D printing. Further, the integration of various production processes, such as in existing research projects, calls for special regulatory frameworks tailored for leading-edge production processes. The integration of additive and subtractive manufacturing methods to create molding inserts calls for regulators to examine hybrid approaches extensively. Each method has its own merits and demerits and thus necessitates individual investigation to balance their safety and efficiency for application in medical contexts. The flaws observed in injection molds created through such processes are an indicator of the failure risk without proper regulatory oversight. Rigorous testing and validation protocols can mitigate the possibility of unintended consequences from the use of such emerging materials and techniques in medicine, while ensuring they are up to the level of standards for treating patients. In addition to material safety, the regulation should also consider the dynamic aspect of biomedical applications, particularly for tissue engineering and regenerative medicine. The mechanobiological nature of materials, particularly bone scaffolds, controls their function in healing. The self-healing property inherent in the material used for bone products indicates a focus of regulation on demonstrating efficacy and long-term effects associated with such properties. With the efforts of organizations to establish and employ standards, using computer models to forecast material behavior under loads can make a marked difference to the process of regulation. Through understanding the interaction between mechanical stimulation and material response, it is possible for regulators to establish standards that ensure these new materials are dependable, thereby ensuring safe integration into practice in addition to merging research findings, as noted in recent research (Eberl et al., 2019) (Figure 3.16).

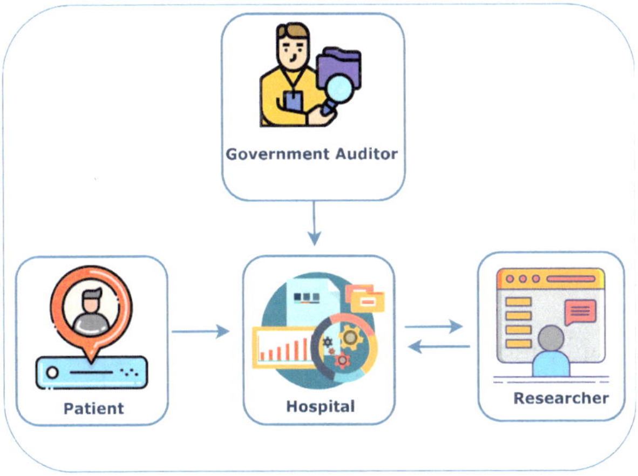

Figure 3.16. Adhering to rigorous testing and validation protocols can help mitigate potential risks associated with the use of such innovative materials and processes in medical applications, ensuring they meet the requisite standards for patient care.

Source: https://www.mdpi.com/sensors/sensors-23-07604/article_deploy/html/images/sensors-23-07604-g007.png.

3.6.2. Cost and Availability

The cost and availability factors are a huge determinant of the biomedical 3D printing landscape, with direct implications for the technology's viability in various healthcare settings. Although the potential of additive manufacturing (AM) to revolutionize the production of customized implants and medical devices is enormous, the price of high-quality material and special machinery can be outside the reach of most organizations. This financial barrier will naturally restrict the use to smaller hospitals and clinics, which may not be able to afford to purchase advanced 3D printing technology. For these advances to penetrate more areas of medicine, less expensive materials and production methods are required which reflect the financial status of existing healthcare delivery. Hence, ongoing research is crucial to justify processes that have the potential to provide cost-efficient biomedical components without compromising quality or functionality, as highlighted in recent research on AM technology (Dehghanghadikolaei et al., 2019). Also, a contributing factor in terms of cost and availability is to acquire raw materials employed for 3D printing in biomedical devices.

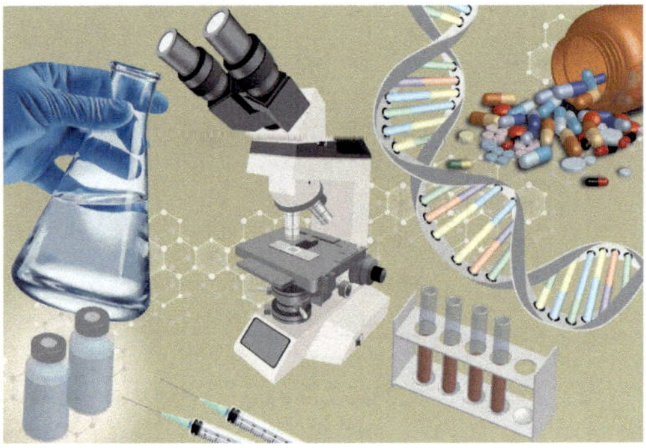

Figure 3.17. Manufacturers are challenged to produce high-quality materials that are both affordable and readily available, necessitating an investment in research and development focused on material science and manufacturing techniques.

Source: https://www.cbo.gov/sites/default/files/2021-04/57025-home-cover.png.

Currently, the variety and accessibility of suitable biocompatible materials, such as thermoplastics and bio-inks, are still limited in comparison to traditional manufacture materials. The technicality of regulatory compliance, or for medical-use materials in particular, contributes to this shortage, further mounting costs. Research into low-cost molding insert process methods indicates the merit of combining additive and subtractive methodology to manufacture specialist components in a cost-reducing approach. This approach also highlights how innovation in production techniques can offer some relief from financial constraints and boost the availability of needed materials, paving the way for wider applications of 3D printing technologies in medicine (Ewart et al., 2019). As the biomedical industry continues to advance, the integration of low-cost methods will be essential in making sophisticated 3D printing technologies more affordable. Manufacturing is a challenge that requires high-quality, affordable, and accessible materials to be made available, which demands a research and development investment in material science and processes. Overcoming these challenges is crucial because it not only guarantees the economic viability of medical devices printed in 3D but also guarantees patient outcomes by ensuring that customized solutions can be made available efficiently and effectively. The transition to an even more sustainable model is reliant on overcoming cost and availability issues by effective management, making an even wider number of institutions, such as rural areas, able to benefit from the advantages that biomedical 3D printing has to offer. Thus, continued research into enhancing new materials and methods will be invaluable (Dehghanghadikolaei et al., 2019) (Figure 3.17).

3.6.3. Material Performance in Biological Environments

Functional suitability of materials in biological environments is critical for effective 3D printed biomedical devices in biomedical engineering. Materials should not only withstand the particular physiological conditions found within the human body but also be biocompatible and functionally functional. As new 3D printing technologies advance, they enable the fabrication of intricate forms and shapes tailored precisely to the patient's individual requirements. This tailoring is particularly important in fields like tissue engineering, where the scaffolds designed need to be capable of mimicking the mechanical and biological properties of native tissues. New developments in various 3D printing technologies, including Fused Deposition Modeling and Stereolithography, highlight the ongoing efforts to overcome material limitations, thereby advancing the field of regenerative medicine and enhanced patient recovery in the case of organ reconstruction (Chia et al., 2015). Also, the integration of biomaterials with the 3D printing technology has raised interest regarding their performance under physiological conditions. All such critical parameters like degradation rates, mechanical properties, and biocompatibility with the surrounding tissues must be carefully considered. Hydrogels, ceramics, and bioactive glasses are also being aggressively studied because of their potential to support cell adhesion and proliferation and to carry out beneficial functions within the body. The issue is to create materials that not only help in healing but also possess adequate strength and toughness to resist the physiological stresses. For instance, the use of titanium alloys in particulate injection molding is restraining in the form of surface finish and part removal defects, which must be addressed to render the devices functional. Such a blend of material science and engineering holds the key to shattering the current limitations in 3D printed biomedical devices (Ewart et al., 2019). In the future, continued progress in material science stands on the verge of revolutionizing the potential of 3D printed biomedical implants. The studies mention engaging in optimizing the manufacturing processes and designing new materials that ensure maximum integration of the implant within the body for patient safety and effectiveness. Also, future trends such as the combination of additive and subtractive manufacturing techniques enhance design flexibility and accuracy, which can have significant effects on material performance. Clarifying and optimizing the interaction between these materials in biological systems is most critical for creating technologies for use in drug delivery systems and personalized implants. Ultimately, ongoing research into material performance in biological environments will not only provide the enabling opportunities for novel biomedical applications but also fill the gap between engineering principles and clinical needs (Chia et al., 2015).

3.7. CONCLUSION

In conclusion, the development of biomedical 3D printing materials is a significant leap in medical technology and patient treatment. The universality of 3D printing has enabled accurate construction of medical devices, implants, and tissue scaffolds in a personalized way that is tailored to meet individual patients' needs. This customization permits more effective fitting, reduced time in surgery, and improved outcomes of recovery, highlighting the convergence of creative material science with practical application in medicine. As researchers continue to advance biocompatible materials, the potential for personalized medicine grows, paving the way for therapies that not only succeed but also save time and money. Besides, the integration of new materials such as nanogels in 3D printing provides new paths for developing drug delivery systems that are optimized to suit particular biopharmaceutical needs. Nanogels, owing to their unique composition, can hold various therapeutic products, thereby enhancing the specificity and efficacy of treatment. Their use in different applications, including tissue regeneration and wound healing, emphasizes the value that material innovation can add to patient results. With this technological progress, there is a need to pay attention to the role that 3D printing plays in the production of specialized medical solutions that go beyond traditional methods and support the growing need for customized healthcare solutions (Cho et al., 2018). In addition, the design of evaluation systems for particular designs, such as 3D printed ankle foot orthoses (AFOs), demonstrates the potential of advanced modeling approaches in providing functional medical devices. The verification of finite element models with respect to experimental data proves the accuracy of 3D printed solutions in maximizing patient-specific applications. These technologies not only enhance manufacturing but also ensure that these technologies can adapt to the specific needs presented by each patient, fortifying the significant connection between materials science innovation and practical application in medicine. The future will witness continuous enhancement of 3D printing materials as a fundamental driver for the transformation of healthcare standards and the enhancement of the potential for successful medical intervention (Beule et al., 2019).

3.7.1. Summary of Key Points

The intersection of additive manufacturing (AM) and biomedicine has transformed medical device production. With technologies experiencing Industry 4.0 paradigm shifts, AM is increasingly emerging as a credible rival in terms of optimizing design efficiency in addition to facilitating expediting prototyping of customized goods. The complex designs that can be achieved with 3D printing technology enable the manufacture of complex parts that are not only functional but also tailored to the precise needs of a single patient. Additionally, material efficiency is greatly improved, addressing the long-existing challenges of reducing waste in the manufacturing process. As the review states, new developments in AM technology acknowledge its significant role in economic, environmental, and social sustainability of the biomedical sector, which recognizes the different benefits of embracing AM processes in health care programs (Dehghanghadikolaei et al., 2019). The study of hybrid production processes realizes the capability of creating biomedical devices that meet stringent industry standards. A case in point is the combination of additive and subtractive methods, which is an effective method to offset the drawbacks presented by each process. By application of both modalities, producers are able to acquire better surface finishes and take full advantage of material properties, which are important in the delicate nature of biomedical applications. The study on mold inserts for particulate injection molding demonstrates the combined method effectively. Tests showed that while such problems as brittleness and part removal defects were encountered, it was with fixes initiated by the synergetic use of both the fabrication processes, leading to innovation in reducing costs and increasing the biomedical production capacity (Ewart et al., 2019). The future of 3D printing in the biomedical industry is thus one of continuous development and exploring new materials. Advancements in bio-compatible materials and composites will definitely expand the horizon of medical application, leading to the generation of implants, prosthetics, and tissue engineering scaffolds not only efficient but sustainable as well. One of the major drivers for these innovations is integration of science and technology, allowing research and application to synergize. Further studies on material properties and processing techniques will play a key role in determining the role of AM in biomedicine. In conclusion, with every advancing success in design and materials science, the possibility that AM has to revolutionize biomedical manufacturing becomes increasingly defined, paving the way for paradigm-shifting applications that are centered on patient-centric solutions (Dehghanghadikolaei et al., 2019).

3.7.2. Future Trends in Biomedical 3D Printing Materials

The future of 3D printing materials in biomedicine appears to have significant breakthroughs that will redefine the majority of medical applications. Biocompatible material advancements, particularly those intended for regenerative medicine and tissue engineering, take center stage. Researchers are focusing more on materials that can copy the complicated structure and mechanical properties of tissues in nature. For instance, incorporating nanomaterials into traditional polymers enhances not just the durability and toughness of constructs but also their biocompatibility, which enables them to create an optimal condition for cell growth and integration into tissues. Further advancements in developing these materials further open up the possibility of making more efficient prosthetics and implants that can better address individual patients' requirements, thus lessening risks associated with rejection as well as overall clinical success. With this field changing, the concerns are greater than simply utility, with the need for regulatory frameworks capable of keeping up with such rapid progress (Pinkerton et al., 2015). The potential of smart materials to biomedical 3D printing is increasing as well, and it is a revolutionary movement to revolutionize patient care. Smart materials are designed to respond dynamically to physical stimuli, such as temperature, pH, or biochemical signals. These responsive features enable the creation of smart implants that can respond to changing physiological conditions, thus optimizing their performance and longevity. This development is particularly relevant in the areas of drug release systems and tissue scaffolding, where controlled release processes have pivotal roles to play in therapeutic action. Moreover, the intersection between materials science and biotechnology is leading to new combinations of biologically active agents in 3D-printed matrices. This convergence holds potential for personalized medicine, where treatments can be designed to individual patient profiles and therefore boost therapeutic interventions and outcomes (Amrollahi et al., 2016). As such directions evolve, business organizations and research institutes are increasingly focusing on multidisciplinary approaches that combine materials science with engineering, biology, and computation modeling. This collaboration advances the development of bespoke materials designed specifically for specific biomedical applications. Furthermore, advancements in bioprinting technology, including the incorporation of living cells and bioactive molecules into the printing process, are a move towards the potential for more sophisticated tissue regeneration. The capacity to create intricate structures that closely replicate natural tissue not only maximizes the efficacy of 3D-printed implants but also optimizes their acceptability by the body. Forward, the future of biomedical 3D printing materials is bound to be characterized by continuous innovation, regulation, and the need for breakthroughs in patient-relevant solutions that propel the sector into unprecedented realms of healthcare (Pinkerton et al., 2015).

3.7.3. Final Thoughts on the Impact of Material Innovation

The revolutionary impact of material innovation on biomedical 3D printing is immense, not just on the production processes but also on the variety of applications in the field. Additive manufacturing (AM) makes it possible to fabricate complex, patient-specified anatomical models that traditional manufacturing technologies cannot. This capacity makes the design process simpler without sacrificing customization that is tailored to a patient's requirements, which is particularly valuable across industries such as orthopedics and dental. Adding AM to the healthcare sector is indicative of the broader trend in industry that is called industry 4.0 in which smart manufacturing promotes efficiency and reduces waste. These advancements are part of the shift toward personalized medicine, where the quality of the healthcare can be significantly enhanced by new materials and manufacturing techniques (Dehghanghadikolaei et al., 2019). Furthermore, the combination of additive and subtractive processes, such as what is being seen in recent studies, holds promise for the production of high-complexity biomedical devices. The development of low-cost molding inserts for particulate injection molding (PIM), with a combination of AM and conventional machining, implies the increasing likelihood of strategic material use in manufacturing. With the optimization of processing techniques and circumventing inherent limitations such as surface finish and geometrical intricacy, scientists pave the way for efficient production procedures. This combined approach not only increases the promise of biomedical applications but also reduces the cost of manufacture, hence making sophisticated medical solutions accessible to many. Such innovations exhibit the potential of transcending existing limitations and expanding the boundaries of material utilization in medicine (Ewart et al., 2019). Ultimately, the future of material development in biomedical 3D printing is dependent on continuous research and development of new materials up to rigorous medical standards. As research continues, it is crucial that sustainability and biocompatibility come first in the development of these materials. To be able to transition new materials into clinical applications seamlessly while also reducing harm to the environment is crucial. Achievement of these goals will most likely speed up innovations to create materials that not only contribute to the care of patients but also beneficially impact the health of the environment. Overall, material innovation and biomedical 3D printing are converging into an exciting frontier that can revolutionize healthcare and enhance the human way of life worldwide (Dehghanghadikolaei et al., 2019).

REFERENCES

1. Abalymov, A., Parakhonskiy, B., & Skirtach, A. (2020). Polymer- and hybrid-based biomaterials for interstitial, connective, vascular, nerve, visceral and musculoskeletal tissue engineering. https://core.ac.uk/download/299792280.pdf (accessed on 14th October 2025).
2. Aguilera Velázquez, J. R., Alcudia Cruz, A., Begines Ruiz, B., He, Y., et al. (2019). Design of highly stabilized nanocomposite inks based on biodegradable polymer-matrix and gold nanoparticles for inkjet printing. https://core.ac.uk/download/286564742.pdf (accessed on 14th October 2025).
3. Almeida, L. E., Dashtimoghadam, E., Fahimipour, F., Jazayeri, H., et al. (2017). A current overview of materials and strategies for potential use in maxillofacial tissue regeneration. https://core.ac.uk/download/213072267.pdf (accessed on 14th October 2025).
4. Amrollahi, P., Seifi, A., Shah, B., Tayebi, L., et al. (2016). Recent advancements in regenerative dentistry: A review. https://core.ac.uk/download/213080485.pdf (accessed on 14th October 2025).
5. Ask, B., Bhure, S., Bibb, R., Cai, H., Castner, H., Chaki, S., Chang, Y., et al. (2014). Functionalization of Ti6Al4V components fabricated using selective laser melting with a bioactive compound. https://core.ac.uk/download/84637053.pdf (accessed on 14th October 2025).
6. Bakhshinejad, A., & D'Souza, R. M. (2015). A brief comparison between available bio-printing methods. http://arxiv.org/abs/1502.04991 (accessed on 14th October 2025).
7. Carvalho, C., Landers, R., & Mülhaupt, R. (2004). Soft and hard implant fabrication using 3D-Bioplotting TM. https://core.ac.uk/download/287648471.pdf (accessed on 14th October 2025).
8. Chen, Q. (2007). Bioglass®-derived glass-ceramic scaffolds for bone tissue engineering.
9. Chia, H. N., & Wu, B. M. (2015). Recent advances in 3D printing of biomaterials. https://core.ac.uk/download/323078409.pdf (accessed on 14th October 2025).
10. Cho, H., Jammalamadaka, U., & Tappa, K. (2018). Nanogels for pharmaceutical and biomedical applications and their fabrication using 3D printing technologies. https://core.ac.uk/download/212859248.pdf (accessed on 14th October 2025).
11. Clark, E. A., Evangelista Barreiros, M. I., Greco, F., Hart, A., et al. (2020). A 3D printed drug delivery implant formed from a dynamic supramolecular

polyurethane formulation. https://core.ac.uk/download/322487176.pdf (accessed on 14th October 2025).

12. Concheri, G., Meneghello, R., Rosso, S., Savio, G., et al. (2018). Geometric modeling of cellular materials for additive manufacturing in biomedical field: A review. https://core.ac.uk/download/154326170.pdf (accessed on 14th October 2025).
13. Costa, P., Dios, J. R., Lanceros-Méndez, S., et al. (2021). High deformation multifunctional composites: Materials, processes, and applications. https://core.ac.uk/download/372700344.pdf (accessed on 14th October 2025).
14. Cristóvão, A. F. M. (2018). 3D printing of biocompatible materials for biomedical applications. https://core.ac.uk/download/187233556.pdf (accessed on 14th October 2025).
15. De Beule, M., Deckers, J. P., Forward, M., Ielapi, A., et al. (2019). A validated computational framework to evaluate the stiffness of 3D printed ankle foot orthoses. https://core.ac.uk/download/237010383.pdf (accessed on 14th October 2025).
16. Dehghanghadikolaei, A., Emamian, S. S., Fotovvati, B., Gisario, A., et al. (2019). The potential of additive manufacturing in the smart factory industrial 4.0: A review. https://core.ac.uk/download/231748826.pdf (accessed on 14th October 2025).
17. Eberl, C., Fratzl, P., & Weinkamer, R. (2019). Mechan regulation of bone remodeling and healing as inspiration for self-repair in materials.
18. Ewart, P. (2019). A comparison of processing techniques for producing prototype injection molding inserts. https://core.ac.uk/download/322841895.pdf (accessed on 14th October 2025).
19. Farahi, E., Gibbons, G. J., Lv, Y., Purnell, P., & Williams, R. (2010). 3D printing of cement composites. https://core.ac.uk/download/44217.pdf (accessed on 14th October 2025).
20. Hansen, H. N., Hofstätter, T., Pedersen, D. B., Tosello, G., et al. (2017). State-of-the-art of fiber-reinforced polymers in additive manufacturing technologies. https://core.ac.uk/download/84005855.pdf (accessed on 14th October 2025).
21. Hossain, M. (2023). Additive manufacturing of sustainable biomaterials for biomedical applications. https://core.ac.uk/download/564441786.pdf (accessed on 14th October 2025).
22. Macwan, I., Patra, P., Shinde, D., Tavares, L., et al. (2018). 3D printed hyaluronic acid hydrogels using free form fabrication technique for tissue engineering. https://core.ac.uk/download/156902195.pdf (accessed on 14th October 2025).

23. Pinkerton, A. J. (2015). Lasers in additive manufacturing. https://core.ac.uk/download/42415986.pdf (accessed on 14th October 2025).
24. Rosa, A., & Salaris, F. (2019). Construction of 3D *in vitro* models by bioprinting human pluripotent stem cells: Challenges and opportunities. https://core.ac.uk/download/231747057.pdf (accessed on 14th October 2025).
25. Schneider, S. (2022). Organ-on-a-Disc: A scalable platform technology for the generation and cultivation of micro physiological tissues. https://core.ac.uk/download/539565751.pdf (accessed on 14th October 2025).
26. Torrecillas, R., Moya, J. S., Díaz, L. A., Bartolomé Gómez, E., et al. (2009). Nanotechnology in joint replacement. https://core.ac.uk/download/pdf/36093046.pdf (accessed on 14th October 2025).

CHAPTER 4

DESIGN AND MODELING FOR BIOMEDICAL DEVICES

Contents

INTRODUCTION

The rapid evolution of technology has significantly influenced various fields, particularly in biomedical engineering, where 3D design and modeling have become pivotal. The incorporation of three-dimensional design not only enhances the aesthetic appeal of biomedical devices but also optimizes their functionality and patient compatibility. By utilizing advanced modeling techniques, engineers and designers can create intricate structures that mimic biological systems, leading to improved device integration within the human body. This shift is critical since it simplifies the development of customized solutions that respond to specific medical needs. Further, 3D modeling allows for iterative design processes that enhance innovation and efficiency in the prototyping phase. In this way, the use of 3D design in biomedical devices represents a convergence of cutting-edge technology and health science with massive potential for future advances in medical interventions and device performance. With the growing demand for personalized medicine, one cannot overemphasize one's role in applying 3D modeling to tailor-made biomedical devices. Such devices are typically subjected to great amounts of precision engineering to accommodate individual anatomical variation, and hence traditional manufacturing techniques are less favorable. With the help of sophisticated modeling software, engineers are able to produce devices that closely simulate the patients' individual physiology, thereby improving the quality of fit and function precision. Moreover, these technologies provide potential gains over traditional materials and manufacturing techniques, achieving enhanced durability and function under intricate conditions. This is particularly true in applications such as prosthetics and implants, where a more individualized approach can greatly enhance patient function. The ability to see and manipulate device schematics in a three-dimensional space offers unparalleled scope for innovation and progress in the biomedical sector. Challenges that are attributed to 3D design and modeling, however, must be scrutinized attentively. While there are some advantages that are attributed to 3D printing and modeling, there are also intricacies, such as the requirement of possessing accurate computational tools and reliable material that will withstand biological stress. For instance, effective communication networks in these technologies must be attained to enable devices to function when used in real conditions. The latest advancements in material science and integration technologies are crucial to overcome the above-discussed problems and enhance the performance of biomedical devices. According to recent literature, addressing the communications requirements of sophisticated systems can lead to better clinical outcomes (Manohar et al., 2018). In addition, the environmental aspects engaged during design, such as noise interference in imaging, emphasize the requirement for robust modeling techniques (Ahmad et al., 2018). Therefore, ongoing 3D design and modeling development is defined by a complex interplay of innovation, challenge, and revolutionary potential within the biomedical context.

Definition of 3D Design and Modeling

The power of 3D modeling and design lies in the ability to create three-dimensional object models from specialized software. It entails the conceptualization, visualization, and development of complex shapes, which can be very important to medical fields such as biomedical engineering. In this case, 3D modeling enables designers and engineers to create sophisticated structures that mimic biological systems or medical devices. The precision delivered by such models enables simulation and analysis, which can significantly enhance product development. With increasing use of new technologies in modern medicine, the specificity and adaptability delivered by 3D design are significant to design devices catering to diverse patient needs and ensuring more positive outcomes of healthcare. Advanced 3D design techniques compel innovation in the biomedical device market by adopting elements like computer-assisted orthopedic surgery (CAOS) systems.

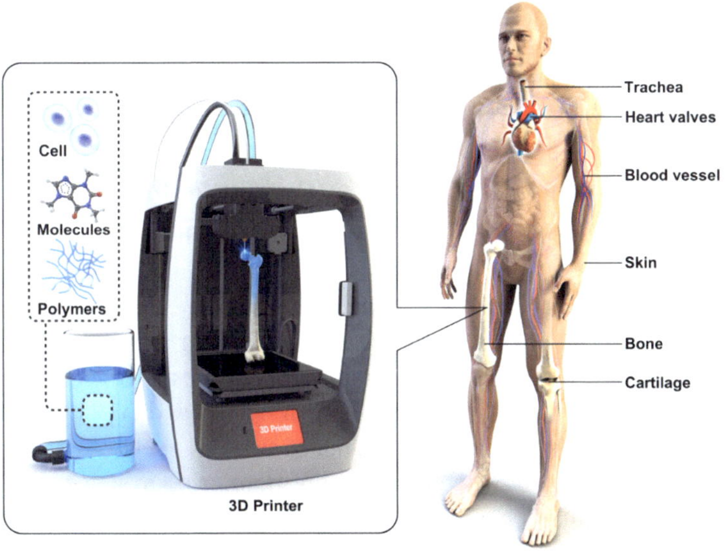

Figure 4.1. 3D modeling enables designers and engineers to construct intricate structures that mimic biological systems or medical devices.

Source: https://images-provider.frontiersin.org/api/ipx/w=1200&f=png/https://www.frontiersin.org/files/Articles/586406/fbioe-08-586406-HTML/image_m/fbioe-08-586406-g001.jpg.

These systems employ volumetric imaging and kinetic information for enhanced planning and conduct of surgery, delivering accuracy in treating musculoskeletal conditions. Facilitating such surgeries through tailored 3D models is a sign of the convergence of technology and medicine, where design not only constitutes an introductory phase but is a crucial component of treatment solutions. The mixing of high-end modeling with therapeutic applications points towards the utilitarian importance of 3D design since it translates conceptual designs into functioning machinery that can be utilized by health practitioners in real-world applications (Kalová et al., 2019). The development of additive manufacturing (AM) has also fundamentally altered the landscape of 3D design and modeling for biomedical applications. This technology allows for the creation of complex, custom-made parts that fit the needs of the individual patient without wasting material and resources. Engaging AM in the design process is consistent with Industry 4.0 principles, where the role of smart manufacturing and data-driven methods enhances efficiency and innovation. Through effective prototyping and quick iteration, designers can easily perfect and fine-tune models quickly in response to feedback, driving innovation in device performance and patient compatibility. With advancements in 3D design emerging hand in hand with AM, its potential to enhance biomedical devices becomes increasingly clear, driving future potential for patient care and treatment modality (Dehghanghadikolaei et al., 2019) (Figure 4.1).

Importance of Biomedical Devices in Healthcare

Biomedical devices play an important role in modern healthcare by enhancing the ability to diagnose, monitor, and treat disease. Biomedical devices range from the most straightforward devices such as thermometers to highly complex systems such as pacemakers and implantable sensors that provide real-time feedback regarding body states. Their importance lies in their capability to improve patient outcomes by enabling early diagnosis and ongoing monitoring of health status. For instance, ubiquitous sensing technologies signal a seamless transition to more advanced health monitoring systems, which offer continuous data acquisition and analysis with minimal disturbance to patients. The breakthrough opens the door to various healthcare possibilities, ranging from customized treatment protocols to preventive interventions aimed at preventing the development of chronic diseases. The integration of such devices into clinical practice is an ideal expression of the intersection that is so crucial between technology and medicine, depicting their promise to speed new healthcare solutions (Perez et al., 2015). Biomedical devices are critical in precision medicine since they offer individualized treatments from patient-specific information. The advent of 3D modeling and designing transforms the construction of these devices to a large degree through enabling the production of customized implants and prosthetics that closely replicate patients' anatomical requirements. Not only does the personalization improve medical device fit and function, but it also results in better patient compliance and satisfaction. For instance, the application of 3D-printed orthopedic devices facilitates a patient-specific approach that considerably reduces recovery periods and enhances outcomes through rehabilitation. Furthermore, the application of innovative modeling methods facilitates easier exploration of materials and designs that can ensure maximum device performance with the additional advantage of reducing negative effects. Hence, biomedical device design with the application of 3D modeling is vital to attaining personalized health care and improving the overall quality of medical procedures (Berger et al., 2017). Besides, the uses of biomedical devices extend beyond addressing personal health problems because they help advance public health initiatives as well. Devices such as implantable devices and wearable health monitors play a critical role in generating big data that may assist in directing health policy and preventive care interventions. By analyzing complete data that is being generated from these monitors, clinicians are in a position to discover more about disease patterns and outcomes, thereby making more accurate medical interventions possible. Besides, such devices are required for the treatment of chronic diseases due to their ability to allow constant monitoring and instant adjustments of the treatment regimen. This aspect captures the essence of the aims of the emerging pervasive health model, which aims at preventive, predictive, personalized, and participatory medicine. In this case, the significance of biomedical devices is more than their immediate therapeutic utility, highlighting their critical contribution to shaping sustainable healthcare systems (Perez et al., 2015).

Overview of the Role of 3D Design in Biomedical Applications

Within biomedical applications, 3D design has been an innovative approach that significantly enhances the performance and fabrication of medical devices. With the capability to produce complex geometries and patient-specific models, 3D design facilitates precise fabrication of implants, prostheses, and scaffolds tailored to particular anatomical features. This customization has resulted in improved surgical outcomes, with 3D-printed models being utilized in pre-surgical simulation and planning to improve the safety and efficacy of surgeries. Furthermore, the use of 3D design in biomedical engineering has improved manufacturing, making rapid prototyping and iterative testing possible, which can contribute to device design and performance innovation. It is evident that the further advancement of 3D design technologies will continue to shape the landscape of biomedical applications in meaningful ways. One interesting application of 3D design is its role in tissue engineering, wherein the construction of biocompatible scaffolds is central to enabling cell growth and tissue regeneration. With the advancement in 3D printing technology, researchers are able to produce intricate scaffold geometries that mimic the nature of the extracellular matrix of tissues. Scaffolds can be produced with a specific design tailored to the individual structural and mechanical requirements of the target tissues, and this can optimize the possibility of successful integration and function. In addition, recent advancements in 3D printing materials such as bioinks with embedded living cells predict an age when fully functional tissues are fabricated via additive manufacturing. Future research on such technologies will definitely give more scope to regenerative medicine and therapeutic intervention in patients suffering from extreme tissue deficiencies, thus marking the innovative impact of 3D design in biomedicine.

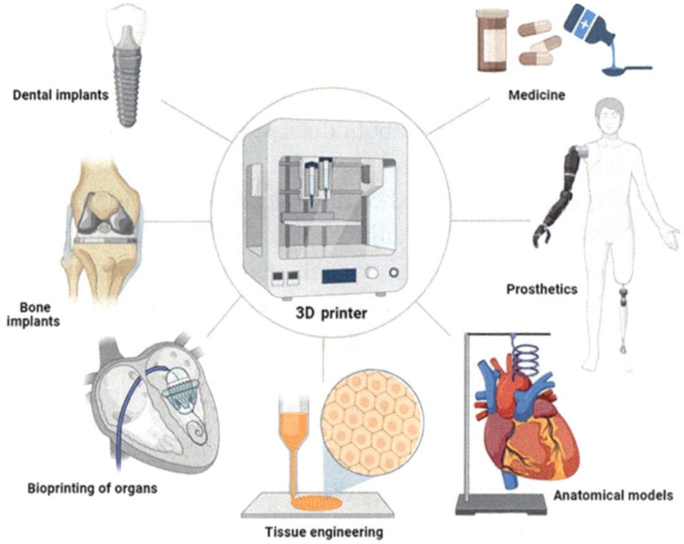

Figure 4.2. With the capability to create complex geometries and patient-specific models, 3D design allows for the precise fabrication of implants, prosthetics, and scaffolds tailored to individual anatomical structures.

*Source:*https://www.explorationpub.com/uploads/Article/A1001200/em-04-1001200-g000.jpg.

With ongoing research, the application of nanogels combined with 3D designing is becoming increasingly important in the biomedical field. Nanogels, as micellar networks capable of holding both hydrophilic and hydrophobic molecules, are new delivery platforms for drug delivery and tissue engineering. Involvement of 3D printing technology during the production of nanogels provides a new way of designing targeted drug delivery systems according to the requirement of patients. Based on recent studies, 3D printing has been found to be precise and customizable, and therefore it is the optimum method of producing nanogels with controlled release and enhanced therapeutic effect. With applications that range from wound healing to complex drug delivery, the incorporation of advanced 3D designing in nanogel manufacturing would revolutionize treatment regimens and pave ways to novel biomedical applications, emphasizing the tremendous potential of 3D technologies in modern medicine (Cho et al., 2018) (Figure 4.2).

4.1. HISTORICAL CONTEXT

The past of 3D modeling and design in biomedical devices borrows from significant historical events that have impacted technology and medicine. The computer-aided design (CAD) was brought into the biomedical industry in the 1970s, which marked a significant shift from labor-intensive hand prototyping to more efficient and precise modeling. This transition allowed for the development of complex devices such as prosthetics and implants, wherein engineers began employing computer-aided tools to mold anatomical data and design custom solutions. With increasing computing capacity and software capabilities, rapid prototyping in the 1980s allowed faster iteration and testing of biomedical devices. This background is indicative of how technological advancements synergistically have influenced the design and fabrication of devices that are more customized to serve the needs of patients individually. In particular, the field of soft robotics and intelligent materials has led the frontiers of 3D design in biomedicine. Soft robotics, unlike traditional stiff mechanisms, is concerned with compliance and flexibility, which are essential in applications to healthcare. Recent developments in magnetic soft materials demonstrate this tendency, wherein actuators are responsive to environmental stimuli and provide more sophisticated interactions with biological organisms. The unique benefits of these materials suggest that they can revolutionize how devices such as surgery instruments or prosthetic limbs are designed, making their operation even more similar to that of the biology. The growing amount of literature on magnetic soft robotics, as outlined in most scientific reviews, highlights the need for partnership between engineers, biologists, and doctors to push the boundaries of 3D design within the biomedical field (Kim et al., 2022). Secondly, the historical context of wound healing treatments proves the immense impact that advances in 3D modeling can make to medical practices. Traditional therapy for chronic wounds has hitherto been limited by the efficacy of the therapy available. Novel therapies on the basis of activated biocompatible scaffolds, however, hold the potential for a paradigm shift with increased accuracy of modeling. Personalized therapy design made possible by 3D printing and modeling aims to address the complexities of wound healing through the integration of cellular engineering and tailored biomaterials. Such an evolution in strategy not only ensures enhanced patient outcomes but also highlights the pivotal role of technological advancement in addressing persistent medical challenges. In the future, the meeting point of 3D design with emerging biomedical needs will increasingly redefine the health space (Tottoli et al., 2020) (Figure 4.3).

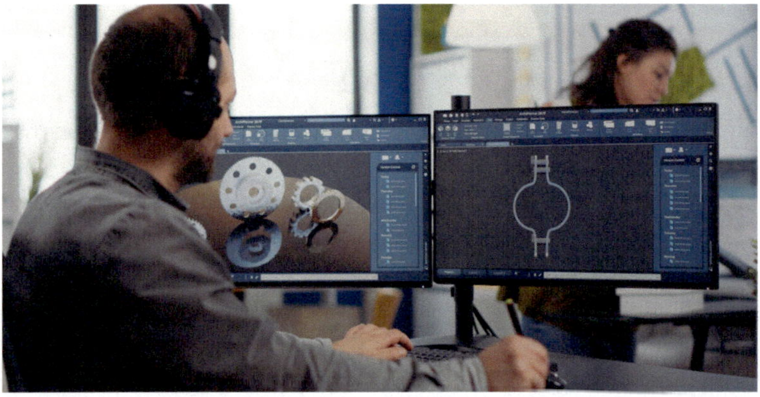

Figure 4.3. As computing power increased and software capabilities expanded, the concept of rapid prototyping arose in the 1980s, allowing for faster iteration and testing of biomedical devices.

Source: https://breinerco.com/wp-content/uploads/2024/04/20240410_BRI_RapidPrototyping.png.

4.1.1. Evolution of Biomedical Devices

The evolution of biomedical devices has been one of revolution, with spectacular technological breakthroughs that have dramatically enhanced patient care. From rudimentary equipment used in ancient times to the sophisticated devices of today, such advancements are largely the result of the confluence of engineering, biology, and materials science. Above all, the development of implantable devices has been a landmark stage in this evolution, allowing for minimally invasive procedures that achieve improved patient outcomes. The design and modeling of such devices increasingly rely on state-of-the-art techniques, allowing simulation of complex interactions within the human body. Such advancements not only improve the efficacy of biomedical devices but also reduce dangers of surgical intervention. With such technologies advancing, the necessity for precise, patient-specific solutions is all-important, paving the way for further advancements within the field. One of the most significant advancements within the field of biomedical devices is the utilization of advanced 3D modeling techniques. These techniques have allowed healthcare professionals to change the way device design is developed, with full preclinical simulations and assessments being achievable that were undreamed of previously. Specifically, the simulation of implantable devices such as stents has progressed with the use of dynamic mesh methodology that simulates the dynamics of such devices in real time. The ability to pre-simulate stent deployment, for instance, is crucial in the prediction of clinical outcomes and enhancing procedural safety. The method does not only increase the accuracy of designs but facilitates the study of varied cases of deployment. The understanding gained through these sophisticated modeling techniques is invaluable, ultimately leading to improved designs that more effectively meet both clinical and patient needs (Spranger et al., 2014). With increasing technology in biomedical devices, the application of novel materials and biosensors is growing more prominent, particularly in targeted therapies. Interestingly, DNA aptamers are emerging as key constituents in the development of new biosensing technologies with advantages of low cost and reusability over traditional antibody-based systems. The creation of aptamer-based biosensors is marked by the need for precise 3D modeling to predict and maximize their functionality. Advanced computational aids of recent times have enabled the creation of realistic three-dimensional structures of aptamers, a key necessity for their application in real biomedical environments. This achievement is very important since the enhancement of the consistency and predictability of biosensors has the potential to greatly transform diagnostic and therapeutic methods in medicine (Jeddi et al., 2017). With ongoing research to enhance these devices and methods, the future of biomedical device design stands poised to make a revolutionary quantum leap, held out with greater efficiency and efficacy in patient care solutions (Figure 4.4).

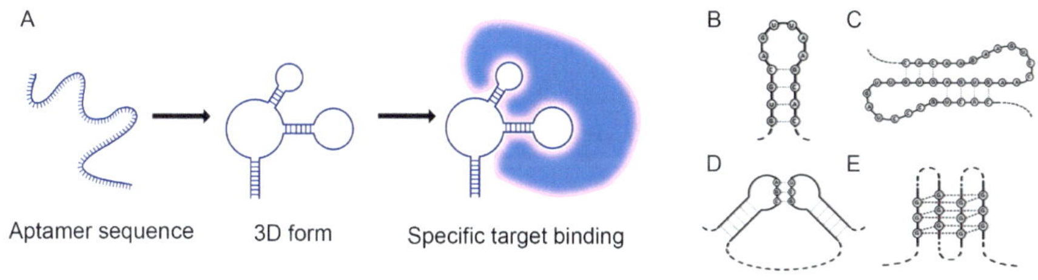

Figure 4.4. DNA aptamers are emerging as vital components for the development of new biosensing technologies, offering advantages such as affordability and reusability over traditional antibody-based systems.

Source: https://pub.mdpi-res.com/ijms/ijms-25-06833/article_deploy/html/images/ijms-25-06833-g001.png?1718961770.

4.1.2. Early Uses of 3D Modeling in Medicine

The use of 3D modeling in medicine has significantly evolved various healthcare branches, particularly surgical planning, and education. Early applications of this technology allowed for the creation of patient-specific anatomical models, which established a better understanding of complex geometries within the human body. For instance, doctors began to utilize 3D printed models acquired from CT and MRI scans to view anatomical variations, thereby improving preoperative planning. These models enabled surgeons to simulate intricate procedures, anticipate defects, and subsequently improve operating outcomes. The verification feedback from these models allows physicians to prepare for actual surgeries more effectively, ultimately reducing the duration of operating and complications.

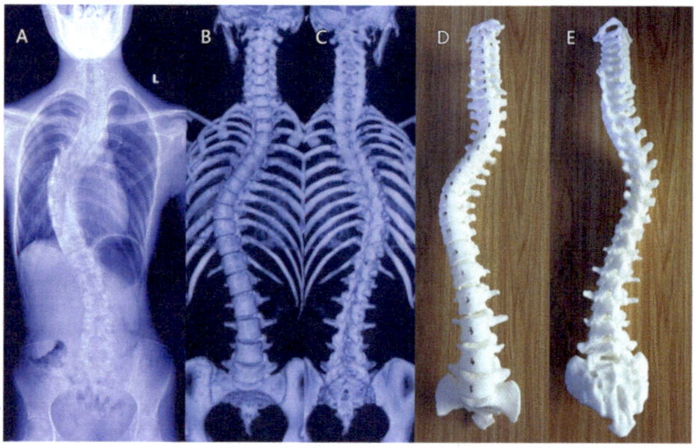

Figure 4.5. Medical students and residents benefit immensely from the ability to engage with detailed 3D reproductions of human anatomy.

Source: https://media.springernature.com/lw1200/springer-static/image/art%3A10.1186%2Fs12909-024-06617-2/MediaObjects/12909_2024_6617_Fig1_HTML.png.

Such application of 3D modeling is a significant shift in the practice of the medical profession and paves the way for further integration of technology in medical disciplines. Furthermore, early 3D modeling technology has demonstrated exceptional capability in the treatment and management of cardiovascular diseases. Based on the interdisciplinary studies of coarctation of the aorta, 3D modeling appeared as an optimal means of hemodynamics comprehension among patients. Computational fluid dynamics (CFD) enabled more in-depth investigations of the blood flow pattern characteristics and shear stress indexes among abnormal vascular anatomy patients. Such findings, drawn from 3D models, contribute to critical surgical decision-making and the creation of customized interventions. By modeling various forms of surgical interventions and stent structures within a virtual environment, medical professionals can examine the likely outcome of various strategies and hence optimize treatment regimens. Such early applications of 3D modeling not only enhanced individualized patient treatments but also increased the general understanding of cardiovascular pathology. Early uses of 3D modeling have also come far in academic settings, where they are superb instructional tools. Residents and medical students benefit greatly from the ability to work with high-fidelity 3D representations of the human body. Models offer an improved understanding of complex anatomical relationships and physiological processes over more traditional 2D imaging methods. Most notably, the experiential learning developed through these interactive models enhances retention and understanding, paramount in a field where precision is necessary. Such educational application sets forth the revolutionary capability of 3D modeling, as it prepares the next generation of physicians to make use of cutting-edge technologies responsibly and effectively. The collaboration of the engineers and healthcare professionals in this innovative approach demonstrates the power of multidisciplinary integration to medicine, which can lead to future advancements of biomedical devices (Figure 4.5).

4.1.3. Technological Advancements Leading to Modern 3D Design

The land of technological advancements has had a significant impact in modern 3D design, especially in the case of biomedical devices. Technologies such as computer-aided design (CAD) and three-dimensional printing have transformed the way scientists and engineers design and realize intricate geometries. CAD software can be used to accurately model intricate geometries for the purpose of extensive visualization before physical models are constructed. Moreover, the enhanced computing power has also made it possible to process big data, which is critical for medical applications requiring an inordinate amount of detail and accuracy. Improvements to software tools enhance user productivity and experience, with the added benefit of an intuitive interface for designers. Therefore, biomedical professionals are able to seek novel solutions quicker than ever before and have breakthroughs like personalized prosthetics or implants developed and experimented on in a rapid manner, propelling the industry into a new age of medical engineering. Additionally, the integration of artificial intelligence (AI) in 3D design pipelines has pushed biomedical innovation further. AI can analyze large databases of data from patient images and clinical results to create optimized iterations that will better address specific needs. For instance, machine learning programs can predict the behavior of new materials under diverse physiological conditions and guide the choice of materials for their most appropriate use. This not only reduces development time but also optimizes the performance of biomedical devices, rendering them functional and biocompatible. With these advancements, AI enables devices to be personalized, making them better suited to individual patient needs. This marriage of AI and 3D design is a perfect example of an advancement in biomedical engineering, demonstrating how new tech tools can best address the evolving healthcare needs. Digital twin technology also overhauls modern 3D design in the biomedical industry by enabling real-time monitoring and simulation of device functionality. Digital twins are virtual replicas of physical devices, not only their design specifications but also information on how they function. The technology provides critical information on interactions among designed components and physiological conditions, allowing for correct adjustments and optimal results in device functionality. Through the use of Internet of Things (IoT) and augmented reality (AR), designers are able to emulate complicated scenarios and make adjustments in real time. Such functionality has the potential to vastly streamline the design and testing stages of device production. In general, digital twin application is able to raise 3D design process efficiency in the development of biomedical devices in order to respond to the evolving measures of patient care and operation performance (Afridi et al., 2024; Yanto et al., 2024) (Figure 4.6).

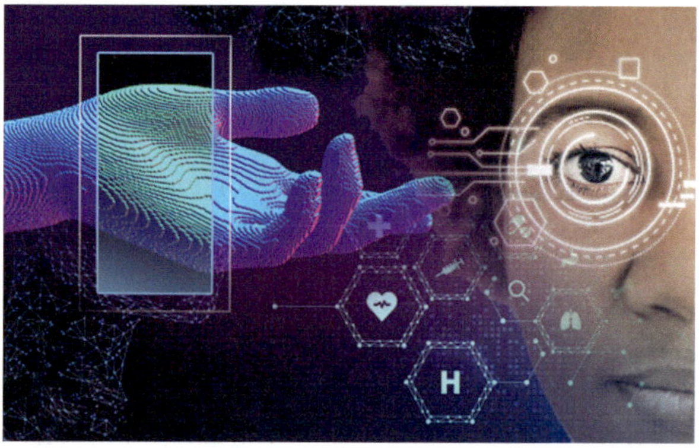

Figure 4.6. AI can analyze vast amounts of data from patient imaging and clinical outcomes, allowing for optimized designs that better meet individual needs.

Source: https://www.aha.org/sites/default/files/2023-05/How-AI-Is-Improving-Diagnostics-Decision-Making-and-Care.png.

4.2. 3D DESIGN SOFTWARE AND TOOLS

The advancement of 3D design software has revolutionized the field of biomedical devices, with precision and innovation at the forefront. The software provides a platform to designers and engineers to create accurate models that can replicate the complex structure found in the human body. With tools such as SolidWorks and AutoCAD, professionals are able to create accurate digital models of devices such as surgical tools, implants, and prostheses. These models also make visualization and analysis of mechanical properties and their interaction with the biological tissues possible. Also, the integration of computational modeling offers the possibility of optimizing the design so that it reduces errors and enhances performance in actual devices. Due to increased growth in the biomedical field, the role of 3D design software is increasing day by day so that the devices meet the demanding criteria of functionality, safety, and patient compatibility. The use of advanced 3D model software is not only during the initial design process; these programs allow rapid prototyping and validation of biomedical devices. Techniques such as 3D printing take advantage of computer models' precision to generate physical prototypes rapidly, with the option of creating iterative modifications based on empirical testing. This facilitates a smoother innovation process, with design changes readily being addressed in response to test results, thereby reducing the time to market for new devices. As stated, advancements in memory technology in recent years can facilitate these processes via optimized data management and integration, allowing designers to manage higher numbers of data and intricate simulations without affecting performance (Manohar et al., 2018). Hence, the relationship between 3D design software and modern design-to-manufacturing technology is critical to further pushing the limits of what can be achieved in designing biomedical devices. Moreover, the new trend of incorporating artificial intelligence (AI) within 3D design software has the potential to further enhance biomedical device design. Designers can utilize AI to identify the most suitable configurations and even suggest possible improvements not necessarily understood through traditional design methods. For instance, AI algorithms may process vast amounts of data to predict how a device will behave under diverse conditions and thus provide vital information before physical prototypes are constructed. Besides, these technologies promise to automate part of the design work, which eventually results in higher efficiency and allows designers to concentrate more on innovative ideas and challenging problem-solving. This integration of AI reflects the broader move towards autonomous medicine, where better accuracy and functionality are of key importance (Das et al., 2017). With the increasing convergence between 3D design software and AI, the effect on biomedical device innovation is profound, with the potential to revolutionize the medical technology sector.

4.2.1. Popular Software used in Biomedical Design

Software tools take a vital role in the process of developing medical devices in the fast-paced arena of biomedical design. Most widely used among them is SolidWorks, a software that is most preferred because of its powerful parametric modeling feature. Biomedical engineers can use this software to develop complex designs that can be easily changed according to project requirements. SolidWorks flexibility enables designers to analyze the stress and strain experienced by devices under various situations, as it is vital for ensuring safety and efficiency. For instance, pre- and post-treatment procedures in medical devices can be plotted extensively in three-dimensional space, such that intricate concepts are conveyed visually with greater potency. Such software not only enhances innovation but also facilitates collaboration among multidisciplinary teams, making the overall design process more effective in biomedical fields.

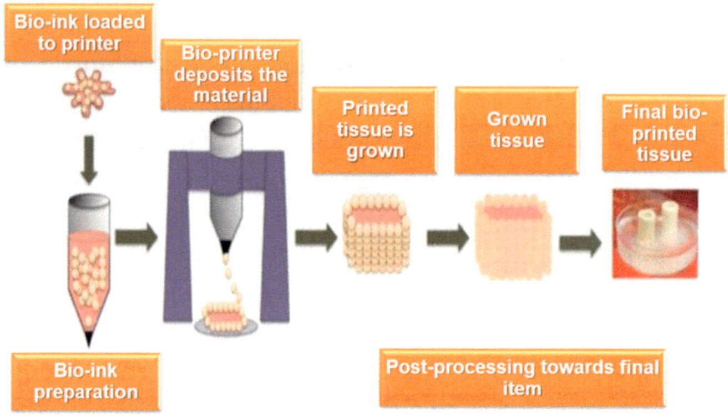

Figure 4.7. BioCAD allows for the manipulation of bio-relevant prototypes, enabling researchers to specify the materials and structural integrity required for various biomedical applications.

Source: https://www.mdpi.com/bioengineering/bioengineering-12-00076/article_deploy/html/images/bioengineering-12-00076-g001.png.

Autodesk Fusion 360 is another extremely popular software suite utilized in biomedical design. It is equipped with parametric, direct, and surface modeling functionality, which is well-suited for creating accurate prototypes of medical devices. Its cloud-based platform facilitates real-time collaboration among designers, engineers, and stakeholders simultaneously, important in integrated product development. With simulation support for device functionality, the users can conduct finite element analysis (FEA) for mechanical testing without even requiring physical prototyping, thus both time and resources saved. Visualization of design component dependencies also facilitates optimization of the final product before fabrication. As much as there is a demand for customized biomedical solutions, companies like Autodesk Fusion 360 are at the center of embracing the challenges of rapid prototyping and personalized medicine. Software designed to specifically respond to 3D printing technologies has attracted a huge following among the biomedical design fraternity over the last couple of years. Software packages like Creo and BioCAD are designed to optimize the design of structures for additive manufacturing, particularly in areas like tissue engineering and personalized implants. For instance, BioCAD allows for the manipulation of prototypes that are bio-relevant so that researchers can set the material and strength of structure required for biomedical applications. Furthermore, the integration of nanogel characterization and drug delivery modeling is enabled by software that supports such innovative design capabilities. Complementarity between the capabilities of software and biomedical innovation is seen through 3D printing's ability to revolutionize the production of complex geometries, thus making it easier to achieve better wound healing, surgical tools, and tailored therapies (Cho et al., 2018). Furthermore, design strategies for nanotechnology in biomedical applications continue to benefit from these advancements, in line with the central position of software in future biomedical device design (Figure 4.7).

4.2.2. Features and Capabilities of 3D Modeling Tools

The evolution of 3D modeling software has opened the doors to great advances in the field of medicine, particularly in biomedical device design and production. The software yields excellent features that enhance the accuracy and efficiency of device development methods significantly. Advanced 3D modeling software makes it possible for users to create highly intricate and detailed geometries, which is of paramount importance within the biomedical community where minute variations influence functionality and safety. Moreover, integration of the simulation capabilities allows designers and engineers to test devices virtually before production is undertaken. Time and resources are not only saved but also the risk of design failure, thus prompting innovation in the medical solutions. The capabilities of these tools allow for simple collaboration among multidisciplinary teams through design iteration by shared knowledge and feedback. In addition to accuracy and simulation functionality, 3D modeling tools are now being augmented with automation and artificial intelligence (AI) advancements. Such features simplify the design workflow through the automation of repetitive tasks and predictive analytics, which enhance decision-making. For instance, AI algorithms can suggest ideal design improvements based on a predefined set of parameters and learning from previous projects. This promotes innovation as it reduces the design burden on designers so that they can focus on more complex design problems. In the case of biomedical devices, this enhancement is particularly important because products are likely to need to comply with stringent standards of regulation. The ability of 3D modeling software to track design modifications and generate detailed documentation to support it also facilitates compliance, providing traceability and transparency to every stage of the design process and eventually leading to quality assurance. Another prominent feature of modern 3D modeling technology is its capability to support additive manufacturing technologies such as 3D printing. This convergence presents new possibilities for personalizing biomedical devices to the specific requirements of individual patients or target application. Practitioners can therefore create patient-specific models that enhance outcomes, for example, implants or prosthetics customized to precisely fit the anatomy of the individual.

The access to the tools also brings democratization of the design process in a way that enables smaller groups and institutions to create innovations within the biomedical field without the need for enormous resources. Greater collaboration is another benefit as the platforms facilitate sharing of concepts and designs, leading to greater innovation in the creation of biomedical technology. With regard to this, the impact of 3D modeling software in the creation of sophisticated medical devices cannot be overemphasized, as they present opportunities for future development in healthcare delivery and treatment of patients (Figure 4.8).

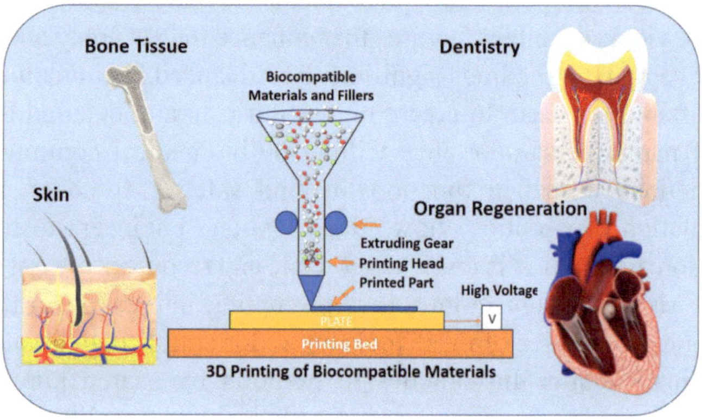

Figure 4.8. Advanced 3D modeling software enables users to create highly detailed and complex geometries, which is essential in the biomedical field where even minor variations can impact functionality and safety.

Source: https://media.springernature.com/lw1200/springer-static/image/art%3A10.1007%2Fs43939-024-00115-4/MediaObjects/43939_2024_115_Figa_HTML.png.

4.2.3. Comparison of Software Options for Different Applications

Comparison of software for 3D design and modeling of medical devices is required because of the unique requirements of this industry. Various packages are employed to meet various elements of design, from CAD packages like SolidWorks and AutoCAD that are famous for precision and engineering to elaborate modeling packages like ANSYS and COMSOL Multiphysics that accommodate intricate simulations and analysis. There are advantages to each program; for instance, SolidWorks is intuitive and widely used in business, so a favorite among students and professionals alike. But when developing complex devices such as implantable technologies, simulation programs such as ANSYS are required because they can model material characteristics and behavior under different conditions. In the end, the choice of software will need to serve the purpose of the application, balancing usability, functionality, and accuracy. Moreover, emerging biomedicines technologies point to specialized software facilitating new materials and methods of introduction, such as 3D printing. Specialized software for additive manufacturing, such as Ultimaker Cura and Materialise Magics, makes digital prints less complicated to convert into physical prototypes. These software packages feature user-friendly interfaces and can accept various file types needed in 3D printing, which is critical in the fabrication of medical devices. Besides, with the advancements in nanotechnology in devices, as is clear with the advancements in the formulation of nanogels for drug delivery systems, software functionalities must incorporate a complex understanding of material behaviors at the microparticle level (Cho et al., 2018). The fusion of 3D modeling with advanced manufacturing techniques bears testimony to the state of advancement in software solutions in this context. This software integration also extends to collaboration and workflow management among biomedical device development teams. Software like Autodesk Fusion 360 provides nuanced cloud-based solutions that allow various stakeholders to interact and update designs in real time, promoting communication and aligning all stakeholders on the same page. These collaborative environments are invaluable when rapid iteration of design is required, as is often the case in biomedical breakthroughs. Furthermore, as mandated by new neural network architectures, artificial intelligence incorporation in design programs is becoming more of a trend (Manohar et al., 2018). This renders modeling and predictive analytics more intuitive during the design phase, thus more likely to reduce time to market and enhance device functionality. As software adapts to keep pace with the vast applications in 3D modeling for biomedical devices, judicious consideration of potential will be the most important factor in successful application in this developing field.

4.3. APPLICATIONS OF 3D DESIGN IN BIOMEDICAL DEVICES

Inclusion of 3D design in biomedical devices has had a monumental effect on medical device development and customization. The most significant advantage of 3D modeling is that it is able to make copies of patient-specific anatomy. The replicas aid pre-surgical planning, allowing surgeons to model complex structures prior to performing intricate surgeries. For instance, 3D-printed models from imaging data enhance patient outcomes and accuracy of surgery by providing tactile feedback during procedures. In addition, the precision enabled by 3D printing enables the production of customized devices such as implants and scaffolds tailored to specific anatomical requirements, a factor that is extremely critical in fields such as orthopedics and reconstructive surgery. Thus, the capability for personalization using 3D design significantly enhances the usability and applicability of biomedical devices. In addition to enhancing pre-surgical planning, 3D design plays a critical role in the development of tissue engineering applications. As 3D printing technologies advance, sophisticated structures closely mimicking the anatomy of native tissue can now be produced. 3D-printed scaffolds provide support for cell proliferation and tissue regeneration and therefore are a promising area for regenerative medicine. Advances over the last few years have broadened the application of 3D printing through the incorporation of biocompatible material and living cells into the structure, thereby facilitating the production of bio-printed tissue. As presented in recent research, crossing the technological hurdle in creating intricate 3D microarchitectures is an imperative to fully utilize the capacity of tissue engineering in repairing or replacing damaged tissues and organs (Chia et al., 2015). In addition, beyond the point-of-care tissue and surgical engineering applications, 3D design in medical devices is influencing the design of novel diagnostic platforms and drug delivery systems. The ability to engineer very specialized devices makes it possible to assemble complicated systems capable of sensing or treating in custom manners. Personalized drug delivery implants, for example, can be designed to release medication based on patient-specific states, and this greatly increases efficacy while reducing side effects. Moreover, the availability of 3D-printed diagnostic tools holds potential to advance the efficiency of medical testing and monitoring, decrease healthcare expenses, and enhance access to critical services. As noted in recent studies, the convergence of novel materials and fabrication techniques is unlocking potential for breakthroughs in these applications in the biomedical device domain (Manohar et al., 2018). Therefore, the use of 3D design not only captures its transformative impact but also demonstrates the need for continuous exploration and imagination in the field.

4.3.1. Custom Prosthetics and Implants

The advent of three-dimensional (3D) design and modeling software has revolutionized the field of custom implants and prosthetics. They enable the manufacture of tailor-made medical devices to match the very specific anatomical shapes of individual patients.

With information gained from medical imaging technology such as MRI and CT scanning, medical professionals can design prosthetics that not only work towards improved function outcomes but also optimize comfort and aesthetic satisfaction for the user. This is a direct opposition to what used to be done in the past with generic solutions designed that did not take into consideration the needs of individualized patients. According to research, use of 3D printing techniques in surgery has been associated with better surgical outcomes and reduced operative time, observing the efficiency and flexibility of such emerging techniques in prosthetic design and implementation (Annemans et al., 2016). In addition to improving prosthetic apparatus accuracy, 3D modeling also allows for iterative design strategies that enable rapid prototyping. Medical Reverse Engineering (MRE) techniques are to be held accountable for developing accurate 3D models of biological structures and biomedical objects, which ultimately give rise to implants and prosthetics specifically tailored to perfection. MRE is an iterative technique through which engineers and medical physicians can evaluate and update designs via the mechanism of real-time feedback, thereby avoiding any potential complications before production.

This cooperative process not only makes the manufacturing process easier but also minimizes the risk of surgical revision from poor-fitting or dysfunctional material. With continued progress, MRE facilitates the support of an ever-broader variety of applications, ranging from dental and orthopedic implants to individualized surgical instruments, thus propelling the field of biomedical engineering (Jos et al., 2010).

In addition, the application of 3D printing in the development of personalized prosthetics and implants is accompanied by a solid examination of economic aspects in healthcare. While the startup costs for utilizing 3D printing—e.g., advanced scanning technologies and materials—are likely to be high, several studies demonstrate potential cost savings in the long term through better patient outcomes and fewer postoperative complications. The time saved in surgical procedures, along with decreased demand for long-term follow-up care, can lead to decreased overall healthcare expenditure. However, comprehensive cost-effectiveness analyses are required to ensure that the observed benefits with 3D-printed implants and prosthetics are reasonable enough to be in the price range in clinical use. As technology and medicine interface more and more, research continues to be crucial in order to comprehensively value such innovations in maximizing patient quality of life while optimizing healthcare resources (Annemans et al., 2016) (Figure 4.9).

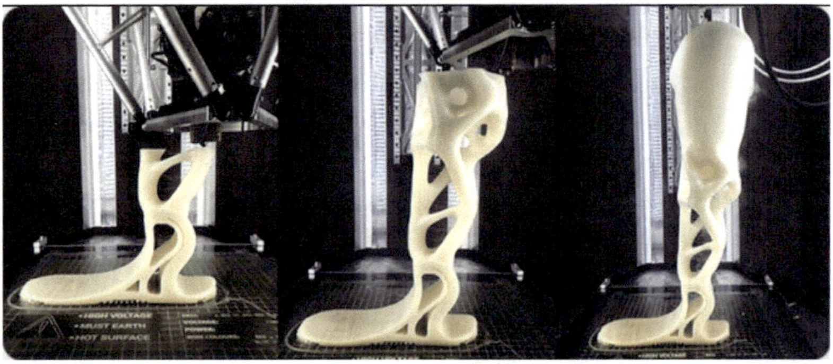

Figure 4.9. The advent of three-dimensional (3D) design and modeling technologies has significantly transformed the landscape of custom prosthetics and implants.

Source: https://pub.mdpi-res.com/applsci/applsci-15-01350/article_deploy/html/images/applsci-15-01350-g008.png?1738672900.

4.3.2. Surgical Planning and Simulation

An essential part of modern surgical practice, surgical simulation and planning are founded upon the establishment of 3D modeling and design technology, which enables precise preoperative assessment. Computer-assisted orthopedic surgery (CAOS) technology is a significant leap forward in this regard. These systems utilize several imaging modalities like computed tomography (CT), magnetic resonance imaging (MRI), and even ultrasound to reconstruct sophisticated 3D models of anatomy. This detailed modeling allows for greater understanding and dexterity in surgery, as professionals are able to view intricate interactions within the musculoskeletal system and make plans for distraction or correction methods based on accurate representations of anatomy tailored to individual patients. The use of these methods not only saves time in surgery but also minimizes the risk of complications, thereby making surgical planning a foundation in contemporary orthopedic procedures (Kalová et al., 2019). In surgical planning, simulation is also involved through rehearsals of the surgical process in a virtual setting. In virtual reality and advanced modeling, surgeons rehearse complicated maneuvers in a secure setting before they actually perform the actual procedure. This element of surgical training significantly contributes to skill acquisition because it provides surgeons with a stage where they can hone their techniques and decision-making without putting patient safety at risk. By simulating potential operative scenarios, clinicians can anticipate issues that could arise during an operation and plan contingencies more effectively. These pre-planning exercises underscore the role of 3D design software in fostering a culture of safety and competence within surgical teams, which, in turn, translates into improved patient outcomes and health effectiveness as they design individualized treatment approaches (Jos et al., 2010). Furthermore, surgical simulation and planning have significant consequences outside the operating room, extending into biomedical device manufacturing and design. One notable application in this regard is Medical Reverse Engineering (MRE), which enables 3D reconstruction of imaging data to create patient-specific implants and surgical instruments. Through MRE techniques, biomedical engineers can enhance the design of implants, such as bone rebuilding and dentistry, by exploring diverse methodologies that achieve optimal fit and function. Such personalized products not only provide increased performance and satisfaction for the patient but also provide a rich challenge for future advances in biomedical technology. With simulation and planning in surgery continuing to evolve with technology in terms of 3D modeling and design, there is great potential for enhancing accuracy in surgery, eventually driving the field of biomedical engineering forward in incredible ways (Jos et al., 2010) (Figure 4.10).

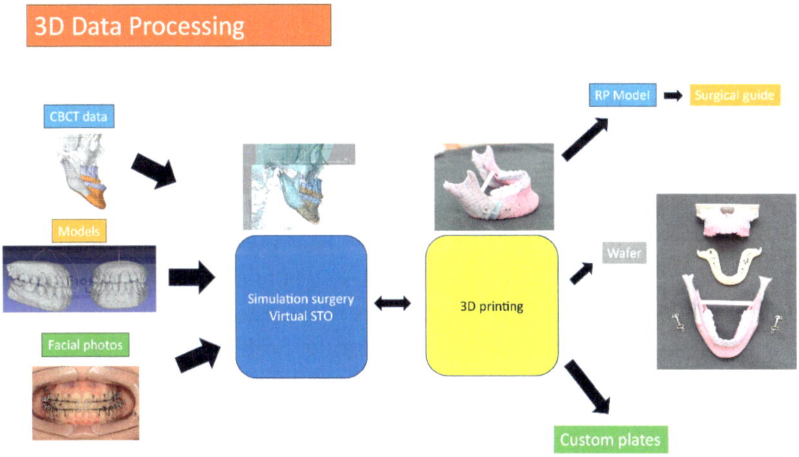

Figure 4.10. Medical reverse engineering (MRE) is a prominent application in this sphere, enabling the reconstruction of 3D models from imaging data to produce customized implants and surgical instruments tailored to individual patients.

Source: https://pub.mdpi-res.com/applsci/applsci-13-09907/article_deploy/html/images/applsci-13-09907-g005.png?1693558593.

4.3.3. Development of Medical Devices and Instruments

The technology of the production of medical devices and instruments has also undergone a very profound change, particularly with the advent of 3D design and modeling technologies. The technologies have changed the way individualized solutions specific to the requirements of patients are produced. For example, additive manufacturing, also known as 3D printing, allows the production of complex geometries with high accuracy that cannot be produced by traditional manufacturing processes. This technology has also enabled the development of patient-specific prosthetics, implants, and surgical devices, further enhancing the efficiency of medical procedures. Moreover, the ability to manufacture designs rapidly enhances innovation since medical experts can implement changes on devices based on instant feedback from clinical practice. Lastly, the integration of 3D design into medical device development ensures that there is an increased level of personalization and efficiency, thereby improving patient outcomes.

The contribution of material selection to the development of medical devices cannot be overstated. There has been enhanced material science, and this has given rise to several biocompatible materials that are usable on 3D printed medical devices and implants. Scaffolding materials, as the literature describes, are critical components that offer a platform to cultivate tissue growth and integration into the human body (Reddy et al., 2021). Both are natural and synthetic polymers, both of which are selected for specific applications because of their physicochemical properties such as porosity, biodegradability, and mechanical strength. By selecting materials that suit their preferred application, manufacturers can produce devices that are not only regulatory compliant but also have the potential to enhance healing. This precise attention to material science during the engineering and design stages additionally emphasizes the revolutionizing potential of 3D modeling for the medical industry. In addition to customization and material creation, bioprinting's role in the design of medical devices is also potentially significant for the future. Bioprinting employs 3D printing technology to print living organs and tissue, which opens the doors to more advanced regenerative medicine. Bio-ink utilization, or the use of materials intended to support cellular activity, allows for the development of intricate tissue architectures that closely mimic natural conditions (Datta et al., 2023). The innovation finds most relevance in tissue engineering and regenerative medicine, where these technologies aim to restore or replace compromised tissues and organs. But bioprinting's limitations, such as vascularization and the incorporation of implanted tissue into the recipient body's systems, must be overcome if full potential for such applications is to be realized. Therefore, today's research in this area not only holds so much promise for future medical applications but also helps illustrate the dynamic, evolving nature of the medical device market as fueled by 3D design and modeling (Figure 4.11).

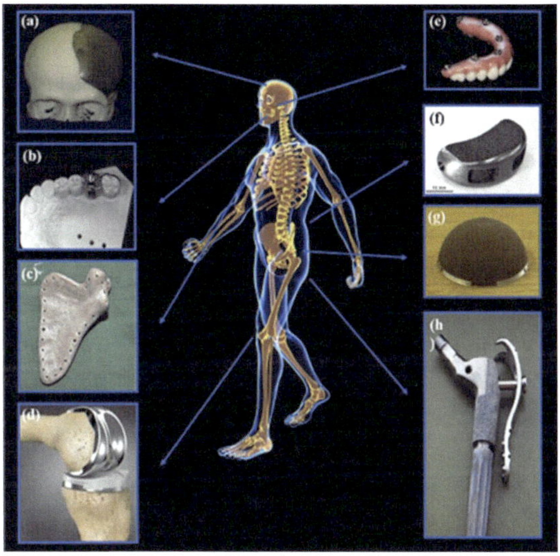

Figure 4.11. Advances in material science have led to the emergence of various biocompatible materials that can be used in 3D printed medical instruments and implants.

Source: https://media.springernature.com/lw685/springer-static/image/art%3A10.1007%2Fs11665-021-05578-7/MediaObjects/11665_2021_5578_Fig1_HTML.jpg.

4.4. BENEFITS OF 3D MODELING IN HEALTHCARE

3D modeling integration in medicine redefines the process of biomedical device design into a highly accurate and customized procedure. 3D modeling technology enables engineers and physicians to observe detailed anatomy of intricate structures, which are impossible with traditional means. Through the creation of accurate digital models of patients' anatomical data, 3D modeling enables customized treatment planning by offering devices that are uniquely designed for unique needs. Such individualization not only improves patient results but also reduces the risk of complications associated with ill-fitting devices. Moreover, such personalization can lead to decreased surgery duration and improved recovery outcomes, ultimately enabling healthcare delivery and optimizing overall patient satisfaction. Therefore, the use of 3D modeling in biomedical device design is one of the most significant advancements in the healthcare sector that balances technology and patient care (Huertas et al.,

2016). Also, cost-effectiveness is one of the biggest healthcare contributions 3D modeling provides. The process reduces the overall cost incurred by biomedical device design and prototype testing. With additive manufacturing techniques, prototypes are produced faster and more cost-effectively, without the need for costly traditional fabrication procedures. For instance, rapid prototyping through 3D printing makes possible fast iteration of device design so that engineers can identify and fix mistakes immediately. Iterative development becomes not just cheaper but also speeds up the process from concept to marketplace. The reduced production cost using 3D models offers the prospect of innovations that would otherwise be economically non-viable through conventional production methods. Such affordability makes the advanced medical technology readily available to both practitioners and patients, facilitating the facile uptake of new solutions (Ewart et al., 2019). Finally, 3D modeling goes a long way in enhancing education and training in the healthcare industry. Medical students and professionals can utilize 3D models to experience interactive learning, where they can learn about complex procedures and devices in a simulated setting. This hands-on learning permits aspiring medical professionals to understand anatomical pathways and device functions much better. Healthcare educators can also utilize these models to deliver complex concepts, making otherwise complex information easy to understand and learn. Such training developments eventually lead to more competent healthcare workers who can provide quality patient care. With healthcare practice still evolving, applying 3D modeling in training demonstrates its numerous benefits. By enhancing the quality of learning processes and outcomes, technology ensures an effective and competent workforce in addressing the complexities of new health practices (Huertas et al., 2016).

4.4.1. Enhanced Precision and Customization

The evolution of 3D modeling and design technologies has laid the ground for a new age of higher precision and customization in the manufacture of biomedical devices. In contrast to traditional manufacturing methods that are commonly restricted by preconceived forms and material limitations, 3D printing facilitates the manufacture of components that are uniquely designed for patient needs. Not only does this ensure optimized therapeutic gain but also results in the creation of complex geometries that optimize functionality. For instance, through the use of additive manufacturing, intricate inner structures can be produced to enable biological integration or improve the mechanical strength of implants, thus transforming patient recovery and device life fundamentally. The advantages cross cost-effectiveness and time saved in the production process, all in accordance with industry 4.0 assumptions where innovative fabrication techniques come under the spotlight. Therefore, adoption of these technologies triggers innovation while ensuring that devices align to personalized healthcare requirements (Dehghanghadikolaei et al., 2019). Apart from patient-specific treatment, precision in biomedical device modeling translates into improved surgical outcomes. Technologies such as the Immunotargeted Nanoparticle Single-Chip Imaging Technology (INSITE) illustrate the benefit of 3D modeling in delivering more sophisticated scale imaging and intervention capability. Because traditional imaging instruments are generally deficient in accessing remote surgical sites, the introduction of advanced nanostructures in a device provides an invaluable tool for minimally invasive surgery. The high-performance imaging efficiency of aUCNPs, along with their compatibility with narrow-band excitations, allows precise targeting of tumors and thereby maximizes the effectiveness of the treatment.

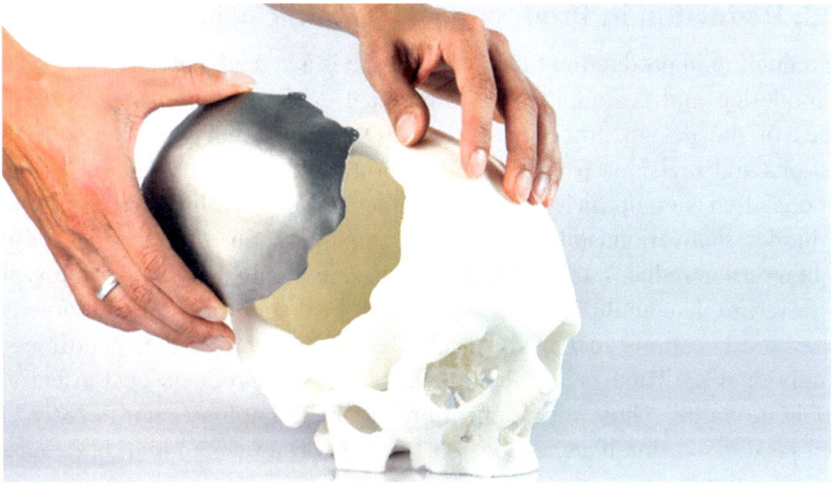

Figure 4.12. 3D modeling allows for the creation of patient-specific implants, prosthetics, and surgical instruments that can be fabricated with high resolution, significantly reducing the risk of complications.

Source: https://www.3dnatives.com/en/wp-content/uploads/sites/2/cover-162-1280x720.jpg.

The engineering of these complex devices serves to illustrate the role of 3D modeling in enabling functionalities that are not possible in traditional designs, demonstrating the critical role that individualized solutions play in the dynamic world of modern medicine (Anwar et al., 2019). Moreover, the value of customization in biomedically engineered 3D devices emerges when considering patient anatomy and pathology variability. Each individual's body shape is quite unique, and thus personalized device requirements need to be compatible and functional. 3D modeling allows for the creation of patient-specific implants, prosthetics, and surgical devices that can be produced at high resolution, significantly reducing the risk of complications. Such advancements not only yield enhanced patient satisfaction but enhance the overall efficiency of healthcare delivery systems as well. The harmonization of precision engineering and customization brings a paradigm that presents the device not as an off-the-shelf item but as a device engineered to meet the specific physiological and pathological complexities of each patient. This is essential in battling the complexities of modern-day healthcare, which ultimately results in a responsive and effective healthcare system (Dehghanghadikolaei et al., 2019) (Figure 4.12).

4.4.2. Reduction in Production Time and Costs

The reduction in production time and expense is a key advantage of employing 3D modeling and design for the biomedical devices market. By putting all phases of the design process together, 3D printing makes possible quicker iterations and revisions from concept to prototype. Traditional manufacturing methods often encompass lengthy setup times and high tooling expenses, which can hinder innovation and increase costs of operation. Conversely, additive manufacturing reduces these impediments and facilitates rapid prototyping and faster implementation of customized medical solutions. Since biomedical devices are becoming increasingly complex and tailored to the specific needs of individual patients, being able to produce these products cost-effectively is of huge value. Thus, the application of 3D technology significantly cuts down production timelines, enabling faster response rates to market demands, thereby achieving significant cost savings in the entire development process (Dehghanghadikolaei et al., 2019). Furthermore, material efficiencies that accrue from 3D printing advancements significantly contribute to overall cost savings. Conventional manufacturing techniques have a tendency to result in much wastage because extra material is trimmed or taken off. With additive manufacturing, manufacturers and engineers can construct parts layer upon layer, using only the necessary materials, making the best use of resources. In addition to conserving material costs, it contributes to sustainable practice, which is increasingly popular in the biomedical field. The less waste from 3D printing directly serves to reduce costs, and thus advanced manufacturing makes economic sense for developers. As 3D design technologies continue to mature, where decreasing the cost of production meets sustainable approaches, there is potential for increased economic feasibility of mass production of biomedical devices (Chia et al., 2015). Moreover, as production is further decentralized through 3D printing, localized production becomes a potential game-changer in terms of cost-saving. In contrast to relying on large central manufacturing facilities, which have significant shipping and handling costs, 3D printing allows biomedical devices to be produced at or near health care facilities. Not only is this less expensive, but it reduces production lead times because devices can be made on-demand based on patient-specific requirements. Thus, this ability to adjust manufacturing to actual clinical demands enables quick response in healthcare settings, enhancing patient outcomes. With further advances in technology, the integration of localized manufacturing and 3D modeling presents a revolutionary shift in the biomedical industry, mirroring the mutual dependency of cost reduction and better provision of service (Dehghanghadikolaei et al., 2019) (Figure 4.13).

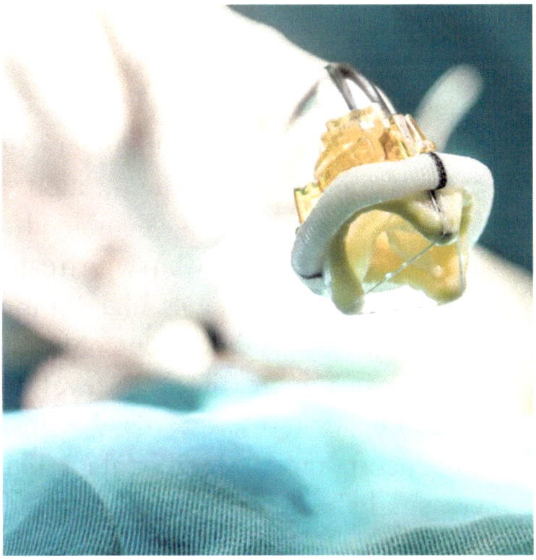

Figure 4.13. As biomedical devices become more complex and tailored to individual patient needs, the ability to efficiently produce these items becomes indispensable.

*Source:*https://www.exponent.com/sites/default/files/styles/fifty_media_large/public/media/images/GettyImages-1182458826.jpg.webp?itok=_7QtJR9E.

4.4.3. Improved Patient Outcomes and Satisfaction

The integration of 3D modeling and design into the development of biomedical devices has led to improved patient satisfaction and outcome. These advanced techniques enable the fabrication of highly personalized medical implants and prosthetics that match the specific anatomical characteristics of the individual. Thus, customization not only enhances the efficacy of such devices but also minimizes complications associated with ill-fitting medical interventions. Greater personalization leads to quicker recovery time and improves functional results following surgery, enabling patients to recover more easily and confidently to resume their daily activity. Moreover, favorable results obtained due to customized devices enhance patient satisfaction, leading to increased compliance with medical therapy and follow-up interventions prescribed. The combined effect underscores the importance of integrating patient-centered approaches in biomedical device design, thus ensuring that technological benefits are translated into actual health advantages. In addition to bettering physical health, 3D designs, and modeling also have an important role in boosting patient participation in their healthcare process. The visualization ability found in 3D modeling allows patients to better think about the devices and treatments they will undergo.

This understanding can reduce stress and provide a sense of control, which can then translate to greater participation in their own care. Moreover, such educated patients tend to be better informed while interacting with healthcare professionals during visits, enhancing communication and collaborative decision making. Enhanced communication, combined with empowering patients, was proven to have a positive relationship with treatment adherence and health outcomes. Therefore, using technologies like 3D modeling, healthcare professionals are not only improving clinical outcomes but also improving patients' experience overall, thus increasing the level of care in modern medicine. Moreover, as healthcare turns towards the greater application of advanced technologies, the incorporation of artificial intelligence (AI) together with 3D modeling is increasingly beginning to redesign models of patient care.

AI-powered medical imaging and diagnosis applications are a classic example of this convergence, enabling rapid and accurate detection of medical conditions that could easily be integrated in 3D models in order to plan treatments that are customized according to the patient. AI automates processes such as maintenance of electronic health records and virtual patient care, thereby making delivery of healthcare more efficient and keeping medical professionals away from unnecessary workload. The combination of AI and 3D design not only improves accuracy in treatment planning but also addresses important ethical and regulatory challenges, ensuring patient safety and gain trust with technological innovation. An effective combination of the two technologies confirms that a future of increased patient outcomes and satisfaction is not only an aspiration but an achievable goal as the healthcare sector continues to unfold (Kuwaiti et al., 2023; Luo et al., 2023).

4.5. CHALLENGES IN 3D DESIGN FOR BIOMEDICAL DEVICES

3D modeling and design of medical devices face a myriad of challenges that have the potential to hinder progress in this rapidly advancing area. One of the most prevalent challenges is the complexity of human anatomy, which enforces highly complex and precise models. Tailoring devices for unique patient anatomies requires high-resolution imaging modalities, such as MRI or CT scans, which, although useful, can create variability in such a way that makes it difficult to model. For instance, even small mistakes in the scans have a likelihood of inducing drastic differences in the end product, which may influence device performance or patient safety. Secondly, integrating patient-specific information into the design process poses challenges related to data standardization and interoperability. Ensuring that the modeling tool has the capability of accommodating diverse datasets and analyzing them efficiently becomes the hallmark in rising above the initial challenges in 3D design. Moreover, the selection of material for 3D-printed biomedical devices comes with complications.

Biomaterials not only must satisfy mechanical requirements but also biocompatibility, allowing proper integration into the human body. Conventional materials limit design possibilities as they are either too stiff or unable to simulate the properties of the elasticity of human tissue. Current developments in the field of materials science demonstrate the potential for using biodegradable polymers and composites, but these are mostly special processing methods not readily accessible. According to recent studies, for the best harnessing of the potential of 3D printing in biomedicine, it is required to actively pursue and further develop these materials as a matter of urgency (Chia et al., 2015). These challenges can be overcome, clearing the ground for even more innovative solutions to address patient-centered care. Beyond material challenges, production process itself can be a huge stumbling block.

3D printing technologies, such as Selective Laser Sintering and Fused Deposition Modeling, each possess inherent constraints that could affect the fidelity of the resultant device. For instance, issues related to layer adhesion, resolution, and surface finish influence the performance and lifespan of the devices that are being produced. Moreover, with the ever-growing demand for customized medical solutions, the scalability of these processes' gains importance. Being able to have efficient workflows in hand that guarantee quality and allow for customization will be the way forward for meeting future demands. Researchers have been increasingly going towards developing precision techniques like nanogel production via 3D printing, which has promising potential for more customization options in addressing these challenges (Cho et al., 2018). With this new field, continuous innovation in processes as well as techniques will be the solution to surmounting the many challenges in 3D design of biomedical devices.

4.5.1. Regulatory and Compliance Issues

The convergence of 3D modeling and designing technologies in biomedical devices is a huge regulatory and compliance challenge that has to be addressed for public safety and efficiency. The use of additive manufacturing techniques, for instance, allows for rapid prototyping and customized medical device manufacturing, but such new developments also call for strict regulation by regulatory bodies such as the Food and Drug Administration (FDA). As these kinds of organizations strive to bridge their architectures to accommodate new technology, companies must navigate shifting landscapes of law governing materials, methods of production, and device function overall. Effective compliance requires a keen understanding of local and global legislation, with standards such as ISO 13485 for quality management systems playing an extremely crucial role in guaranteeing device performance and safety across global markets. Complimenting traditional compliance concerns are the newer ones created by advances in 3D design and modeling. As these advances occur, there are special intellectual property and data security concerns. When biomedical companies utilize advanced digital design tools, intellectual property violations are more possible; protecting trade secrets is essential to remaining competitive. Moreover, as greater numbers of medical devices become networked, data privacy and security are concerns. Regulatory frameworks are not yet prepared to address these new risks, and institutions are thus compelled to put in place proactive controls that can address both regulatory compliance and data integrity.

Collaboration between industry stakeholders and regulation players is essential in defining standards that can keep pace with technological development as well as defend intellectual property and patient data. Moreover, the regulatory environment for 3D-printed healthcare devices is also shrouded by varied standards and requirements for clinical trials. Whereas traditional manufactured alternatives rely on established clinical trial protocols, their 3D-printed counterparts may have novel strategies necessary to demonstrate safety and efficacy. This is best exemplified in instances like total arthroplasty, where customized artificial joints offer dramatic improvements in outcomes for patients but are subjected to harsh criticism in order to minimize the complications that accompany the procedure, such as the probability of multiple interventions (Pakhaliuk et al., 2020). As exemplified by the visionary literature, incorporating new technologies in addressing current compliance issues demands a futuristic regulatory framework that encourages innovation without compromising on safety and efficacy (Cippitelli et al., 2017) (Figure 4.14).

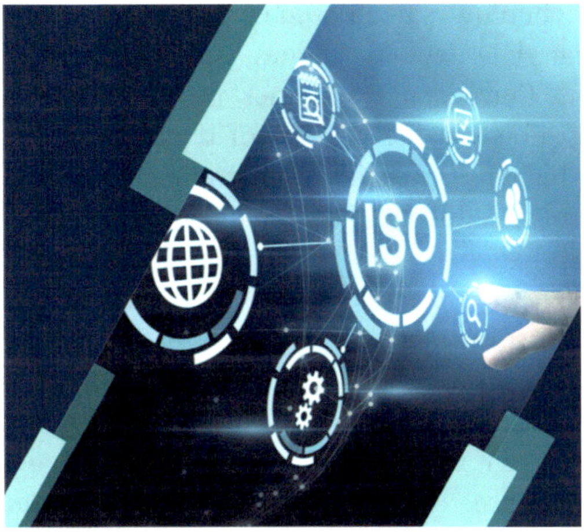

Figure 4.14. Effective compliance requires a comprehensive understanding of both local and international regulations, as standards such as ISO 13485 for quality management systems play a crucial role in maintaining device safety and effectiveness across global markets.

Source: https://media.licdn.com/dms/image/v2/D5612AQED5NyZxsr2RQ/article-cover_image-shrink_720_1280/article-cover_image-shrink_720_1280/0/1733526200030?e=2147483647&v=beta&t=7SZelmxiu7W4AlWntj-i3aLA59yxofOKA-OfmazS6PVk.

4.5.2. Material Limitations and Biocompatibility

The growth of 3D modeling and design of biomedical devices has been influenced greatly by material limitation and the issue of biocompatibility. As researchers develop increasingly complex biomedical devices, the selection of materials becomes a more critical factor in order to ensure the success of the devices. Titanium alloys, for example, are used widely since they have good properties, including strength and resistance against corrosion; however, they generally suffer from problems related to their biocompatibility. The interaction between the implant material and surrounding biological environment can induce destructive reactions that compromise the functionality and lifespan of the device. Understanding these material limitations and principles of biocompatibility is essential in a bid to improve scaffold and implant design for better integration with the human body. With the advancement of 3D printing technology, solving these issues will take center stage to improve clinical applications and patient outcomes (Chia et al., 2015). Material behavior in the processes of 3D printing contributes to the challenges in creating biocompatible devices. Printing technologies like Fused Deposition Modeling and Bioprinting provide varying material selection avenues, yet each material produces varying biological reactions. For instance, polymer materials used in the manufacture of scaffolds can exhibit varying degrees of biodegradability and mechanical property, both of which influence tissue integration and mechanisms of healing. Experiments have revealed that the choice of raw material impacts directly on how scaffoldings can support cellular activity and facilitate tissue growth. As defined in Finite Element Method analysis-based research (FEM), the elasticity and structural integrity of diverse material combinations are key determinants of device performance in response to physiological stress (Bramanti et al., 2018). Thus, improving 3D printing technology while ensuring top-of-the-line material choice is imperative in mitigating biocompatibility concerns encountered in biomedical device use. In the coming future, the promise of 3D-printed biomedical devices is to unravel the intricate trade-off between material limitations, biocompatibility, and the new technology that can be used to propel their manufacture. Scientists are continually looking for new biomaterials and composite materials that combine the best properties of the available alternatives while minimizing their drawback. An example is the addition of bioactive glass or ceramics to polymeric matrices that yield osteoconductivity and healing potential in orthopedic treatment. Also, enhancement in surface modification techniques can increase protein adsorption and cellular adhesion to attain better integration with host tissues. With the growing demand for personalized medicine solutions, it is the need of the hour to highlight such interdisciplinary approaches that merge materials science with innovations in 3D printing engineering. Through the implementation of this strategy, the field can ultimately fulfill the promise of creating sophisticated, patient-specific biomedical devices that more accurately meet personal health needs with continued biocompatibility over the entire device lifetime (Chia et al., 2015).

4.5.3. Integration with Existing Medical Technologies

The integration of 3D modeling and design with modern medical technology is slowly changing the landscape of biomedical device manufacturing. Conventional methods do not meet the demands of the growing need for individualized and complex medical devices, yet 3D printing, or additive manufacturing, may be the answer. With this technology, it is possible to create custom-made parts that cater to individual patient requirements, significantly enhancing the performance and efficiency of medical devices. For instance,

3D printing allows for quick prototyping of prostheses and implants custom-shaped to fit the specific anatomy of each patient, enhancing both surgical success and patient satisfaction. As highlighted in more recent studies, the implementation of emerging manufacturing technologies is consistent with Industry 4.0, highlighting their capability to enhance innovation and efficiency in healthcare (Dehghanghadikolaei et al., 2019). Integrating 3D modeling into existing medical technology architectures also paves the way for more cross-disciplinary interaction.

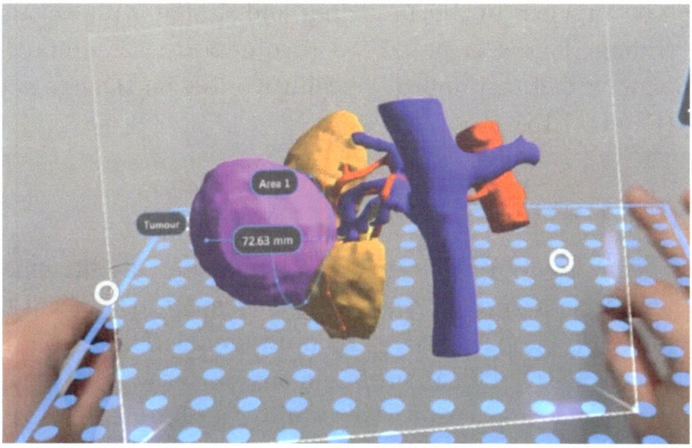

Figure 4.15. 3D printing allows for the rapid prototyping of prosthetics and implants that fit each patient's unique anatomy, thereby improving surgical outcomes and patient satisfaction.

Source: https://appinventiv.com/wp-content/uploads/2025/06/extended_reality_xr_in_3d_planning.webp.

For example, the coupling of photonics and biomedical applications is one of the best examples of how light technologies can be integrated with 3D-printed devices to improve diagnostics and treatment. The Boston University Photonics Center is itself a product of such interdisciplinary research, promoting the convergence of micro/nanofabrication techniques with biological translation to advance medical innovation (N/A, 2013). As researchers merge the power of 3D design with photonics, they are better poised to tackle pressing health problems, such as the development of point-of-care diagnostics and minimally invasive therapeutic interventions. This cooperative approach not only accelerates the innovation process but also facilitates the sharing of experience and resources between stakeholders in the biomedical industry. Moreover, the integration of 3D design into the existing medical system enhances the sustainability and availability of biomedical devices. Minimization of waste embedded in additive manufacturing reduces the generation of unhealthy practices all over the healthcare supply chain. By making effective use of materials and allowing for localized production, 3D printing can help decrease the environmental impact of traditional manufacturing. Furthermore, as technology continues to evolve, the opportunities for affordable medical solutions in low-resource settings emerge. The access benefits are particularly relevant to creating devices tailored to specific populations, with the aim of making advanced health solutions accessible to individuals of varying socioeconomic backgrounds. Overall, the convergence of 3D modeling and design with existing medical technology without lapses is poised to revolutionize the biomedical arena, driving innovations that can improve health worldwide (Dehghanghadikolaei et al., 2019) (Figure 4.15).

4.6. CONCLUSION

Overall, the integration of 3D design and modeling in the production of biomedical devices is a groundbreaking advancement in medical technology. Being able to create precise, patient-specific models has revolutionized the way doctors and other medical professionals perform diagnosis, treatment planning, and surgical preparation. This ability not only enhances the degree of personalization in healthcare but also streamlines the process of device fabrication. High-fidelity 3D models allow for better visualization of the anatomical structures and replicate many medical conditions, ultimately leading to better patient results. As demand for customized medical solutions increases, the position of 3D modeling in the same will become increasingly robust. While the benefits of 3D design are huge, there are certain challenges left. Scalability and integration of technology into existing medical platforms are some of those issues that need lengthy research and innovation. Studies indicate that emergent technologies, particularly nanoscale memory systems, may offer viable avenues towards enhancing the efficiency of computation in medical devices. Constructing high-performance on-chip communication networks that are able to provide additional connectivity without being limited by the inherent constraints of current architectures is critical to the development of biomedical devices (Manohar et al., 2018). Future studies on such network paradigms shall become instrumental in de-mystifying the complexities involved in the operation of 3D models. Finally, one has to admire the persistent image quality and data accuracy problems that can have direct implications for the efficiency of biomedical devices, especially in sub-optimal operating environments. For instance, it has been proven through research that environmental conditions can damage image data, thus affecting important tasks such as iris recognition (Ahmad et al., 2018). In the future, there is a need to improve image processing techniques alongside the development in 3D design to ensure that the best performance is realized for real-world applications. This concurrent focus on modeling and imaging will ultimately advance the quality and reliability of biomedical equipment, paving the way for new developments in healthcare technology.

4.6.1. Summary of Key Points

The progress of 3D modeling and design in the biomedical field is a quantum leap in the design and production of medical devices. Initially applied for pre-surgical visualization, the technologies have seen their application extended to include complex biomedical devices tailored to specific anatomical needs. The key feature, however, is the integration of patient-specific data to create personalized implants and scaffolds, significantly enhancing the efficiency and precision of medical interventions. With advancing technology, 3D printing has moved from basic tooling molds to sophisticated constructs used in tissue engineering and drug delivery systems. More research into such advancements has the potential for increased accessibility and customization in regenerative medicine, but there are tremendous amounts of technological challenges that must be addressed before such universal application becomes feasible (Chia et al., 2015). Based on this, recent advances in several of the 3D printing technologies have highlighted the possibility and the constraint inherent in the development of complex biological architectures. Three-Dimensional Printing, Fused Deposition Modeling, and Stereolithography are at the forefront of this advancement with each having distinctive capabilities that improve the fabrication of sensitive biomedical devices. For instance, the rapid rate of progress in material science has broadened the range of materials that are biocompatible and enhanced the structural integrity of printed devices. However, there still persist challenges in replicating the intricate microarchitecture necessary for the regeneration of highly complex tissues and organs. Overcoming these challenges is essential for the future of 3D printing in medicine, with researchers and clinicians aiming to utilize such advances for practical applications in health care (Chia et al., 2015). The convergence of emerging technologies with 3D modeling and design is central to the creation of next-generation biomedical devices. Specifically, the emergence of advanced computational methods is improving device manufacturing and design process efficiency. The combination of artificial intelligence and machine learning with 3D modeling is providing a platform where optimization and rapid prototyping are facilitated, and the ability to iteratively design rapidly based on real-time data is allowed. The potential for integration of neuromorphic computing systems also offers an alternative model for increasing the processing power of biomedical devices. The systems have different architectures from the normal ones, potentially resolving issues of communication built into conventional designs. Lastly, these developments give emphasis on the central interface between technology and medicine, with the potential for a future holding individualized, effective, and efficient solutions to a broad spectrum of medical conundrums.

4.6.2. The Impact of 3D Design on the Future of Healthcare

The coming of 3D design has transformed the future of healthcare to a large degree, bringing with it an age of medical innovation and rationalization. By allowing for the exact modeling of biomedical devices, technologies in 3D design enable the customization of devices and implants according to the anatomy of particular patients. This customization not only enhances the efficacy of medical therapy but also minimizes adverse responses that have mostly to do with ill-fitting devices. For instance, the capacity to produce patient-specific orthopedic implants using computer-aided design (CAD) software and additive manufacturing is likely to lead to improved surgical outcomes. Moreover, the utilization of intelligent materials in 3D designs, as highlighted in recent research, has the ability to develop adaptive biomedical devices with dynamic responses to fluctuations in the body environment, thus delivering increased functionality and comfort for patients (Oliver et al., 2009). In addition to customization, the impact of 3D design also extends to the cost-effectiveness of medical product development. Traditional manufacturing techniques of medical devices tend to cause significant material loss and lengthy processes. But with new methods such as particulate injection molding (PIM) and additive manufacturing, complex geometries can be produced with minimal wastage. The study of various processing methods, like a hybrid method combining additive and subtractive methods, illustrates the potential to make the manufacturing of molds and prototypes more efficient, ultimately leading to lower entry costs for manufacturers (Ewart et al., 2019). Not only does it increase competitiveness in the market but also compresses the concept-to-clinical time, making new medical solutions available to patients and clinicians promptly. Apart from that, 3D design plays a priceless role in health when it comes to personalized medicine and patient-centered care. Using 3D modeling to simulate and model the development of disease, care providers are better positioned to personalize treatment choices according to individual patient needs. This proactive intervention enables providers to engage in shared decision-making with their patients, leading to better health results and increased patient satisfaction. Three-dimensional printing, fused deposition modeling, and stereolithography are at the forefront of this advancement, with each having distinctive capabilities that improve the fabrication of sensitive biomedical devices. The development of smart bandages and digital theranostics, for instance, is indicative of how 3D design can be employed in the preemption of patient health monitoring and management. Thus, the future of health care is increasingly reliant on the union of technology and artistry offered by 3D design, essentially bridging gaps in current medical procedures.

4.6.3. Call to Action for Further Research and Development

The rapidity of 3D design and modeling technology development for biomedical devices presents both great opportunities and severe challenges that call for additional research and development. As 3D printing has grown from producing simple prototype models to facilitating the production of sophisticated biomedical devices, there is an immediate need for focused research into material selection and engineering processes. The prospect of producing patient-specific implants and scaffolding for tissue regeneration is especially promising, but technological limitations such as the precision of microarchitectures and material compatibility with the biological system must be addressed. As in recent literature has been suggested, significant improvements in a number of printing technologies like Stereolithography and Fused Deposition Modeling have been made to overcome such hurdles but there is a necessity for more research to further enhance the efficiency and reproducibility of these biomedical solutions (Chia et al., 2015). Moreover, interdisciplinary collaboration involving engineering, material science, and biomedical research is an urgent necessity. The convergence with advances in neuroscience, particularly in brain-computer interfaces (BCIs), will most probably enhance the effectiveness of 3D-printed technology in human health improvement. With the application of knowledge gained from BCIs, researchers can develop neurotechnological devices that do not only improve the function of prosthetics but also extend the capability of 3D-printed biomedical implants. This integrative approach is required to bridge the gap between technology advancement and practical use, expanding the reach of 3D modelling and design to therapeutic and diagnostic intervention (Kerick et al., 2012). A collaborative strategy for knowledge and resource exchange between sectors can stimulate advancements addressing the complexity of human-system interaction. Finally, societal pressure for 3D printing application in customized medicine calls for increased emphasis on new biomedical technology regulatory channels and ethical concerns. As 3D-printed devices increasingly invade clinical settings, it is critical for investigators and developers to get together with policymakers to guarantee that innovation is not only in compliance with safety requirements but also with ethical requirements. This dialogue can provide a setting where research and development can further proceed without jeopardizing patient well-being. By placing very high value on such collaboration with regulating organizations, biomedical and engineering communities can ensure that 3D designs not only fulfill technical specifications but also end up meeting patients' needs. A concerted effort across the board towards the creation of integrated frameworks will ultimately enhance the impact of such revolutionary technologies on health care.

REFERENCES

1. Afridi, F., Alaoui, C. H., Chigr, M., Fatimi, A., et al. (2024). Recent progress in hydrogel-based bioinks for 3D bioprinting: A patent landscape analysis and technology updates. https://core.ac.uk/download/620924710.pdf (accessed on 14th October 2025).
2. Ahmad, A. S., Ahmar, A. S., Asmuni, A., Hishamudin, H., et al. (2018). Iris segmentation. https://core.ac.uk/download/19162806.pdf (accessed on 14th October 2025).
3. Al Kuwaiti, A., Nazer, K., Alreedy, A. H., AlShehri, S. D., Almuhanna, A., Subbarayalu, A. V., Al Muhanna, D., et al. (2023). A review of the role of artificial intelligence in healthcare. *Journal of Personalized Medicine, 13*, 951–951. https://doi.org/10.3390/jpm13060951 (accessed on 14th October 2025).
4. Aloba, C. O. (2025). Organ-on-a-chip in regenerative medicine: Advancing tissue repair and personalized therapies. *International Journal of Research Publication and Reviews*. https://www.semanticscholar.org/paper/3e7c984e8aea2df8e66a8a0f2a3d33a7bf55bd42 (accessed on 14th October 2025).
5. Andreu-Perez, J., Ip, H., Leff, D., Yang, G. Z., et al. (2015). From wearable sensors to smart implants–towards pervasive and personalized healthcare.
6. Annemans, L., Gemmel, P., Tack, P., Victor, J., et al. (2016). 3D-printing techniques in a medical setting: A systematic literature review. https://core.ac.uk/download/84043719.pdf (accessed on 14th October 2025).
7. Anwar, M., Cohen, B. E., Najafiaghdam, H., Papageorgiou, E., et al. (2019). A 25 micron-thin microscope for imaging upconverting nanoparticles with NIR-I and NIR-II illumination. https://core.ac.uk/download/287623956.pdf (accessed on 14th October 2025).
8. Barcena, A. J. R., Dhal, K., Kundu, S., Patel, D., et al. (2023). Current biomedical applications of 3D-printed hydrogels. https://core.ac.uk/download/619413273.pdf (accessed on 14th October 2025).
9. Berger, M. S., Chang, S. M., Crane, J. C., Elkhaled, A., et al. (2017). Metabolic profiling of IDH mutation and malignant progression in infiltrating glioma. https://core.ac.uk/download/323074384.pdf (accessed on 14th October 2025).
10. Bramanti, E., Campolongo, F., Cervino, G., Cicciù, M., ct al. (2018). FEM and Von Mises analysis of OSSTEM® dental implant structural components: Evaluation of different direction dynamic loads. https://core.ac.uk/download/188826859.pdf (accessed on 14th October 2025).

11. Carpio Huertas, J., Claramunt Alonso, R., Díaz Lantada, A., Jiménez Fernández, A., et al. (2016). CDIO experiences in biomedical engineering: Preparing Spanish students for the future of medicine and medical device technology. https://core.ac.uk/download/148688486.pdf (accessed on 14th October 2025).

12. Chia, H. N., & Wu, B. M. (2015). Recent advances in 3D printing of biomaterials. https://core.ac.uk/download/323078409.pdf (accessed on 14th October 2025).

13. Cho, H., Jammalamadaka, U., & Tappa, K. (2018). Nanogels for pharmaceutical and biomedical applications and their fabrication using 3D printing technologies. https://core.ac.uk/download/212859248.pdf (accessed on 14th October 2025).

14. Cippitelli, E., Fioranelli, F., Gambi, E., Spinsante, S., et al. (2017). Radar and RGB-depth sensors for fall detection: A review. https://core.ac.uk/download/80842153.pdf (accessed on 14th October 2025).

15. Das, N., & Yip, M. (2017). Robot autonomy for surgery. http://arxiv.org/abs/1707.03080 (accessed on 14th October 2025).

16. Datta, S., Barua, R., & Prasad, A. (2023). Additive manufacturing for the development of artificial organs. https://doi.org/10.1002/9781394166985.ch16 (accessed on 14th October 2025).

17. Dehghanghadikolaei, A., Emamian, S. S., Fotovvati, B., Gisario, A., et al. (2019). The potential of additive manufacturing in the smart factory industrial 4.0: A review. https://core.ac.uk/download/231748826.pdf (accessed on 14th October 2025).

18. Ewart, P. (2019). A comparison of processing techniques for producing prototype injection molding inserts. https://core.ac.uk/download/322841895.pdf (accessed on 14th October 2025).

19. Feinstein, J. A., LaDisa, J. F., & Taylor, C. A. (2010). Aortic coarctation: Recent developments in experimental and computational methods to assess treatments for this simple condition. https://core.ac.uk/download/213079154.pdf (accessed on 14th October 2025).

20. Goldberg, J. R., & Malassigné, P. (2016). Lessons learned from a 10-year collaboration between engineering and industrial design students in capstone design projects. https://core.ac.uk/download/213084681.pdf (accessed on 14th October 2025).

21. Jeddi, I., & Saiz, L. (2017). Three-dimensional modeling of single stranded DNA hairpins for aptamer-based biosensors. https://core.ac.uk/download/323070928.pdf (accessed on 14th October 2025).

22. Kalová, M., Kubíček, J., Oczka, D., Tomanec, F., et al. (2019). Recent trends, technical concepts and components of computer-assisted orthopedic surgery systems: A comprehensive review. https://core.ac.uk/download/287649034.pdf (accessed on 14th October 2025).
23. Kerick, S. E., Lance, B. J., McDowell, K., Oie, K. S., et al. (2012). Brain computer interface technologies in the coming decades. http://arxiv.org/abs/1211.0886 (accessed on 14th October 2025).
24. Kim, Y., & Zhao, X. (2022). Magnetic soft materials and robots. *Chemical Reviews, 122*, 5317–5364. https://doi.org/10.1021/acs.chemrev.1c00481 (accessed on 14th October 2025).
25. Luo, Y., Abidian, M. R., Ahn, J. H., Akinwande, D., Andrews, A. M., Antonietti, M., Bao, Z., et al. (2023). Technology roadmap for flexible sensors. *ACS Nano, 17*, 5211–5295. https://doi.org/10.1021/acsnano.2c12606 (accessed on 14th October 2025).
26. Manohar, R., & Moradi, S. (2018). The impact of on-chip communication on memory technologies for neuromorphic systems. http://arxiv.org/abs/1809.06016 (accessed on 14th October 2025).
27. Mathur, V., Gadre, M., Amrutha, H. K., & Vasanthan, K. S. (2025). A micro physiological systems approach to design gastrointestinal system. *Journal of Biomaterials Science. Polymer Edition*. https://www.semanticscholar.org/paper/3f4f13026ad4202540e1260539f9a0edea4b4c99 (accessed on 14th October 2025).
28. N/A. (2013). *The Boston University Photonics Center Annual Report 2013–2014*. https://open.bu.edu/bitstream/2144/29752/1/Photonics-Center-Final-Annual-Report-2013-2014-v2.pdf (accessed on 14th October 2025).
29. Oliver, R., Tillotson, J., & Toomey, A. (2009). Bioengineered textiles and nonwovens–the convergence of bio-miniaturization and electroactive conductive polymers for assistive healthcare, portable power and design-led wearable technology. https://core.ac.uk/download/9587153.pdf (accessed on 14th October 2025).
30. Pakhaliuk, V., Poliakov, A., & Popov, V. L. (2020). Current trends in improving of artificial joints design and technologies for their arthroplasty. https://core.ac.uk/download/322793610.pdf (accessed on 14th October 2025).
31. Reddy, M. S. B., Ponnamma, D., Choudhary, R., & Sadasivuni, K. K. (2021). A comparative review of natural and synthetic biopolymer composite scaffolds. *Polymers, 13*, 1105–1105. https://doi.org/10.3390/polym13071105 (accessed on 14th October 2025).

32. Spranger, K., & Ventikos, Y. (2014). Which spring is the best? Comparison of methods for virtual stenting. https://core.ac.uk/download/29413340.pdf (accessed on 14th October 2025).

33. Tottoli, E. M., Dorati, R., Genta, I., Chiesa, E., Pisani, S., & Conti, B. (2020). Skin wound healing process and new emerging technologies for skin wound care and regeneration. *Pharmaceutics, 12*, 735–735. https://doi.org/10.3390/pharmaceutics12080735 (accessed on 14th October 2025).

34. Vander Sloten, J., Lam, K., Le, C., Le, L., et al. (2010). Medical reverse engineering applications and methods. https://core.ac.uk/download/42389848.pdf (accessed on 14th October 2025).

35. Yanto, D. T. P., Novaliendry, D., Saragih, F. M., Febrianti, N., Saputra, R. F. Y., Rahiman, W. M. Y., et al. (2024). Development of a digital twin prototype for industrial manufacturing monitoring system using IoT and augmented reality. https://core.ac.uk/download/616998179.pdf (accessed on 14th October 2025).

CHAPTER 5

TISSUE ENGINEERING AND BIOPRINTING

Contents

INTRODUCTION

The synergy between bioprinting and tissue engineering is perhaps one of the most groundbreaking innovations in the medical world, with the potential to provide answers to restore or replace damaged tissues and organs. Tissue engineering integrates biological and engineering principles to create functional tissue substitutes for biological structure, while bioprinting entails the use of advanced printing techniques to build defined tissue constructs in three dimensions. This groundbreaking method allows researchers to replicate the complexities of human tissue, architecturally and in cell organization. With organ failure and tissue injury on the rise, it has become most important to discover ways to produce useful bioengineered tissue. With 3D bioprinting's inherent advantages, scientists are capable of identifying novel pathways for therapeutic applications and creating scaffolds that can ultimately lead to the regeneration of functional organs and improved patient outcomes. The key to 3D bioprinting is the careful selection and development of the bioinks used, which need to closely mimic the native ECM in order to support cell survival, proliferation, and differentiation. Advancement in various bioink materials that are biocompatible and are able to mimic cellular milieus has significantly enhanced the versatility of bioprinting. Advanced technology, such as co-axial wet-spinning extrusion, has become a promising technique that enables the generation of cellularized hydrogel fibers for tissue constructs. This technique not only improves printing resolution and accuracy in shape but also allows for the bioink properties to be separated from the printing process, thus simplifying the development of bioinks. These developments are a significant milestone towards closing the current gaps and expanding the diversity of the tissue types that can be successfully engineered (Barbetta et al., 2019). Furthermore, the application of pluripotent stem cells, such as human embryonic and induced pluripotent stem cells, holds great promise in the application of bioprinting. These cells provide a pluripotent platform for the development of heterogeneous cell types needed for complex tissue structures, including hepatic, cardiac, and vascular tissues. Researchers have increasingly employed this method to mimic the heterogeneity of cells and cytoarchitecture present in native tissues. By exploring the potential of differentiation and functional integration of these stem-derived cells in tissue models, the field stands at the precipice for huge advances. However, challenges do exist, particularly in bioprinting more complex cell types like neurons, which consist of overcoming issues with respect to cell survival and functional assessment (Rosa et al., 2019). With continuing progress, bioprinting and tissue engineering stand to radically transform regenerative medicine, paving the way for the fabrication of completely functional organ substitutes.

Definition of Tissue Engineering

Tissue engineering is an interdisciplinary field that combines biology, materials science, medicine, and engineering in an attempt to regenerate or replace damaged tissues and organs. The complexity of biological systems demands close understanding of cellular action and interaction in a biocompatible matrix. Essentially, tissue engineering aims at creating living tissue constructs by combining cells, biomaterials, and growth factors to stimulate tissue regeneration.

There have also been significant advances in the manufacture of biomaterials that closely mimic the extracellular matrix, allowing for the enhancement of cell adhesion, proliferation, and differentiation. This sophisticated blend of materials and living cells serves as the foundation for new methodologies, where the potential uses of tissue engineering in the treatment of disease and injury are underscored. During the last few years, bioprinting has been a core technology of tissue engineering where cells and biomaterials can be deposited layer by layer with great control.

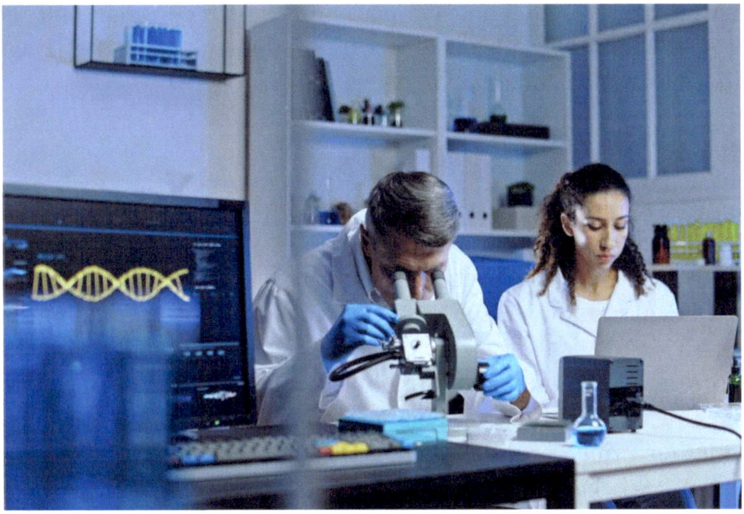

Figure 5.1. Tissue engineering emerges as an interdisciplinary field that converges biology, materials science, engineering, and medicine to regenerate or replace damaged tissues and organs.

Source: https://thelifesciencesmagazine.com/wp-content/uploads/2024/02/1.1-How-do-tissue-engineering-and-regenerative-medicine-work-Image-by-Synthetic-Exposition-from-Getty-Images.jpg.

Automated systems when implemented in bioprinting enable complex three-dimensional configurations to be fabricated that can emulate native tissue microenvironments. Utilization of biocompatible materials as bioinks is most essential in order to facilitate imparting desired physiological functions to printed structures. As observed in more recent studies, methods such as co-axial wet-spinning extrusion exhibit promising development in printing resolution and shape fidelity, enhancing the ability to fabricate heterogeneous multi-materials with the capability to approximate native tissue behavior, with potential for regenerative medicine and transplantation applications (Barbetta et al., 2019). Besides, integration of stem cell technology with tissue engineering has provided new opportunities for the field, particularly through use of human embryonic and induced pluripotent stem cells. The cells possess a remarkable capability of differentiating into various forms of specialized cells necessary for designing functional tissues. Recent reports demonstrate the potential for utilizing differentiated stem cells as the building blocks of bioprinted models of complex organs like hepatic and cardiac tissues (Rosa et al., 2019). These advances capture the lofty hopes of tissue engineering: to replicate not only the architecture but the intricate cellular dynamics and vascular networks present in human tissue. By combining the possibilities of bioprinting and stem cell technology, the future of tissue engineering is brighter, with broad potential for personalized medicine and organ regeneration (Figure 5.1).

Overview of Bioprinting Technology

Bioprinting technology innovations are unfolding to revolutionary uses in tissue engineering and regenerative medicine. The new technique allows for high-precision deposition of the bioinks, living cells and biomaterials, into intricate tissue architectures. Among the most crucial aspects of bioprinting is bioink selection, as rheological properties and gelation mechanisms directly affect the print process and function of the printed construct. Among the stimulating approaches in this field is co-axial wet-spinning extrusion, which enhances high-resolution print capability while ensuring shape fidelity. The method separates bioink behavior from print precision, hence expanding the range of bioink formulations at one's disposal for successful application to bioprinting, eventually resulting in the creation of more advanced, heterogeneous tissue constructs mimicking native physiological environments (Barbetta et al., 2019). The multidisciplinary nature of bioprinting goes beyond tissue constructs to the creation of personal biomedical devices, an essential aspect of personal medicine. Three-dimensional (3D) printing found early applications in surgical modeling and scaffolding, but current advancements now make it possible to produce complex biomedical devices adapted to a patient's specific requirements. As patient-specific anatomical information are integrated in the design, bioprinting facilitates the production of individualized implants, scaffolds, and even drug-delivery systems. Furthermore, the combination of stem cells with 3D scaffolds expands the possibilities of personalized regenerative therapy, which is increasingly needed to address the issue of complex tissue regeneration. Nevertheless, along with the promising developments, some severe issues still linger regarding regeneration of complex tissues and organs, which require further research and technological advancement to overcome current barriers in biofabrication processes (Chia et al., 2015). Looking into the future, the market of bioprinting is ready to experience significant growth as ongoing research manages to overcome its current limitations and unveil newer prospects. New materials and techniques are being designed continuously, which enhance the range of applications in tissue engineering. For instance, there may be advancements in the biocompatibility and properties of bioinks towards better integration with host tissue for superior overall results. Furthermore, as researchers explore the creation of vascular and innervated tissue constructs, the realistic modeling of organ microarchitecture is becoming more feasible. Co-axial bioprinting systems are demonstrated in research to have a hopeful line of approach to circumvent certain of these limitations by encouraging diverse multi-material and multicellular constructs that are more representative of native tissues. With maturing technology, it is crucial to develop a deeper understanding in these technologies in order to utilize their advantage to improve regenerative medicine and provide functional tissue solutions to the clinic (Barbetta et al., 2019) (Figure 5.2).

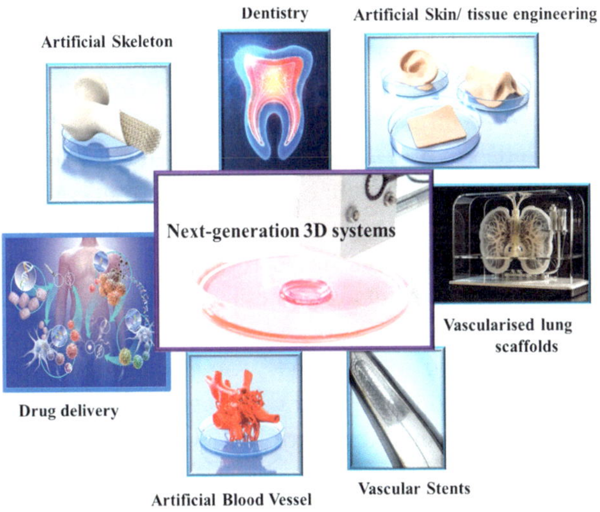

Figure 5.2. With the integration of patient-specific anatomical data into the design process, bioprinting facilitates the generation of unique implants, scaffolds, and even drug delivery systems.

Source: https://www.tandfonline.com/action/showGraphicalAbstractImage?doi=10.1080%2F10667857.2025.2530639&id=ymte_a_2530639_uf0001_oc.jpg.

Importance of the Field in Modern Medicine

The field of tissue engineering and bioprinting holds a significant role in modern medicine, overcoming substantial deficiencies of traditional forms of treatment. In accordance with conventional therapies, such treatments normally are not able to completely cure complex health issues, such as organ failure or severe tissue damage. Tissue engineering makes an appearance as a groundbreaking method that not only tries to reestablish function in damaged or ill tissue but also devises innovative ways of creating biological substitutes tailored to suit every patient's requirement. For instance, the advancement of bioprinting allows for precise layering of cells and biomaterials, ultimately creating functional tissues that can mimic natural shapes. This customized strategy improves outcomes for patients through the provision of tailored therapies, thereby supporting the fundamental position of tissue engineering in contemporary healthcare application. Beyond structural replacement, the significance of tissue engineering goes to address the limitations of organ transplant availability, as it can quite profoundly influence regenerative medicine. The latter aims to repair or regenerate human organs, tissues, and cells, thereby providing the potential to transcend the boundaries of organ transplant availability. With biocompatible materials and advanced scaffolding processes, researchers can engineer environments to foster cellular growth and activity. It is by synthesizing composite materials with different properties that they need to be used because a single material would be incapable of fulfilling the broad spectrum of mechanical and biological needs for proper tissue integration, indicative of the complexity of today's medical problems (Geyter et al., 2009). These technologies have the promise of revolutionizing treatment procedures, creating opportunities for previously impossible therapeutic approaches in ailments like cardiovascular disease or spinal cord damage. In addition, developments in processing techniques for low-cost insert molding fabrication, as reported in recent studies, reflect ongoing interest in improving tissue engineering application (Ewart et al., 2019). This achievement promises that the bioprinted organs and tissues could be manufactured at low costs, a necessity for mass clinical application. The integration of both additive and subtractive manufacturing processes together enables the transference of complex tissue geometries into products for marketability in response to the varied demands for medical application. With the advancing technology, emphasis on material optimization, biocompatibility, and manufacturing efficiency speaks volumes of deep respect for the requirements of contemporary medicine. While creating and propelling forward both the methodologies and the technologies, tissue engineering and bioprinting are going to remain at the frontline of medical innovation, initiating a new age in paradigms of treatment.

5.1. HISTORICAL BACKGROUND

The history of tissue engineering dates back to where biology and engineering converged and the fundamental concepts of regenerative medicine began to take shape. During the latter half of the 20th century, researchers started conceptualizing the idea of integrating living cells with synthetic materials to create functional tissue constructs. It was a significant shift from traditional organ transplant procedures to new approaches toward addressing the growing organ shortage issue. Early experiments primarily consisted of the application of three-dimensional scaffolds that would serve as a basis for cell development, ultimately giving rise to innovation that established the foundation of modern approaches in tissue engineering and bioprinting.

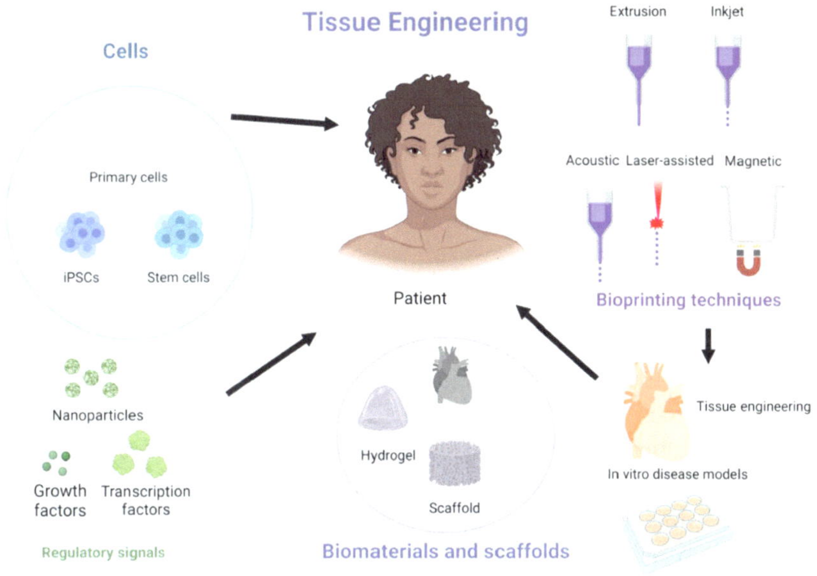

Figure 5.3. Early experiments primarily involved the use of three-dimensional scaffolds to support cell growth, ultimately fostering advancements that paved the way for modern techniques in bioprinting and tissue engineering.

Source: https://media.springernature.com/lw1200/springer-static/image/art%3A10.1007%2Fs43939-025-00286-8/MediaObjects/43939_2025_286_Fig3_HTML.png.

As technology developed, a sophisticated appreciation of material science and cellular biology was required to develop effective tissue engineering products. Breakthrough studies by visionary scientists revealed basic parameters that influence cellular behavior, such as biochemical cues and mechanical properties of scaffolds. This refined understanding encouraged interdisciplinary interaction, which resulted in new approaches to building complex tissue architecture. In innovation, moves like the Centennial Challenges initiated by NASA were a testament to a greater commitment to technological advancement, driving public investment and interest in allied areas of tissue engineering, including materials and structures, and applications in nanotechnology (Brewer et al., 2025). The transition to bioprinting itself was a consequence of these advancements, moving the frame of tissue engineering. Using 3D printing technologies, researchers were able to precisely produce biomimetic structures that closely resembled native tissues. This innovation was not simply technological but was also a paradigm shift in the way regenerative therapies can be created and used. As technology progressed, the use of additive and subtractive processes for manufacturing picked up popularity, enabling fast prototyping of complex tissues and organs. Research on various processing methods emphasized quality control and functional outcomes, indicating the potential of bioprinting to revolutionize therapeutic strategies and overcome the limitations of traditional transplantation (Ewart et al., 2019) (Figure 5.3).

5.1.1. Early Developments in Tissue Engineering

The advent of tissue engineering, as a discipline that stood at the intersection of biology, engineering, and materials science, was as early as the initial 1990s. It represented a landmark milestone in regenerative medicine, fueled by greater understanding of the need for artificial scaffolds that had the ability to effectively restore or replace damaged tissues. The initial work was on the premise of using natural biomaterials and scaffolds that would guide cellular development. Researchers began to explore the potential of synthetic polymers and biocompatible materials to develop the foundation upon which future progress would be achieved. This foundation paved the way for an explosion of research to discover cellular interactions in engineered environments, a distinguishing characteristic that would define the function of tissue. These early developments not only highlighted the importance of material selection but also underscored the importance of having engineering principles congenially merged with knowledge of biology. Advances in the early stages of tissue engineering led to the creation of crude models that aimed at replicating the function and form of the original tissues. In particular, researchers focused on creating scaffolds that would allow cell proliferation and adhesion. Such scaffolds were intended to replicate the extracellular matrix, which provides important structural cues related to cellular behavior. The arrival of biocompatible hydrogels during this time made them significant since they could be physically soft enough to confine living cells and therefore provide a more dynamic and responsive environment for tissue growth. Hydrogels are ideal materials since they mimic the naturally occurring extracellular matrices, which provide better nutrient retention and higher cell migration. The discovery of these materials represents a major step towards the development of more sophisticated and functional tissue constructs, thus progressing considerably in the field. Concurrent with these technological developments, the appreciation of the limitations inherent in conventional surgical approaches underpinned the need for novel solutions towards tissue regeneration. Surgical procedures tended to be insufficient in restoring or replacing damaged tissues effectively and thereby pointing to an important lack of medical treatment alternatives. As a result, regenerative medicine began picking up steam as researchers searched for options that could meet the growing demands of transplants and tissue repair. The discovery of 3D bioprinting became a revolutionary tactic at this early phase by offering unparalleled accuracy in the construction of scaffolds. This process made the actual inclusion of cells and biological cues in printing directly, thereby allowing for enhanced complexity and function of engineered tissues. Not just did 3D bioprinting open up new avenues for producing viable tissue constructs but also pave the way for other innovations that are central to patient-specific tissue engineering solutions (Birchall et al., 2016) (Figure 5.4).

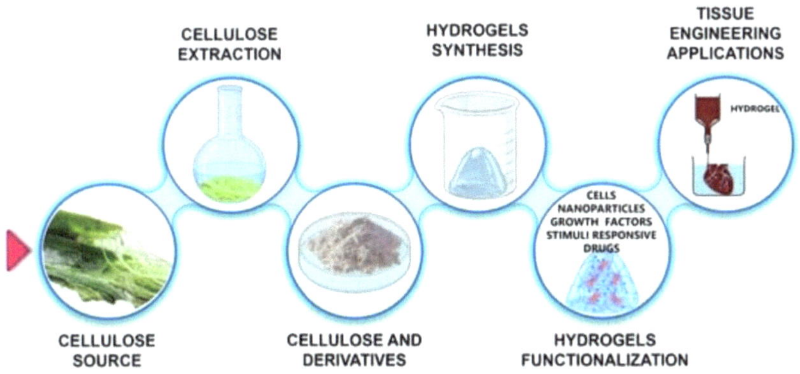

Figure 5.4. Hydrogels are ideal materials due to their similarity to naturally occurring extracellular matrices, which enhances nutrient retention and promotes cell migration.

Source: https://pub.mdpi-res.com/gels/gels-11-00438/article_deploy/html/images/gels-11-00438-ag-550.jpg?1749783907.

5.1.2. Milestones in Bioprinting Technology

The evolution of bioprinting technology has been marked by milestones that transformed the landscape of tissue engineering. Early progress entailed creating seed technologies for initiating printing methods, like inkjet and laser-guided bioprinting. These technologies enabled controlled deposition of living cells into ordered patterns, leading to more complex tissue models. As the scientists developed these methods, specific focus was laid on the development of biomaterials that resembled human tissue properties and therefore enhanced biocompatibility. Innovation in the advancements of three-dimensional (3D) bioprinting techniques has led to the development of intricate cell-holding biomaterial structures, leading to the establishment of tissue grafts and organs with possible regenerative medicine applications (Plana et al., 2017). One of the first advances in bioprinting technology is the employment of decellularized extracellular matrix (dECM) scaffolds. As a source material for dECM, human donor organs have been used to create scaffolds with highly native-like characteristics. Such scaffolds are capable of being seeded with many different cell types and provide a promising route for recellularization with human pluripotent stem cells (hPSCs). The ability to effectively repopulate dECM scaffolds with appropriate cell sources is crucial, as it allows for the production of autologous grafts that can be transplanted into patients with minimal risk of rejection (Plana et al., 2017). This multi-scale approach is an enhancement in bioprinting technology, as it marries the principles of tissue engineering and the stem cell regenerative properties. Furthermore, the inclusion of competition-based innovation models, such as the Centennial Challenges (CC) program by NASA, has significantly promoted innovation in bioprinting technologies. This program, designed to engage external innovators, has promoted a platform where diverse approaches to solutions can thrive. By incentivizing the competitors to fill important technological gaps within competitions, the CC program has encouraged the development of novel bioprinting materials and solutions, as witnessed in various fields of technology related to bioprinting, including materials and structures. With the progress of the field, these achievements highlight the importance of interdisciplinary and greater appreciation for bioprinting as a critical component of the future of regenerative medicine and organ production.

5.1.3. Key Figures and Their Contributions

On the field of tissue engineering and bioprinting, there have been many influential figures who have made a great contribution to the development of the fields and application of advanced technology. Among the trendsetters, one can isolate the activity of researchers who have focused on the development of three-dimensional (3D) models of the skin. For instance, the transformation from simple skin biopsies to intricate vascularized organotypic full-thickness skin equivalents represents an important advance in biofabrication. These developments not only improved *in vitro* tissue culture methods but have also aimed at achieving physiological relevance in reconstructed skin models. Difficulty is still present, however, as more complex structures like glands and sensory components are still in the process of research, proving that research and investment must continue to be made on this rapidly growing field (Jüngel et al., 2018). One of the most important names in tissue engineering and bioprinting is that of the advocate of additive manufacturing technologies, which have revolutionized tissue printing and fabricating processes. The shift from rapid prototyping to industrial manufacturing processes provides evidence of a major turn to production processes, enabling the fabrication of complex biological structures. With the growing trend of 3D printing, exploring its potential disruptiveness in mainstream manufacturing processes becomes increasingly critical day by day.

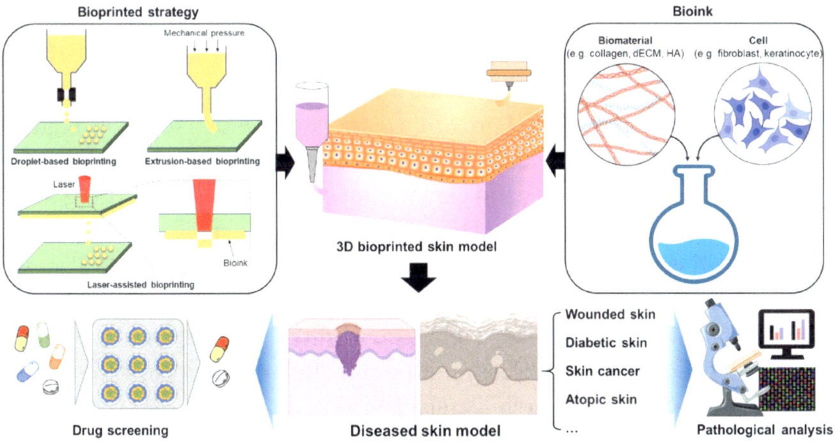

Figure 5.5. The transition from simple skin biopsies to sophisticated vascularized organotypic full-thickness skin equivalents marks a notable advancement in bio-fabrication.

Source: https://spj.science.org/cms/10.1186/s40824-023-00415-5/asset/b0db57c7-df36-4217-90fc-b0edd185bc3f/assets/graphic/s40824-023-00415-5.fig.003.png.

The input flexibility and efficiency of this input technology not only facilitate tissue construct development but also its application in a variety of industries, including healthcare. Analyses of the dynamics of the market for 3D printing and a description of its condition circumstances enable players to adjust better to tissue engineering's changing environment so as to maintain its growth and uptake into medical care (Bechthold et al., 2015). Finally, the collaboration between scientists, doctors, and policymakers also plays a key role in maximally utilizing the potential of tissue engineering and bioprinting technologies. Researchers, entrepreneurs, and policymakers have joined hands to develop frameworks that promote innovation while surmounting ethical and regulatory challenges. Their ideology is to encourage advances in bioprinting techniques that will potentially form functional tissue for treatment. With this collaborative work in progress, the potential to engineer tissues as a way to create personalized medicine forges ahead. In the process, all inputs here not only enhance scientific knowledge but also impact patient care and treatment strategies, and in doing so, illustrate the long-term significance of collaboration in the scientific endeavor of enhancing human health (Bechthold et al., 2015; Jüngel et al., 2018) (Figure 5.5).

5.2. FUNDAMENTAL PRINCIPLES OF TISSUE ENGINEERING

The tools of tissue engineering are three primary elements: scaffolds, cells, and signaling molecules. Scaffolds provide the structural skeleton that supports cell attachment, migration, and growth, mimicking the extracellular matrix of native tissue. Scaffolds may be composed of various materials including natural polymers, synthetic polymers, and ceramics and are selected according to their biocompatibility and mechanics. The architecture of such scaffolds is critical, as it must facilitate diffusion of nutrients and removal of waste while also being mechanical in nature to provide mechanical integrity for tissue regeneration. Upon seeding with appropriate cells, the ability of the scaffold to induce tissue repair efficiently increases, promoting cellular functionalization toward restoration of native tissue architecture and function. Cells, the second pillar of tissue engineering, are derived from various sources, i.e., primary tissues, cell lines, and pluripotent stem cells. Pluripotent stem cells, such as human embryonic stem cells (hESCs) and induced pluripotent stem cells (hiPSCs), are of particular interest due to their potential to differentiate into many specialized cell types. These cells can be incorporated in bioprinting techniques, which lead to the production of advanced 3D tissue constructs exhibiting enhanced cellular diversity and organization of native tissues. Recent developments in techniques of bioprinting have demonstrated that microstructure and porosity of the scaffold have a significant influence on cell behavior, including migration, differentiation, and survival. Hence, cell-scaffold interaction plays a crucial role in the development of successful tissue-engineer strategies. Finally, signaling molecules are in charge of regulating cell function and behavior in engineered constructs. Growth factors, cytokines, and hormones are some of the examples of these molecules, which can regulate various cellular activities, such as differentiation, proliferation, and extracellular matrix synthesis. Spatial positioning and controlled release of these molecules in the scaffold are required to guide the regeneration process. In hybrid bioprinting advancements, growth factors can be blended with scaffold materials to enhance the chondrogenic differentiation of stem cells, with more precise tissue formation, as evidenced by more recent studies with higher glycosaminoglycan (GAG) and collagen production in differentiated chondrogenic constructs through judicious modulation of hydrogel attributes (Asadian et al., 2020). Where cell dynamics, biomaterials, and biochemical cues meet is the complexity of tissue engineering with its potential to revolutionize regenerative medicine procedures (Rosa et al., 2019).

5.2.1. Cell Sourcing and Types of Cells Used

In bioprinting and tissue engineering, cell sourcing is a make-or-break element for regenerative therapies. Cells of various types can be employed, ranging from autologous cells of the patient, allogeneic cells from donors, and stem cells with the capacity to differentiate into multiple cell lineages. Autologous cells are the most frequent because they reduce the risk of immunogenicity, but availability and quality of cells may be a problem. Allogeneic cells provide a broader selection but may necessitate the administration of immunosuppressive treatments to prevent rejection. Besides, the finding of induced pluripotent stem cells (iPSCs) has revolutionized tissue engineering as they can be derived from somatic cells and can exhibit pluripotent characteristics, expanding the scope of available cells to be employed in order to produce tissues in bioprinting technologies. Tissue engineering cells are largely dependent on the tissue that needs to be regenerated. For instance, mesenchymal stem cells (MSCs) are well recognized for their ability to differentiate into many cell types including osteoblasts, chondrocytes, and adipocytes, and thus are best suited for bone and cartilage engineering. Endothelial cells also play a role in vascularization, a significant aspect of any engineered tissue to ensure proper nutrient supply and waste removal. Integration of the cell types into bioprinting platforms is central to printing functional tissues that mimic the native microenvironment. Integration of such heterogeneous cell types allows for the recapitulation of the complex architecture and function required for tissues, although challenges remain in achieving maximum cell viability and function post-printing. Recent developments in bioprinting technology have also highlighted the significance of not just choosing the right cells but also making use of those complex scaffolding materials that enable cellular attachment and growth. Scaffolds with different porosity, stiffness, and surface properties can play a critical role in affecting cell behavior such as proliferation and differentiation. The best scaffold should be able to give structural support, enable diffusion of nutrients, and permit tissue ingrowth and hence necessitate a custom approach for each application. For example, in tracheal prostheses development, scaffolds must be biocompatible and exposed to mechanical stress while promoting epithelial cell growth to prevent complications and infection (Birchall et al., 2016). With ongoing research, combinations of synthetic and natural biomaterials and various cell types are expected to produce clinically relevant tissue constructs. The multi-disciplinary approach will tackle the key unmet clinical needs for effective regenerative therapies (Martins et al., 2014) (Figure 5.6).

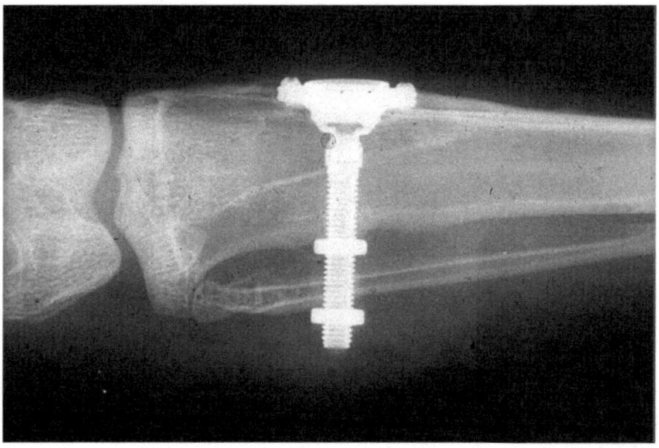

Figure 5.6. The advent of induced pluripotent stem cells (iPSCs) has revolutionized tissue engineering, as they can be generated from somatic cells and exhibit pluripotent characteristics, expanding the potential cell repertoire for crafting tissues in bioprinting applications.

Source: https://upload.wikimedia.org/wikipedia/commons/4/47/Branemark's_initial_radiograph.jpg.

5.2.2. Biomaterials and Their Properties

The production of biomaterials is also a basic procedure in tissue engineering and bioprinting, as the biomaterials give scaffolds to support cell adhesion, growth, and differentiation. The biomaterials must possess certain properties, such as biocompatibility, bioactivity, and biodegradability, to facilitate easy interaction with living tissues. Biocompatibility is the cause of ensuring that the materials will not initiate any negative reactions from the hosts immune system, whereas bioactivity refers to how well the biomaterials can intermingle with surrounding tissues and provoke cellular responses that are essential for tissue regeneration. Moreover, biodegradability is crucial as it will allow the scaffold to degrade progressively and be replaced by the body tissue so that surgery will be minimized. With the increased demand for such complex and functional tissue constructs, studies also continue to focus on developing improved biomaterials that fulfill such vital demands. The inclusion of 3D printing technologies has revolutionized the way biomaterials are addressed in tissue engineering, and it currently enables one to manufacture tailor-made scaffolds for a patient's individual anatomical needs. This degree of personalization is particularly clear in the creation of implants and tissue constructs that are closely analogous in structure and composition to native tissue. Various 3D printing techniques, such as Fused Deposition Modeling and Stereolithography, offer a high level of control over the architecture of the scaffolds, which contributes to their mechanical performance and triggers cell infiltration and vascularization. In addition, incorporating bioactive molecules and growth factors in these biomaterials can further boost their functionality by directing tissue development and supporting healing processes. Such synergy between biomaterials and state-of-the-art manufacturing technology paves the way for new applications in regenerative medicine, culminating finally in better patient outcomes. Recent advances in bioprinting demonstrate the potential for incorporating stem cells with biomaterials to create intricate tissue structures that mimic human tissues. Utilizing human embryonic stem cells (hESCs) and induced pluripotent stem cells (hiPSCs) as bioink facilitates the differentiation of various cell types needed for tissue development, hence improving the complexity of the constructs from bioprinting. With the ability to replicate cellular diversity and cytoarchitecture of real tissues, bioprinting stands to overcome challenges in engineering functional organs for transplant and repair. However, as noted, further research must be conducted to overcome current shortcomings, namely in the bioprinting of more specialized cell types such as neurons. Reversing these technical challenges not only expands the possible applications of bioprinting but also significantly contributes to further advancement of the tissue engineering sector (Chia et al., 2015; Rosa et al., 2019).

5.2.3. Scaffolding Techniques and their Significance

With the new field of tissue engineering and bioprinting, scaffolding techniques are essential to provide structural support for cell growth and proliferation. The scaffolds are designed to mimic native extracellular matrix so that cells can attach, grow, and differentiate effectively. Their significance lies in their ability to create three-dimensional (3D) niches that closely mimic the native tissue, thus facilitating more realistic *in vitro* models. With varied biomaterials—ranging from natural polymers to hydrogels that are synthetically produced—researchers have the ability to tailor the characteristics of scaffolds such as porosity, biodegradability, and mechanical strength to meet particular tissue engineering requirements. Such tailoring is important because it not only affects cellular behavior but also the success of bioprinting processes in constructing functional tissues and organs. Moreover, the development of scaffolding techniques is greatly influenced by the need to have better models in virology, particularly for the study of viral infections. Traditional models do not work because they cannot replicate human tissue complexity. For example, techniques used from tissue engineering enable scientists to develop scaffolds that better match the *in vivo* environment, greatly making it easier to study hepatotropic viruses and other viruses. The capacity of scaffolding to marry complexity of biological process with ease of use operates to transcend the limitations of existing viral models.

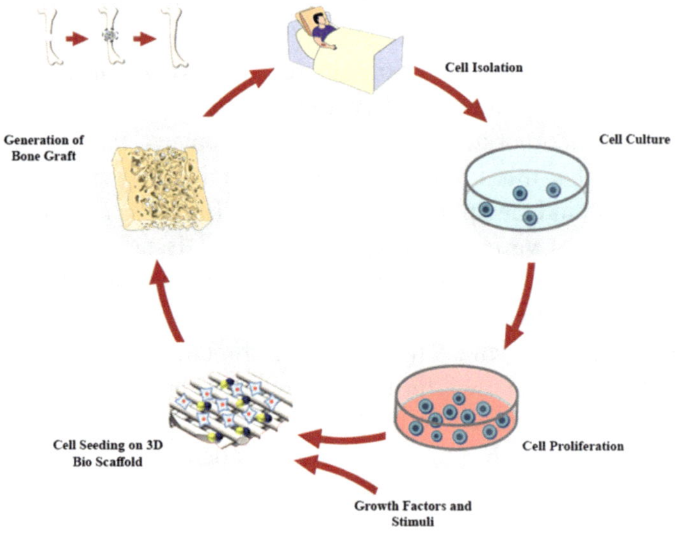

Figure 5.7. The potential of scaffolding to integrate biological complexity with ease-of-use aids in overcoming the limitations of existing viral models.

Source: https://media.springernature.com/lw1200/springer-static/image/art%3A10.1186%2Fs13036-021-00282-5/MediaObjects/13036_2021_282_Fig3_HTML.png.

Not only do such new approaches generate new mechanistic understanding of virus-host interactions, but they also enable the design of therapeutic interventions that can be interrogated in a more biologically relevant context than existing models allow for, as discussed by Bhatia et al. (2014). In addition to improving models of viral infection research, scaffolding techniques have implications on cultured meat production through bioprinting techniques. The growing interest in alternative sources of protein is complemented by the utilization of 3D bioprinting to create constructs that replicate the texture and structure of meat. The ability to fabricate scaffolds on which muscle cell growth and viability occur is central in the formation of cultured meat products that retain the sensory qualities of meat. However, problems remain in the printability and biocompatibility of the material being used, such as seen in the complexity of edibility and biocompatibility (Zanderigo et al., 2022). Solving these issues through creative design of scaffolds can facilitate scaling and optimization of cultured meat production, thus contributing significantly to sustainable food provision and low environmental impact (Figure 5.7).

5.3. BIOPRINTING TECHNIQUES

The arrival of bioprinting technologies has transformed tissue engineering by providing the potential for printing complex biological structures that mimic natural tissues. With three-dimensional (3D) printing technologies, bioprinting allows for the controlled printing of bioinks that consist of living cells and biocompatible materials. This aspect is crucial in generating constructs with well-defined architectures that can attain functionality *in vivo*. Notably, various bioprinting methods, e.g., Fused Deposition Modeling and Stereolithography, possess individual strengths depending on the purpose. These technologies have improved vastly, surpassing previous constraints inherent in traditional tissue engineering, e.g., the reproducibility of tissue architectures and custom-fit according to patient-specific needs (Chia et al., 2015). As such, bioprinting not only enhances the capability to regenerate tissues but also the potential for personalized medicine through the capacity to generate bespoke solutions that may be designed to match individual patient anatomies. In bioprinting, arguably one of the most intriguing avenues of research is the utilization of pluripotent stem cells, such as human embryonic stem cells (hESCs) and induced pluripotent stem cells (hiPSCs), as simple building blocks. The application of these stem cells enables the bioprinting of numerous cell types, thus reconstructing the intricate cellular populations within natural tissues. The novelty of this idea has been brought about by recent studies, which have created bioprinted constructs with the characteristics of hepatic, cardiac, and vascular tissue, testifying to the variability and potential of bioprinting for regenerative medicine (Rosa et al., 2019). These developments not only emphasize the likelihood of functional tissue regeneration but also indicate the ongoing research necessary to optimize cell behaviors within printed environments, ultimately enhancing the viability and efficiency of engineered tissues. Despite the dramatic progress developed in bioprinting techniques, there remain several challenges that exclude their universal application in clinic settings. Critical challenges include creating proper bioinks that are able to maintain cell viability and function, as well as the creation of vascularization within printed tissue constructs. Adequate perfusion is critical to tissue survivability, particularly as sizes increase where diffusion limitations of nutrients and waste products pose a problem. Finally, regulatory challenges towards the clinical translation of bioprinted tissue demand strict validation and testing processes (Chia et al., 2015). As the researchers continue to innovate on both the bioprinting methods and materials science, addressing such issues will become crucial towards advancing the field of tissue engineering and making the full potential of bioprinted organs a reality for therapeutic applications.

5.3.1. Inkjet Bioprinting

Inkjet bioprinting is an advanced tissue engineering technique that enables precise deposition of biomaterials to construct three-dimensional tissue models that are similar to human tissues. It employs a specialized inkjet printer that extrudes bioink comprising living cells and biocompatible elements in a layer-by-layer fashion. High-resolution construct fabrication is possible in this approach, which is critical in precisely reconstructing tissue structure and function. Besides, inkjet bioprinting is particularly preferred for its ability to produce detailed geometry and patterns required in tissue scaffolding. With advancing research, the innovative method is on the cusp of transcending current limits in producing viable tissues for drug screening and regenerative medicine, suggesting profound implications for individualized solutions in healthcare (Chia et al., 2015). The use of stem cells in inkjet bioprinting enhances the ability to generate customized tissue constructs. By employing human embryonic stem cells (hESCs) and induced pluripotent stem cells (hiPSCs), researchers have the ability to develop bioinks that mimic the cellular composition of human tissues. Early studies have shown promising results whereby structures printed using these stem cells are capable of mimicking key tissue characteristics, such as cytoarchitecture and cellular heterogeneity. This technology not only facilitates the generation of tissues such as cartilage and blood vessels but also opens up opportunities for the generation of more complex organ models, required for disease modeling and drug screening. But preserving cell function and viability following printing remains a challenge that calls for further research into materials and techniques able to tolerate robust stem cell activity in engineered tissue (Rosa et al., 2019). While significant advancements have been achieved in inkjet bioprinting, several technical challenges need to be addressed in order to realize the full potential of the technique for tissue engineering. Issues such as the need for optimal bioink formulation that can provide cell viability during printing and the necessity for sophisticated bioprinting systems with sustained cell viability are key constraints. Moreover, the applicability of inkjet bioprinting to produce more complex and larger tissues continues to be explored. Future studies aim to advance this technology further through the development of new strategies that enhance material properties and facilitate the integration of vascular networks in bioprinted tissues. Addressing these problems will be essential to advancing inkjet bioprinted constructs from the laboratory setting into the clinic, thereby paving the way for regenerative medicine and tailored therapy treatments (Chia et al., 2015) (Figure 5.8).

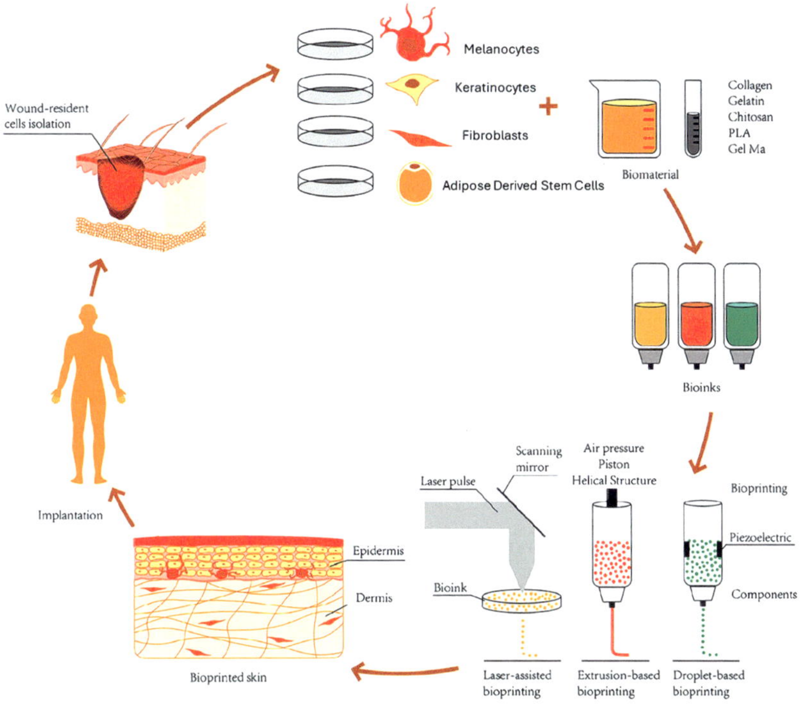

Figure 5.8. Inkjet bioprinting represents a significant advancement in the field of tissue engineering, facilitating the precise deposition of biomaterials to create three-dimensional structures mimicking human tissues.

Source: https://www.mdpi.com/bioengineering/bioengineering-11-00777/article_deploy/html/images/bioengineering-11-00777-g001.png.

5.3.2. Extrusion-Based Bioprinting

Of tissue engineering and bioprinting, extrusion-based bioprinting is becoming more widely known as a method whereby controlled deposition of bioinks results in complex tissue structures. The process involves mechanical or pneumatic pressure to extrude thick bioinks out of a nozzle to create three-dimensional constructs. The rheological properties, including viscosity and gelation, of such bioinks also play a crucial role in determining their printability. Remarkably, advancements in the extrusion systems, e.g., co-axial wet-spinning units, have demonstrated enhanced resolution as well as shape integrity, which are factors of significance in replicating the tissue structures. This ability also allows it to easily create new bioinks with precise needs for particular uses, thereby enhancing the versatility and effectiveness of bioprinting techniques in regenerative medicine (Barbetta et al., 2019).

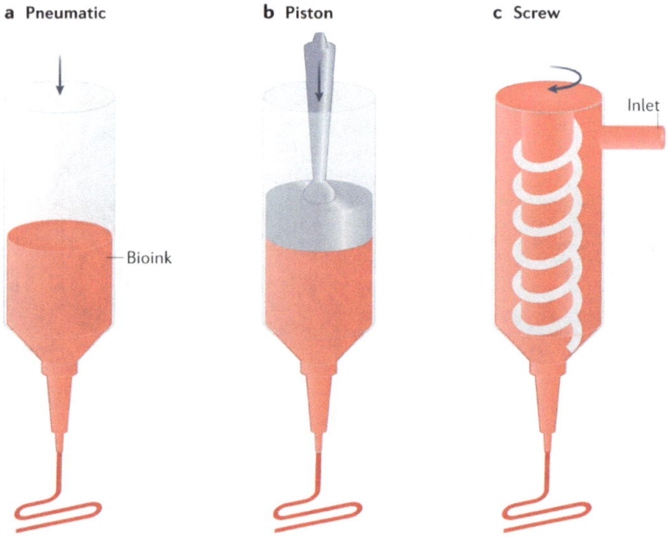

Figure 5.9. Extrusion-based bioprinting has gained prominence as a method that facilitates the precise deposition of bioinks to construct complex tissue structures.

Source: https://media.springernature.com/lw1200/springer-static/image/art%3A10.1038%2Fs43586-021-00073-8/MediaObjects/43586_2021_73_Fig1_HTML.png.

As technology advances in extrusion-based bioprinting, the employment of cellularized hydrogel fibers is at the center of research. Application of human pluripotent stem cell bioinks is a possible route towards the creation of heterogenous multi-material constructs mimicking native tissue. Scientific studies have revealed that such constructs are able to exhibit cellular sophistication and cytoarchitecture of natural tissue, thus pushing the frontiers of 3D models with hepatic, cardiac, and vascular tissue, among others. The incorporation of sophisticated techniques, such as microfluidics into the extrusion platform, allows for control of deposition and flow with accuracy, hence significantly improving the cellular microenvironment during the process of bioprinting. With the continuing progress in technology, applications in the field of complex tissue engineering are significantly enhanced (Rosa et al., 2019). Extrusion-based bioprinting still has to overcome several problems that necessitate further research and development. Remediation of challenges to the mechanical properties of bioinks, such as stress deformation and shape retention after printing, remains crucial. It is also required that knowledge be gained about interactions between various cell types in the bioink in order to achieve functional tissue constructs. These issues will be resolved through an interdisciplinary approach, integrating concepts in materials science, biology, and engineering. Continuing developments in bioprinting technology will eventually enable the production of fully functional, vascularized tissue constructs that will be able to advance regenerative medicine. By breaking past limitations, scientists can pave the way for creating personalized therapeutic solutions and fundamentally understand complex biological systems (Barbetta et al., 2019) (Figure 5.9).

5.3.3. Laser-Assisted Bioprinting

Laser-assisted bioprinting is a sophisticated new field in the science of tissue engineering that employs high-precision techniques to manufacture intricate biological structures with high accuracy. Laser-assisted bioprinting employs focused laser beams to manipulate bioink—biocompatible materials and living cells—to print the cells in intricate patterns resembling natural tissue structure. Compared to traditional printing methods, which may undermine cellular viability, laser-assisted technology has little impact, preserving the function of cells during printing. It is particularly useful in constructing tissue with multiple layers since the precision of the process enables vascular networks vital for nutrient exchange across engineered tissues to be designed. The ability to print such intricate patterns enhances the prospects of integration of healthy tissue upon implantation, a factor that makes it an essential process in the development of next-generation organ substitutes. The laser-guided bioprinting process is profound, particularly when its root causes are contemplated in tissue regeneration in humans. The technique goes beyond cellular deposition; it entails highly advanced layers in the design of scaffolds that can accommodate complex tissue functions. Studies have established that traditional bioprinting techniques may find it difficult to maintain the desired cell viability, while laser-based techniques effectively retain this fundamental aspect, therefore enhancing the engineering of more intricate tissue models. Furthermore, the technology facilitates the construction of multi-material constructs in which the bioinks may be tailored to create heterogeneous environments that closely reflect the physiological biological environments. Accordingly, research indicates that such developments would make it possible to bioprint functional tissues, ranging from cardiac to neural constructs, opening the doors for regenerative medicine and making substantial contributions to the progresses in tissue engineering (Rosa et al., 2019). Along with the potential of laser-assisted bioprinting, there are a number of challenges that lie ahead. The bioink formulation, such as rheological behavior, can critically influence print quality and cell behavior. For instance, both gelation and bioink viscosity optimization are crucial for the achievement of consistent printing resolution and accuracy. Co-axial wet-spinning extrusion has emerged as a potential solution to these problems, allowing improved deposition techniques that enhance print accuracy and simplify bioink design (Barbetta et al., 2019). Solving these issues will not only improve the quality of printed constructs but also pave the way for a higher degree of versatility of bioengineering applications. With researchers continuously improving techniques and exploring novel bioinks, laser-guided bioprinting is extremely prospective for the production of viable and functional tissues that can play a groundbreaking function in clinics (Figure 5.10).

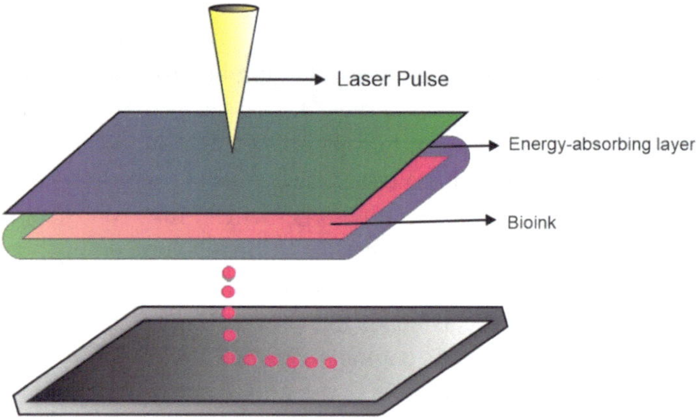

Figure 5.10. Laser-assisted bioprinting represents a sophisticated frontier within the domain of tissue engineering, leveraging high-precision techniques to create complex biological structures with remarkable accuracy.

Source: https://pub.mdpi-res.com/jfb/jfb-13-00214/article_deploy/html/images/jfb-13-00214-g005.png?1667645135.

5.4. APPLICATIONS IN MEDICINE

The advent of tissue engineering and bioprinting has revolutionized the landscape of medicine, particularly in the development of organ and tissue substitutes. With the aid of cutting-edge bioprinting technologies, researchers can print complex three-dimensional structures with structure and function similar to that of human tissues. This capability is particularly valuable in regenerative medicine, where there exists a high demand for organ transplant but scarce donor organs. For instance, tissues can be printed using human embryonic stem cells (hESCs) and induced pluripotent stem cells (hiPSCs) and developed into patient-specific tissues such as hepatic, cardiac, and vascular systems, which are biologically relevant to patient-specific needs. As stated, the development of such tissues has the capability to advance the effectiveness of drug testing and disease modeling, eventually resulting in improved patient outcomes in clinic settings (Rosa et al., 2019). Besides, the ability of bioprinting technologies presents new opportunities in individualized medicine. Tailoring bioinks composed of varied cell types, including differentiated progenies of hESCs and hiPSCs, allows physicians to construct tissues harmonious to a person's specific biological design. This method makes way for more specialized therapy, as patient cells can be used to build functional and anatomically precise tissues, with reduced risk of rejection and complications. Research into methods such as co-axial wet-spinning extrusion further simplified the regulation of bioink properties to respond to the precision with which these constructs can be engineered. The capacity to print heterogeneous, multi-material constructs provides a platform in which engineered tissues are improved in their ability to mimic the physiological behavior of native tissues, overcoming critical problems in regenerative medicine (Barbetta et al., 2019). Beyond organ replacement, bioprinting technologies could transform wound healing and tissue repair. Bioprinted scaffolds, which are densely seeded with bioactive molecules and cells, can be precisely placed at injury sites to aid in healing and rebuild damaged tissue. These emerging scaffolds not only allow for cellular performance but, by engineering, can be made to release drugs as a function of time. These personalized delivery systems allow for more effective healing and reduced risks of infection or complications. Research has already shown that 3D-printed cartilage replacement and skin substitutes obtained by applying bioprinting techniques can significantly improve treatment outcomes and patient recovery times. With further advancement in the technology, joint collaboration will be needed among clinicians, biologists, and engineers to overcome the current bottleneck in bioprinting, thereby making its full potential a reality in clinical translation (Rosa et al., 2019).

5.4.1. Regenerative Medicine and Organ Replacement

The merging of organ replacement and regenerative medicine can revolutionize healthcare, with the most significant advancement expected through tissue engineering innovation and bioprinting. Organ transplantation is severely plagued by limited donors and rejection. Augmenting the scope of regenerative medicine with innovative technologies like 3D bioprinting offers a tool to create functional organ substitutes that bypass such traditional obstacles. For instance, bioprinting methods have the potential to print organs tailored to specific patient needs, essentially removing the dependency on human or animal donors. This technological innovation not only inspires hope in the correction of organ shortages but also fulfills ethical requirements for reducing the need for animal tests and cross-species transplants, as highlighted by Faulkner-Jones et al. (2017). However, the ethical implications of such advancements need careful study and laws to determine the fate of organ replacement therapies. Despite the promise of regenerative medicine, there are many obstacles that prevent engineered organs and tissues from being used.

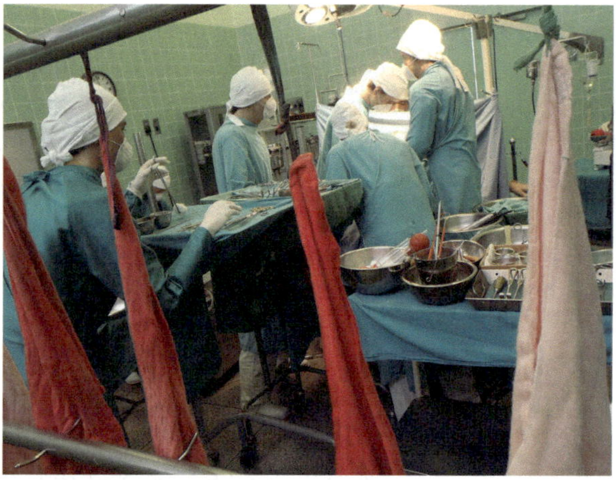

Figure 5.11. Organ transplantation faces significant challenges, including limited donor availability and the risk of rejection.

Source: https://upload.wikimedia.org/wikipedia/commons/thumb/e/e6/Lost_towel_number_15_found.JPG/1200px-Lost_towel_number_15_found.JPG.

The process of human-induced pluripotent stem cells (iPSCs) offers revolutionary tools to combat diseases, but crucial inhibitory factors such as tissue survival, electrical integration, and immune reaction are pointers of concern. The complexity of creating fully viable organs needs not just deep biological understanding but also technical proficiency in the design of 3D scaffolds and bioprinting techniques. Studies highlighted by Abilez et al. (2018) detail these challenges, pointing to the need for new strategies to overcome limitations that slow the realization of mature and scalable solutions. While researchers continue to address such issues, the concept of fusion of interdisciplinary approaches would work to develop effective organ replacements. Organ replacement in the future is closely intertwined with the creation of ethical models to direct regenerative medical treatment. As methodologies such as 3D bioprinting gain prominence, social pressures for access and efficacy of fabricated organs must be managed sensitively. A framework of ethical governance, such as Responsible Research Innovation, is envisioned to solve the problem that advances in tissue engineering do not veer away from ethical standards and public interest. Ongoing debate over the implications of such technologies, as presented by Faulkner-Jones et al. (2017), can help create regulatory systems that center on safety without hindering innovation. The sophisticated challenges of regenerative medicine in the context of organ replacement underscore the necessity to facilitate dialogue among stakeholders, including researchers, ethicists, and patients, to better meet this rapidly evolving environment (Figure 5.11).

5.4.2. Drug Testing and Development

The integration of bioprinting and tissue engineering technologies is revolutionizing the course of drug development and testing. Traditional drug testing methods typically rely on animal models, which are ethically unsound and could also fail to always replicate the human response. Bioprinted tissues provide a more relevant and human-relevant platform to test drugs. Through the creation of three-dimensional cell-based models that mimic *in vivo* environments, researchers are now better able to evaluate the safety and efficacy of medications. Not only is this new paradigm making drug test results more valid but also speeding up the drug development process, thereby bringing the drugs to the market sooner, and reducing the cost of research and development as a whole. With the advancement of the bioprinting field, the selection of appropriate biomaterials is a deciding factor in the effectiveness of drug testing procedures. The biomaterials selected as bioinks—cells that can grow and differentiate—are the foundation for creating functional tissue structures that respond uniformly to drugs. Various materials, such as alginate, collagen, and gelatin, present specific characteristics to the benefit of cellular interaction and tissue growth that are extremely close to meeting individual study objectives. Moreover, developments in bioprinting technique, such as co-axial wet-spinning extrusion, enable the creation of intricate tissue structures that can enhance drug response evaluations (Barbetta et al., 2019). Having the deployed bioinks with the best rheological properties is essential to having high fidelity in tissue architecture, which in turn increases predictive power in drug response *in vitro*. Lastly, the development of useful drug testing platforms utilizing bioprinting and tissue engineering not only fights against the disadvantages of conventional means but also takes on a greener and more ethical approach to research. Enhanced understanding of cell behaviors in bioprinted structures allows researchers to reveal complex drug and target tissue interactions, leading to more personalized therapeutic strategies. Bioprinting flexibility and customization allow the creation of patient-specific tissue models that can revolutionize personalized medicine. Such a message not only sustains a more robust drug pipeline but also emphasizes the potential of bioprinting to transform clinical practice, enabling safer and more effective treatment for future patients (Emanuel et al., 2017).

5.4.3. Personalized Medicine and Patient-Specific Solutions

The process of personalized medicine along with tissue engineering and bioprinting represents a paradigm change in treating patients. By the process of sophisticated bioprinting, clinicians can design patient-specific organs and tissues that possess a more similar simulation of the patient's biological properties. Such a level of personalization reduces the likelihood of organ rejection and improves the likelihood of successful integration with the patient's existing biological systems. For example, use of human organ-derived decellularized extracellular matrix (dECM) scaffolds for application permits a scaffold which not just supports cell growth but also resembles the patient's specific physiological environment. This development underscores the primary importance of personalization in regenerative medicine, demonstrating how technology can be utilized to personalize therapies based on individual needs, thereby augmenting therapeutic efficiency and overall patient outcomes (Plana et al., 2017). 3D bioprinting has also emerged as a primary instrument in generating intricate, patient-specific anatomical models, further advancing the field of personalized medicine. Through the application of patient-specific anatomy, the technology makes it possible to create complicated biomedical devices, scaffolds, and implants that are compatible with the unique biological and structural requirements of each patient. The way toward complete integration of 3D printing into routine clinical practice has already been shown through the creation of personalized implants for bone, cartilage, and a wide variety of other types of tissue. These advances not only open new frontiers for regenerative therapies but also facilitate preoperative planning and personalized diagnostics. The potential for personalized regenerative medicine is vast, given that material and method breakthroughs continue to blaze the trail for patient-specific solutions (Chia et al., 2015). Inclusion of human pluripotent stem cells (hPSCs) within this class of personalized medicine adds further potential in tissue engineering and bioprinting. These hPSCs possess the special ability to differentiate into a variety of cell types and are extremely valuable in recellularizing dECM scaffolds and creating functional tissues that resemble native organs closely. With increasing research on decellularization and recellularization procedures, harmony among hPSCs and 3D bioprinting technologies comes to the fore. The intersection of these fields not only guarantees the future of autologous tissue grafts and tailor-made organs for individual patients but emphasizes the need to overcome existing technological obstacles. This need for innovation is pivotal, as it propels the advancement of personalized medicine, which ultimately leads to effective treatment and improved patients' quality of life (Plana et al., 2017) (Figure 5.12).

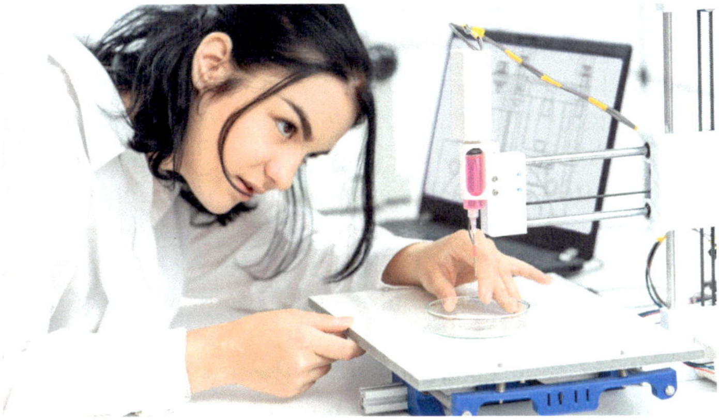

Figure 5.12. By leveraging advanced bioprinting technologies, medical professionals can create patient-specific tissues and organs that more accurately mimic the individuals' biological characteristics.

Source: https://ca-times.brightspotcdn.com/dims4/default/7d1fc46/2147483647/strip/true/crop/2430x1366+0+0/resize/1200x675!/quality/75/?url=https%3A%2F%2Fcalifornia-times-brightspot.s3.amazonaws.com%2F2f%2F75%2F051a7a1f41ce8745bef814d022f8%2F3d-bio-lead.png.

5.5. CHALLENGES AND LIMITATIONS

The field of tissue engineering and bioprinting is full of promise but full of challenges and constraints that keep it from its full realization in therapy. One of the biggest challenges is the inability of bioink materials to closely mimic the native properties of extracellular matrices. Rheological and gelation properties of bioinks have significant effects on printing fidelity but are hard to optimize. Particularly, the preservation of the preferred viscosity without undermining cell viability or biocompatibility remains a thin line that researchers are as yet working to navigate. As literature has touched on, techniques like co-axial wet-spinning extrusion solve problems by decoupling printing precision from bioink properties and simplifying development processes (Barbetta et al., 2019). However, widespread application of such technologies is presently held back by the need for future progress in bioink development and more effective means for the construction of complex structures. In addition to material considerations, the technological limitations of available 3D printing methods effectively constrain their ability to create complex tissue constructs. Even if 3D printing has progressed to produce advanced scaffolds and implants, the development of highly functional tissues with complex 3D microarchitectures remains an even more challenging task. For instance, despite technologies like Stereolithography and Fused Deposition Modeling being promising, they cannot yet succeed in replicating the subtle spatial arrangements and cell-cell interactions of indigenous tissues. Thus, the challenge remains in developing techniques for printing patient-specific designs taking into account the suitability of the scaffolds for cellular incorporation and function (Chia et al., 2015). Progress has been noted, but thorough examination of the limitations of every printing method is essential to further advance the science of tissue engineering to a greater extent. Besides, ethical and regulatory challenges are involved in the creation of bioprinted tissues with further obstacles to translate inventions in the research laboratory to real-world applications. Regulatory agencies require rigorous tests of biocompatibility, mechanical properties, and long-term viability of engineered tissues prior to granting permission to use in humans. Such a sophisticated process is likely to leave large windows between translational research and real-world application, thereby delaying the delivery of potential solutions to patients in need of organ transplantation or new therapies. Moreover, the ethical concerns regarding stem cell application and tissue procurement muddy the waters of how best to move forward with bioprinting responsibly. Though the promise of printing customized tissues is immense for regenerative medicine, balance between innovation and ethical intensity must occur to sustain the credibility and efficacy of this rapidly evolving science. Answers to these multifaceted problems will be crucial to advancing tissue engineering and bioprinting from experimental endeavors to actual clinical applications.

5.5.1. Technical Challenges in Bioprinting

Technical challenges of bioprinting are multifaceted, primarily related to the selection and optimization of bioinks. The properties of bioinks, especially their rheological properties and gelation mechanism, play a major role in determining the success of the bioprinting process. For instance, bioinks must be of appropriate viscosity such that they can easily be extruded while possessing the ability to maintain structure upon deposition. The problem is to reconcile these properties to support precise deposition with minimal loss of cell viability and function. This is compounded by the need to create bioinks that closely mimic the natural extracellular matrix (ECM) because there is a need to offer a suitable microenvironment for cells to thrive in tissue engineering. Hence, researchers are increasingly compelled to explore and develop sophisticated methods, such as co-axial wet-spinning extrusion, which have the capacity to enhance printing resolution and shape retention and overcome the limitations of traditional bioink formulations (Barbetta et al., 2019). Furthermore, the bioprinting method must solve the cellular viability and functionality problem post-printing. After bioprinting, cells must survive the mechanical stress of extrusion and function in the novel tissue.

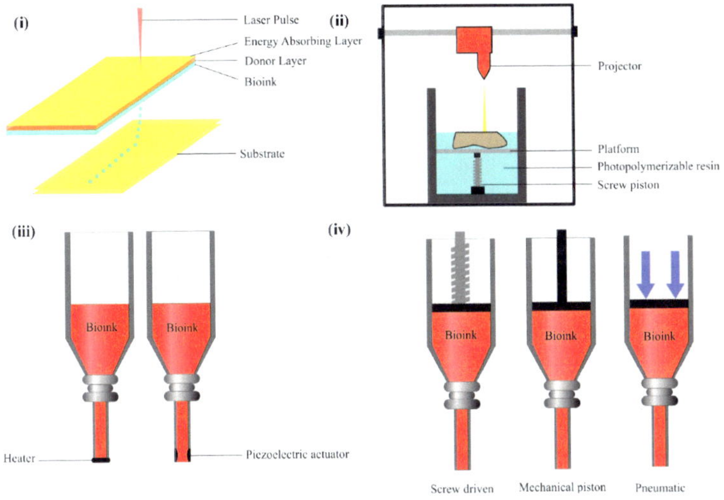

Figure 5.13. The properties of bioinks, especially their rheological characteristics and gelation mechanisms, play a crucial role in determining the success of the bioprinting process.

Source: https://www.mdpi.com/polymers/polymers-17-00917/article_deploy/html/images/polymers-17-00917-g003.png.

This becomes critical for regenerative medicine applications where cell therapies are employed to replace damaged tissues. Recent advances have demonstrated the potential to blend decellularized extracellular matrix (ECM) with human cardiac progenitor cells (hCPCs) to create bioinks that not only exhibit high cell viability but also inducible cardiogenic gene expression (Bejleri et al., 2018). However, uniform cell distribution within the printed construct remains a significant challenge because non-uniform cell distribution can lead to compromised tissue integration and function. Hence, there is a necessity for ongoing research directed at enhancing bioprinting techniques that promote cell viability and foster effective tissue formation. Apart from material characteristics and cellular problems, reproducibility, and scalability of bioprinting are also some of the major challenges. Scale-up from laboratory bioprinting to production demands that there are robust methodologies that replicate high-quality tissue constructs at will. Printer setup variations, environmental conditions, and material variation can lead to inconsistency in the finished product, which can seriously affect clinical use. Moreover, regulatory concerns are additional complicating factors, with bioprinted tissue having to meet strict safety and efficacy tests before it is available for therapeutic application. To address these issues, scientists are currently employing novel next generation bioprinting technologies and integrating artificial intelligence and machine learning to optimize the printing process and predict outcomes to enhance reproducibility and efficiency (Barbetta et al., 2019). With advancements in tissue engineering and bioprinting technologies, addressing these technical issues will be central to realizing the full potential of engineered tissues in the clinic (Figure 5.13).

5.5.2. Ethical Considerations in Tissue Engineering

The field of bioprinting and tissue engineering not just revolutionizes the practice of medicine but also raises grave ethical issues that must be addressed. Among the most serious is the origin of the biological materials used in the process of tissue fabrication. Being that engineered tissue would often take the form of stem cells or other human-derived material, the ethical considerations in terms of consent, procurement, and even commodification of human tissue become highly significant. Such requirements for ethical sourcing are also underscored by the supply gaps between the high demand for tissues and the often-incomplete supply, making it a pressing case for open practice that is donor-conscious. As an example, with the capacity of 3D bioprinting technologies to place cells and scaffold materials with precision, upholding ethical procurement is central to facilitating trust in regenerative medicine as a whole (Birchall et al., 2016). Another moral consideration concerns the regulatory framework of tissue engineering practice, particularly bioprinting. With emerging advancements in 3D bioprinting technology, its compatibility with existing legal frameworks raises safety, efficacy, and regulatory concerns. The regulators must create new mechanisms for adapting to the sophisticated levels of bioprinting capabilities, but not at the expense of compromising on the safety level to protect patients. The emergence of regulations such as the EU Advanced Therapy Medicinal Products (ATMP) Regulation and the Medical Device Regulation (MDR) is an attempt to manage these complexities, yet there is criticism regarding their adequacy (Faulkner et al., 2017). Ethical concerns here include not only compliance with regulations but social effects of technologies advancing at a very fast rate and could possibly surpass existing ethical guidelines and protocols of control. No less compelling is the moral conflict between innovation and access to tissue-engineered solutions. While bioprinting potentially democratizes medicine by allowing for personalized treatment to meet the special needs of individual patients, it may inadvertently widen disparities in healthcare. The price of innovation and implementation of advanced bioprinting technologies will likely be so high that it will only be available for privileged segments of society, leaving the gains from advances in tissue engineering to them alone. Therefore, correcting the equitable distribution of engineered tissues becomes an ethical imperative. Although researchers and practitioners want to innovate, they must consider not just the technological possibility, but also the social implications, so that their innovations benefit the greater good and not exacerbate health care disparities (Birchall et al., 2016).

5.5.3. Regulatory Hurdles and Approval Processes

The shift from the lab innovation process to the clinical utilization process in tissue engineering and bioprinting is disproportionately difficult because of regulatory barriers and the approval process. Regulatory agencies impose strict regulations to ensure safety and efficacy of new biomaterials and products, which is critical because of the intricate nature of human tissue. For instance, long-term safety and stability of tissue-engineered constructs are of utmost concern prior to such constructs being introduced into the clinic. The lack of consensus for best cell sources, scaffolds, and production processes complicates the process of approval. Every one of these factors forces the regulatory agencies to put stringent testing and validation requirements. Thus, this also results in issues in bringing new breakthrough solutions to the market, dampening the possibility of revolutionary medical breakthroughs in reconstructive surgery and other tissue engineering fields (Abbott et al., 2017). Furthermore, the emerging field of additive manufacturing, with top priority within tissue engineering, brings additional regulatory complications. While the developing technologies within 3D printing make them better, the term manufacturing has increasingly more implications of standardization and compliance. Regulatory frameworks lag behind technological advances, creating loopholes that have the potential to disincentivize investment and research collaboration. Regulatory bodies are charged with a duty to incorporate novel modes of work into their existing systems, such as bioprinting technologies that fabricate intricate living tissue structures in a layer-by-layer manner. The process requires an advanced understanding of the technology as well as interdisciplinarity collaboration between engineers, biologists, and regulatory scientists. Therefore, establishing firm guidelines that respect the unique characteristics of bioprinted tissues is critical to facilitating smooth approval and enabling secure clinical use, eventually affecting market dynamics on a greater scale (Bechthold et al., 2015). It becomes increasingly evident for discourse among disciplines with greater complexity in regulatory requirements in tissue engineering. Collaboration between various stakeholders like researchers, clinicians, and regulatory experts is capable of making the approval process easy by starting a rich comprehension of both the scientific and regulatory landscape. For instance, the linking of laboratory findings to clinical relevance in real-time requires all the stakeholders to assist in coordinating research objectives according to regulatory compliance. Such collective effort can open the door to the establishment of standardized procedures that not only ensure efficiency but also enhance faith in the translated versions of tissue-engineered products. Ultimately, addressing these regulatory issues head-on will not only speed up the way towards clinical translation but will also elevate the horizon of tissue engineering and bioprinting as root practices in modern medicine (Abbott et al., 2017).

5.6. FUTURE DIRECTIONS

With the progress of tissue engineering and bioprinting technology, hydrogel-based bioinks have become a key element due to their functional and versatility characteristics. The recent increase in patent applications indicates a vibrant and competitive industry where innovative and new formulations and uses for hydrogel-based structures are being actively pursued. This growth trend signals not just the unveiling of these materials' potential in an array of applications, including regenerative medicine, but outlines the future of bioprinting technology as well. With over an inning of major patent filings since 2018, it is evident that scientists and companies are eagerly committing to developing robust methodologies which can effectively translate laboratory-born innovations into commercially viable solutions. Such work highlights a key trend in the move towards tissue engineering technologies for complex applications and may signal an era when specific patient needs are more easily addressed via personalized regenerative therapies (Afridi et al., 2024). Apart from hydrogels, progress in the field of regenerative dentistry will play a key role in charting the future direction of tissue engineering. The traditional methods of dental restoration are restricted, which the new regenerative processes attempt to overcome, employing recent breakthroughs in material science and stem cell biology. Regenerative dentistry is now planned to regain the function of traumatized dental tissues through novel tissue engineering methods. Specific evaluation of biomaterials, growth factors, and scaffolds has allowed means for improved techniques in dental regeneration. The promise of success in preclinical and clinical trials points toward a necessity for increased utilization of such strategies, and a vision has been sketched where one day the whole-tooth engineering may be possible. The potential for tapping cellular and molecular processes for regeneration possibilities means that the future of tissue engineering is more focused on holistic and personalized patient treatment (Amrollahi et al., 2016). Also, combining the technology of bioprinting with other multidisciplinary fields is likely to yield significant advancements in tissue engineering's future. Through the integration of principles in biochemistry, engineering, and microbiology, researchers are creating complex tissue structures that better mimic the natural environments of human tissue. This multidisciplinary approach fosters groundbreaking methods of developing functional tissue constructs for research and clinical applications. Research on bioprinting in the future will likely focus on enhancing cell-to-extracellular matrix interactions, which are central to enhancing tissue functionality and integration. Researchers by working together and building on what already exists are opening doors to new applications that have the potential to transform healthcare. The advances in tissue engineering and bioprinting have the potential not only to provide enhanced therapeutic interventions but also to replace existing paradigms in medicine and healthcare delivery more broadly (Afridi et al., 2024; Amrollahi et al., 2016).

5.6.1. Innovations in Materials and Technology

The intersection of materials development and technology has been behind the exponentially growing pace in tissue engineering and bioprinting. At the forefront of the growth has been the development of hydrogel-based bioinks, instrumental substances for 3D bioprinting applications. The bioinks are biocompatible and versatile to a high extent, making them capable of printing intricate tissue geometries. Various polymers have been explored to enhance the functionality of bioinks and hence have bred a competitive situation with increased patent submissions. Between 2013 and 2024, there have been 173 published patent reports related to hydrogel-based bioinks, in line with the increasing acceptance of their potential applications for use in regenerative medicine as well as tissue engineering, hence the importance of material formulation innovation in achieving clinically relevant outcomes in bioprinting (Faulkner-Jones et al., 2017). As the technology develops, one finds that technological innovations are central to propelling tissue engineering ability further. 3D bioprinting, in its on-going development, holds revolutionary potential, such as, for example, printing human organs at demand. The technology exists to solve some of the problems organ donation presents, such as ethical dilemmas on live and deceased donors. Though the current level of 3D bioprinting does not yet provide for full organ printing, it has substantial promise for other therapeutic applications, such as the creation of tailored tissues to test drugs and regenerative medicine. The advance of 3D bioprinting technologies demands careful ethical engagement and public debate in order to align its potential with rational realities, ensuring that the developments align with healthcare needs as well as social expectations

(Faulkner-Jones et al., 2017). Also, strategic collaboration among research institutes and industry legends is integral to innovation in tissue engineering and bioprinting technologies. Organovo Inc. and Cellink AB are perfect examples of this collaboration by actively taking part in research and patenting in the area. It allows space for knowledge and skill sharing, eventually speeding innovations from conception to a beneficial application. The broad-based global interest in this area not only highlights the potential of hydrogel-based bioinks but also tracks across a dense tapestry of intellectual property protections and regulatory environments. While stakeholders and researchers both press on with integrating the intricate dance of materials science, technology, and bioethics, potential for revolutionary health solutions remains strong, putting the worth of synergy-driven innovation in tissue engineering front and center (Afridi et al., 2024) (Figure 5.14).

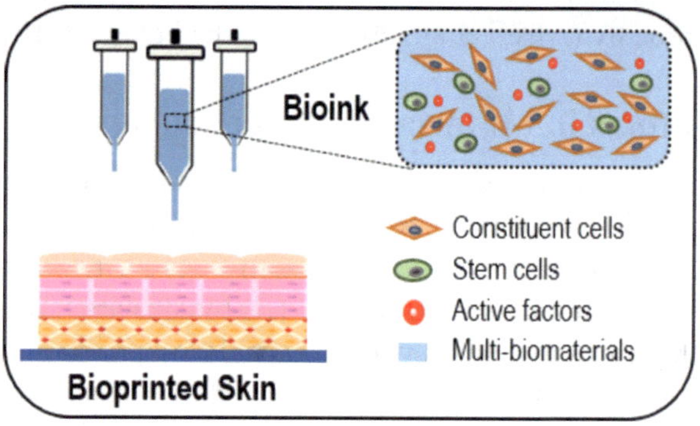

Figure 5.14. Various polymers have been explored to enhance the performance of bioinks, leading to a competitive landscape characterized by a surge in patent activity.

Source: https://pub.mdpi-res.com/polymers/polymers-12-01237/article_deploy/html/images/polymers-12-01237-ag.png?1591151315.

5.6.2. Potential for Integrating AI and Machine Learning

The union of artificial intelligence (AI) and machine learning (ML) with bioprinting and tissue engineering is a visionary leap in the biomedical field. Such technologies involve sophisticated algorithmic functionalities to handle massive datasets, leading to enhanced design and fabrication protocols for bioprinted tissues. For example, AI may be employed for the calibration of parameters of the bioprinting process, such as nozzle temperature, flow rate, and layer thickness, which are critical for the achievement of the desired structural integrity and biological function in engineered tissues. Through the use of machine learning models trained on experimental outcomes, researchers can significantly improve the reproducibility and productivity of the bioprinting processes, which are necessary for clinical applications and regulatory approval. Further, applications of AI and ML are the creation of bioinks that play a crucial part in the efficiency of tissue engineering. Innovations in bioink formulation can take the form of machine learning algorithms that predict printability and cell viability rheological properties. Statistical modeling, for instance, has been employed to determine how variations in bioink composition influence results, such that it is achievable to have more precise and specific ways of developing bioinks. These strategies have been promising in enhancing the performance of complex structures by allowing researchers to maximize properties such as biodegradability and mechanical strength. This intersection of bioink materials and machine learning paves the way towards the development of sophisticated three-dimensional constructs that more closely mimic the biological environment. In addition, predictive modeling of biological response using AI and ML demonstrates profound importance in personalized medicine for tissue engineering. Using past data from various bioprinting studies, machine learning can forecast cellular performance as well as outcome of tissue integration, ultimately guiding the design of tailored treatments. For instance, methods like those that have been recently outlined have demonstrated how such technologies can determine best formulations and processing methods that align with therapeutic objectives. The likelihood of application of AI prediction is guaranteed to provide assurance that bioengineered tissues meet not just the technical specifications but also the biological function needed in patient-specific application. As the field evolves, the marriage of AI and ML is set to enhance both the viability and performance of tissue-engineered products, marking a new dawn for regenerative medicine.

5.6.3. Expanding Applications Beyond Human Medicine

The field of tissue engineering and bioprinting is also rapidly extending from its original focus in human medicine to address a broader range of applications, including veterinary medicine and biological science. This is because there is rising demand for effective solutions to complex biological challenges in animals and the environment. For instance, three-dimensional (3D) bioprinting is under study to produce tissues that will be useful in veterinary surgical procedures and transform animal care. Additionally, possessing the ability to produce tissue models for drug and vaccine testing in non-human organisms can be employed to create species-specific therapies and translate interventions that are effective and ethical. Bioprinting technologies allow for the precise modeling of a wide range of animal tissues, promoting better surgical success and recovery post-surgery, creating synergies between veterinary development and tissue engineering as a whole. In addition, bioprinting has tremendous applications in environmental conservation, presenting an illustrious example of application beyond human-focused initiatives. By creating living systems that can mimic natural processes, researchers can create bioprinted ecosystems that can facilitate the remediation of polluted habitats. Bioprinting can render the process of controlling pollution a whole new experience with the potential to create microorganisms or plant tissues that can remove pollutants or restore ecological balance to devastated ecosystems. Moreover, bioprinting technologies are able to produce bioengineered organisms to enhance food sustainability, address global food security challenges through the creation of tissue in plants with higher yields or nutritional value. Ultimately, this revolutionary technology is bound to make the environment more environmentally resilient in finding sustainable solutions to present-day environmental challenges, ushering in the new field of tissue engineering applications. Finally, increasing application of tissue engineering has significant ethical and regulatory concerns to be addressed so that responsible progress can be guaranteed. With rising advances in bioprinting technology, traditional species boundaries are being challenged and ethical responsibilities towards newly formed organisms are being posed. The potential for creating high-complexity biological systems calls for ethics like Responsible Research Innovation to guide researchers into conducting their work responsibly (Faulkner-Jones et al., 2017). This regulatory caution will enable the examination of bioprinting's promise without inducing adverse effects, like environmental disruption or ethical concern over animal welfare. By addressing these social problems, tissue engineering can establish its credentials and legitimacy, thereby paving the way for penetrating other markets beyond the medical industry. Ultimately, establishing ethical guidelines will be crucial in tapping the full potential of bioprinting to society and the environment.

5.7. CONCLUSION

Finally, the field of tissue engineering and bioprinting is a hopeful medical science field with novel regenerative medicine options. Thanks to advancements in material science, the application of 3D printing technologies has become more and more relevant. Technologies like the synthesis of nanogels, which are of paramount importance to drug delivery and tissue reconstruction, are decent illustrations of the marriage of engineering methodologies and their biological applications. These nanogels, produced using the network of micelles, not only enhance drug delivery but also lead to potential innovations in surgical tools and customized medication. The potential for customized and controlled manufacturing processes makes bioprinting a hub of the future of healthcare. This integration of technology and biology highlights the need for further research in this area to maximize its therapeutic potential (Cho et al., 2018). Moreover, the ethical issues involved with tissue engineering and bioprinting need to be addressed. As 3D bioprinting advances with the capability of producing human organs, issues are posed regarding public expectations, regulatory frameworks, and the socioethical framework of such technology. The possibility of bioprinting living tissues can potentially transform the field of transplantation and reduce the reliance on organ donors. But it is necessary to address this innovation with rigorous ethical examination and sensitivity to its broader social ramifications. Critical discourse of existing literature supports the need for analogous infrastructures as Responsible Research Innovation to steer this new field responsibly. By prior consideration of ethical concerns with accessibility, equity, and potential misuse, the stakeholders can make sense of the complexity of bioprinting and ensure that it derives a positive effect on society (Faulkner-Jones et al., 2017). As this new discipline continues to expand, inter-disciplinary convergence shall play the key role in addressing both the scientific and ethical challenges posed by it. Scientists from bioengineering, medicine, ethics, and policy will have to come together to formulate comprehensive guidelines that not only promote innovation but also safeguard public interest. The rapid rate of advancement in tissue engineering and bioprinting necessitates ongoing debate among scientists, ethicists, and policymakers to ensure that the progress is kept in harmony with values in society and demands of health care. As the debate continues, it will not just define the destiny of regenerative medicine but also mark out the ethical compass of biomedical innovation as a roadmap to sustainable development with a focus on human health and instilling social responsibility in technological progress. The potential benefits are immense, but they will require careful stewardship as the field moves forward.

5.7.1. Summary of Key Points

The intersection of bioprinting and tissue engineering has transformed regenerative medicine as a multidisciplinary answer that aims to overcome the weaknesses of traditional organ transplantation. Of note among developments in the discipline is the application of decellularized extracellular matrix (dECM) scaffolds from human donor organs. These scaffolds provide a natural environment for cellular growth and integration, overcoming the challenge of organ compatibility. Notably, the integration of dECM and hPSCs fosters a healthy recellularization process that lies at the core of generating functional tissues. The importance of these advancements is underpinned by their capacity to generate autologous tissue grafts that translates into optimized outcomes in patient-specific therapies, as well as presenting a novel paradigm in organ engineering in regenerative medicine (Plana et al., 2017). Additionally, three-dimensional (3D) bioprinting offers unparalleled control of tissue architecture and cell placement, allowing biomimetic cell-laden constructs to be fabricated. The technology transcends traditional techniques by providing the ability to reproduce complex tissue structures analogous to native organs. The precision of 3D bioprinting allows researchers to specify the mechanical and biological properties of the constructs in a manner compatible with specific therapeutic needs. Here, the development of bioprinting methods is paramount because it fills the gap between basic tissue scaffolding and the complete production of organ systems, which may solve the pressing problem of organ shortages and organ rejection during transplantations. This new method has a potential to not only produce functional tissues but also organs that can be used for transplantation purposes (Ewart et al., 2019). Overall, the hotspots in tissue engineering and bioprinting show an intensifying trend toward personalized medicine and better patient results. By harmonizing decellularization protocols with new generation bioprinting technology, researchers are opening up new horizons for tissue reconstruction and organ replacement. The ongoing research into different sources of cells as well as bioprinting techniques also reflects the active and ever-evolving nature of the field. With scientists being met with challenges of printed tissue biocompatibility and manufacturing scalability, the quest for successful organ substitutes remains the focus. This intersection of scientific disciplines makes it possible not just to reduce the burden of organ transplantation but also to drive prospective innovation in regenerative methods, ultimately striving to address the needs of patients worldwide (Ewart et al., 2019; Plana et al., 2017).

5.7.2. The Future Impact of Tissue Engineering and Bioprinting

The future of tissue engineering and bioprinting brings about revolutionary developments in regenerative medicine that can revolutionize treatment modalities for a wide variety of medical conditions. Refinement in bioprinting technologies, such as co-axial wet-spinning extrusion, is bound to enhance the production of bioinks and tissue constructs that more closely mimic native tissue function. This strategy not only facilitates higher printing resolution and shape precision but also allows for the generation of multi-material and multicellular heterogeneous constructs that reflect the complexity of human tissues. As highlighted in recent studies, this novel strategy simplifies the design of bioinks via decoupling the printing accuracy from their rheology, thus paving the way for novel tissue constructs that are central to advanced biomedical research and application in customized medicine (Barbetta et al., 2019). As the field advances, hybrid bioprinting is already emerging as a key strategy, notably for the regeneration of complex tissues such as articular cartilage. This approach integrates developmental biology principles with 3D bioprinting, incorporating scaffold-free microtissues to fabricate cohesive macrotissues that replicate the structural and functional properties of cartilage. Human bone marrow-derived mesenchymal stem cell spheroids serve as building blocks, triggering chondrogenic differentiation under specific environmental cues. The ability to culture such spheroids within a photo-crosslinkable hydrogel matrix not only enhances cellular viability but also accelerates the maturation of the extracellular matrix, thereby allowing printed constructs to possess critical phenotypic characteristics necessary for therapeutic functionality (Asadian et al., 2020). Moreover, the implications of these technological advancements extend far beyond cartilage repair to potentially address other degenerative diseases and traumas. With the advancements in bioprinting technologies, focus will more than likely be placed on the optimization of matrix compositions and cellular interactions to realize improved functional outcomes. Future research may likely explore the integration of vascularization into tissue engineering constructs for facilitating greater tissue growth, opening the door for whole organ engineering. Such continued investigation may significantly reduce the need for organ transplantations, enhancing patient prognosis and quality of life through the use of tailored tissue solutions. Thus, the future role of tissue engineering and bioprinting in medicine can be vast with prospects for ushering in a new era where normal tissue regeneration can become a reality (Asadian et al., 2020; Barbetta et al., 2019).

5.7.3. Call to Action for Further Research and Development

The fast-emerging discipline of tissue engineering and bioprinting needs a joint call to action toward enhanced research and development. With its increased maturity, overcoming the existing challenges faced in bioprinting of complex structures is the need of the hour. Combining innovative technologies such as co-axial wet-spinning extrusion has the potential to yield better printing resolution and shape fidelity and facilitates higher versatility in the creation of bioinks. Through focusing on enhancing the properties of bioinks necessary for successful bioprinting, researchers may minimize processes that make the deposition of cellularized constructs complex. In this way, the synergistic approach that integrates cell biology and materials science can significantly promote the creation of functional tissue models that resemble native tissues. The experiences garnered through overcoming these challenges will not only contribute towards the progress of tissue engineering but will also have far-reaching effects on regenerative medicine (Barbetta et al., 2019). Another aspect that needs to be investigated is the use of pluripotent stem cells to bioprinting technologies. Human embryonic stem cells (hESCs) and induced pluripotent stem cells (hiPSCs) are of unparalleled potential as cell-based building materials to produce various types of tissues because they have the ability to differentiate into all human body cell types. The application of the cells in practice in bioprinted structures is accompanied by inherent problems, including ethical considerations and technical complexities of effectively differentiating such cells. Furthermore, the integration of more complicated cell types such as neurons into bioprinter scaffolds is quite an untapped area. Encouraging interdisciplinary research studies that address the nuances of stem cell biology and translate them to tissue engineering will unlock the functionality and utility of bioprinted tissues, thus opening up avenues to tailored regenerative therapies (Rosa et al., 2019). Finally, the intersection of bioprinting technologies and microfluidic systems is a field waiting to be explored. The potential to create heterogeneous multi-material structures with architectures and functional properties similar to those of native tissues can only be achieved by novel ways of merging bioprinting techniques with innovations in microfluidics. The application of the two fields together can provide means to highly sophisticated organ-on-a-chip models that are more realistically representative for biological research and drug screening. Thus, a convergent strategy to resolving these technologies will drive remarkable progress in tissue engineering and bioprinting alike, enabling scientists not only to enhance their experimental models but to generate progressively clinically relevant models for disease and drug response studies. Closing these self-reinforcing challenges will eventually facilitate the maturation of the discipline, allowing the achievement of functional tissue replacements (Barbetta et al., 2019).

REFERENCES

1. Abbott, A., Anderson, J., Asano, M., Atala, A., Baiguera, S., Barnes, C., Berry, D., et al. (2017). Tissue-engineered solutions in plastic and reconstructive surgery: Principles and practice. https://core.ac.uk/download/78862846.pdf (accessed on 14th October 2025).
2. Abilez, O. J., Huang, N. F., Morris, V. B., Nakayama, K. H., et al. (2018). Big bottlenecks in cardiovascular tissue engineering. https://core.ac.uk/download/287623742.pdf (accessed on 14th October 2025).
3. Afridi, F., Alaoui, C. H., Chigr, M., Fatimi, A., et al. (2024). Recent progress in hydrogel-based bioinks for 3D bioprinting: A patent landscape analysis and technology updates. https://core.ac.uk/download/620924710.pdf (accessed on 14th October 2025).
4. Amrollahi, P., Seifi, A., Shah, B., Tayebi, L., et al. (2016). Recent advancements in regenerative dentistry: A review. https://core.ac.uk/download/213080485.pdf (accessed on 14th October 2025).
5. Anwar, A., Barach, B., Bhatla, P., Biglino, G., et al. (2018). 3D printing is a transformative technology in congenital heart disease. https://core.ac.uk/download/212858839.pdf (accessed on 14th October 2025).
6. Asadian, M., De Geyter, N., De Moor, L., Declercq, H., et al. (2020). Hybrid bioprinting of chondrogenically induced human mesenchymal stem cell spheroids. https://core.ac.uk/download/323232718.pdf (accessed on 14th October 2025).
7. Barbetta, A., Colosi, C., Costantini, M., Święszkowski, W., et al. (2019). Co-axial wet-spinning in 3D bioprinting: State of the art and future perspective of microfluidic integration. https://core.ac.uk/download/188825522.pdf (accessed on 14th October 2025).
8. Bechthold, L., Fischer, V., Hainzlmaier, A., Hugenroth, A., et al. (2015). 3D printing: A qualitative assessment of applications, recent trends and the technology's future potential. http://hdl.handle.net/10419/156627 (accessed on 14th October 2025).
9. Bejleri, D., Brown, M. E., Christman, K. L., Davis, M. E., et al. (2018). A bioprinter cardiac patch composed of cardiac-specific extracellular matrix and progenitor cells for heart repair. https://core.ac.uk/download/196295484.pdf (accessed on 14th October 2025).
10. Bhatia, S. N., Ramanan, V., Rice, C. M., Scull, M. A., et al. (2014). New methods in tissue engineering: Improved models for viral infection. https://core.ac.uk/download/78065128.pdf (accessed on 14th October 2025).

11. Birchall, M. A., Bogan, S. L., & Teoh, G. Z. (2016). Tissue engineered airways: A prospects article. https://core.ac.uk/download/79506677.pdf (accessed on 14th October 2025).
12. Brewer, D., Cylar, R., Fiske, M., Herblet, A., et al. (2025). Centennial Challenges Program update: From humanoids to 3D-printing houses on Mars, how the public can advance technologies for NASA and the nation. https://core.ac.uk/download/pdf/161998495.pdf (accessed on 14th October 2025).
13. Campistol Plana, J. M., Fernández Avilés, F., Garreta, E., Montserrat, N., et al. (2017). Tissue engineering by decellularization and 3D bioprinting. https://core.ac.uk/download/83830377.pdf (accessed on 14th October 2025).
14. Chia, H. N., & Wu, B. M. (2015). Recent advances in 3D printing of biomaterials. https://core.ac.uk/download/323078409.pdf (accessed on 14th October 2025).
15. Cho, H., Jammalamadaka, U., & Tappa, K. (2018). Nanogels for pharmaceutical and biomedical applications and their fabrication using 3D printing technologies. https://core.ac.uk/download/212859248.pdf (accessed on 14th October 2025).
16. De Geyter, N., Desmet, T., Dubruel, P., Leys, C., et al. (2009). Nonthermal plasma technology as a versatile strategy for polymeric biomaterials surface modification: A review. https://core.ac.uk/download/55837365.pdf (accessed on 14th October 2025).
17. Emanuel, A., & Ontiveros, F. (2017). Development of a low-cost platform for 3D bioprinting applications. https://core.ac.uk/download/84856783.pdf (accessed on 14th October 2025).
18. Ewart, P. (2019). A comparison of processing techniques for producing prototype injection molding inserts. https://core.ac.uk/download/322841895.pdf (accessed on 14th October 2025).
19. Faulkner, A., & Li, P. (2017). 3D bioprinting regulations: A UK/EU perspective. https://core.ac.uk/download/82914844.pdf (accessed on 14th October 2025).
20. Faulkner-Jones, A., Haddow, G., Seymour, T., Shu, W., et al. (2017). 3D bio prints me: A socioethical view of bioprinting human organs and tissues. https://core.ac.uk/download/80688281.pdf (accessed on 14th October 2025).
21. Jüngel, A., Randall, M. J., Rimann, M., Wuertz-Kozak, K., et al. (2018). Advances in the bio fabrication of 3D skin *in vitro*: Healthy and pathological models. https://core.ac.uk/download/162588741.pdf (accessed on 14th October 2025).

22. Martins, A., Costa, P. F., Endres, S., Jetze, V., Gomes, M. E., Mason, C., et al. (2014). Automating the processing steps for obtaining bone tissue engineered substitutes: From imaging tools to bioreactors. https://core.ac.uk/download/55633366.pdf (accessed on 14th October 2025).
23. Rosa, A., & Salaris, F. (2019). Construction of 3D *in vitro* models by bioprinting human pluripotent stem cells: Challenges and opportunities. https://core.ac.uk/download/231747057.pdf (accessed on 14th October 2025).
24. Wang, J. (2024). Novel 3D bioprinting of biomaterials: Application of statistical modeling & machine learning. https://core.ac.uk/download/603332190.pdf (accessed on 14th October 2025).
25. Zanderigo, G. (2022). Printability assessment of edible bioinks for cultured meat extrusion-based 3D bioprinting. https://core.ac.uk/download/650038392.pdf (accessed on 14th October 2025).

CHAPTER 6

3D PRINTING OF IMPLANTS AND PROSTHETICS

Contents

INTRODUCTION

The rapid rate of technological development has transformed several industries, including medicine, where new ways of caring for patients are ever more required. Of these technologies, the 3D printer has become a critical component in the medical implant and prosthetics industry. Not only does this technology enhance the manufacturing processes of dental and orthopedic implants, but it also changes the way craniofacial reconstruction and prosthetic limb formation is done. As physicians attempt to provide personalized treatment, the adaptability and precision of 3D printing allow for tailored solutions that match individual anatomical needs. The potential for improved patient outcomes through customized implants marks a new era in surgical planning and procedure. This shifting landscape serves to underscore the importance of embracing the interdependence of technological advancement and its impact on medical practice, particularly in terms of safety and efficacy standards set by regulatory bodies. Employing 3D printing technology is not mere fabrication but rather involves sophisticated methodologies that integrate engineering and medical science. As cited in contemporary literature, the use of rapid prototyping techniques has been more forward in medical model preparation, with better implant development and simulation of surgical procedures (Kasturi et al., 2016). This technological intervention enables better preoperative planning since surgeons can visualize each case's anatomy. In addition, the incorporation of 3D-printed prototypes into medical processes contributes to education and training, further solidifying the role of innovation within the medical setting. The research states that a vast number of applications for rapid prototyping in implantology and prosthetics have a significant influence on surgical success through more precision and anatomical detail. These advancements necessitate that medical experts become cognizant of and knowledgeable about these evolving technologies that can potentially redefine the traditional approaches. Secondly, the impact of 3D printing is underscored by studies that explore the effectiveness of combined prosthetic solutions. Researchers have determined that the employment of both fixed and removable prosthetic clements is able to gain greater stability and aesthetic outcomes for patients, minimizing the loading on natural teeth (Lazarova et al., 2018). The hybrid systems demonstrate the potential of 3D printing to facilitate both aesthetic and functional improvements in dentistry, allowing for never-before-seen customization and patient comfort. Additionally, the ability to fabricate removable prostheses highlights the need for hygiene and maintenance in prosthetic construction. These aspects signal a bright future where 3D printing not only helps to bridge the technological divide but also offers creative solutions prioritizing patient requirements and safety. As things develop, ongoing research into these methodologies is required for applications into various clinical situations in the future.

Importance of Implants and Prosthetics in Healthcare

The application of technologies such as 3D printing has revolutionized the method of manufacturing implants and prosthetics, rendering them much more applicable to the medical field. The creation of patient-specific devices that precisely match anatomical structures using 3D printing is among its impressive applications in orthopedic and dental implants. This level of customization enhances fit and function, which may improve patient satisfaction and outcomes. Moreover, such customized implants tend to minimize operation time, as noted in recent research reporting benefits like minimal radiation exposure during the procedure. Therefore, the application of 3D printing technology in the production of orthopedic and dental devices reflects its critical role in modern medicine since it aids in the mission of providing personalized medicine to enhance the efficiency of treatment and the patients' quality of life (Annemans et al., 2016). Moreover, craniofacial reconstruction has become another area where implants and prosthetics play a critical role. The technological progress in 3D printing makes it possible to produce precise anatomical models and surgical guides that can significantly contribute to the planning of complex procedures in reconstructive surgery. These technologies enable the surgeons to practice the operation before the procedure itself, thereby directing important surgical procedures towards fewer complications and improved esthetic outcomes. While their release is also associated with increased expenses to be addressed in terms of the printing process as well as pre-surgery imaging, the potential advantages—e.g., enhanced accuracy in reconstructive surgery—are considerable. The dilemma that persists in this area is how to strike a balance between the economic expenses and the tangible benefits that can be harvested from 3D-printed implants for reconstructive surgery (Annemans et al., 2016). The prosthetics and implant regulatory climate are yet another critical aspect that should not be overlooked. The complexity of approval that is managed by organizations such as the FDA and ISO ensures that the medical devices undergo strict safety and efficacy checks before they can be applied to patients. Such regulation is particularly critical for bio-integrated prosthetics, where mechanical design and biological compatibility are combined. Where technology and patient needs intersect regulatory climates, not only is the priority of safety and efficacy emphasized but also that of additional study to continue to advance implant design and manufacturing techniques. Furthermore, in keeping with emotional and psychological concerns for patients, most especially children who are given prosthetic eyes, catering to the recognition and adaptability of the manufacturing process can further improve user acceptability and overall experience.

6.1. TYPES OF 3D PRINTED IMPLANTS

The progress in implant technology has also ushered in unprecedented breakthroughs in design and production of orthopedic and dental implants through 3D printing. Such sophisticated manufacturing processes offer scope for highly customized implant production, maximizing the harmony of form and function and patient-specific anatomical variations. Orthopedic implants, for instance, can be designed to optimize load-bearing capacity and improve osseointegration, ultimately resulting in more robust healing and long-term stability. Likewise, dental implants also take advantage of custom shapes and surfaces that enhance the speed of bone integration, which results in higher success rates. The application of new materials, such as titanium and bioactive ceramics, further increases the biocompatibility of these implants to which they are more than aptly suited for a wide range of patients with varying degrees of skeletal deficiencies or tooth loss, such as in case studies involving rapid prototyping use in healthcare environments (Kasturi et al., 2016). In craniofacial reconstruction, the potential offered by 3D printing is vast. Custom-made implants which restore the symmetry and function of the face are possible with an accuracy that conventional methods are not able to attain.

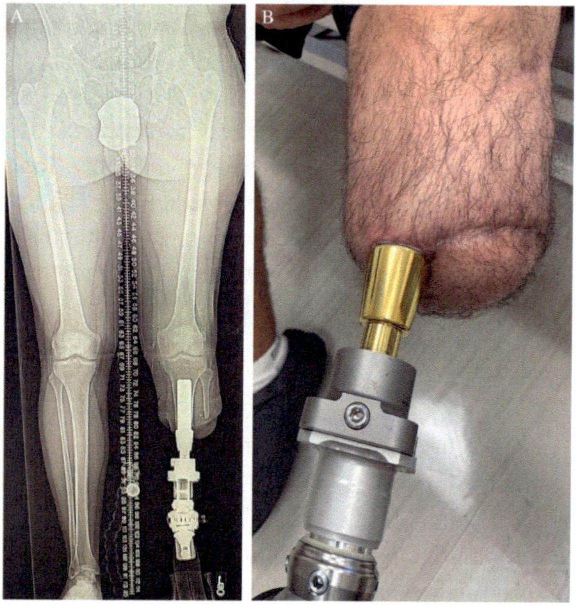

Figure 6.1. Orthopedic implants can be designed to optimize load-bearing capabilities and improve osseointegration, thus enhancing healing and long-term stability.

Source: https://media.springernature.com/lw1200/springer-static/image/art%3A10.1007%2Fs40141-022-00344-9/MediaObjects/40141_2022_344_Fig1_HTML.png.

Through the use of medical imaging data, surgeons create precise models upon which implants are made specifically tailored to fit the patient's own craniofacial structure. Not only do these technologies provide enhanced aesthetic outcomes, but they play a substantial role in enhanced patient comfort and satisfaction. In addition, the degree of customization offered through 3D printing allows for the consideration of biomechanical factors that vary among patients, with a view to having implants enhance successful healing and alignment (Lazarova et al., 2018). This overlap between technology and customization highlights the importance of new fabrication methods for the enhancement of surgical outcomes in craniofacial reconstruction. Prosthetic limbs are the other main application of 3D printing technology, where the shift is done from mechanical to bio-integrated approaches. Prosthetic creation can either be a mechanical approach that focuses on ruggedness or a bio-integrated approach that aims for compatibility with the human body. By 3D printing, prosthetic limbs can be designed to not only the exact measurements of the patient but also to meet their lifestyle requirements, allowing for greater mobility and comfort. Moreover, the capability for rapid prototyping is available for iterative testing as well as real-time feedback loops in alignment with patient input. With growing maturity in the field, control issues, for instance, those exercised by the FDA and ISO, move increasingly center stage, promoting that these new technologies are safe and effective (Kasturi et al., 2016). This careful balance between innovation and regulation is required to build trust and acceptance of 3D printed prosthetic technologies within practitioners and patients alike (Figure 6.1).

6.1.1. Orthopedic Implants

Technological advancements in 3D printing have far transformed the market for orthopedic implants, particularly in terms of enhancing customization and functionality. Orthopedic implants used to be produced in a standardized manner, leading to the disadvantages due to incompatible fit and integration into the patient's anatomy. Through 3D printing, the clinician and engineer can now create patient-specific implants that may be tailored to individual anatomical forms so as to maximize osseointegration—the direct structural and functional interface between implant material and bone, according to recent orthopedic reports. Not only is the mechanical stability of the implants increased by this custom design but also reduced is the risk of ill-advised host reactions. Technologies such as surface modification and bioactive coatings are facilitated by 3D printing that addresses the concerns of aseptic loosening and implant longevity besetting traditional practices, making such next-generation implants a potential solution to achieve optimal orthopedic outcomes (Al-Zeregawe et al., 2025). Integration of artificial intelligence (AI) further optimizes the function of 3D printing for orthopedic implants. By applying AI in design and fabrication phases, orthopedic engineers will be able to optimize the preoperative planning process as well as enhance the accuracy of 3D anatomical modeling. These AI-based systems have the ability to identify minor differences in patients' anatomy and hence a better method of preparing and correcting the complexity of the human body through implant design. Furthermore, robot-assisted surgeries aided by computers with AI power ensure unparalleled precision in implanting such specially designed components, diverging from traditional manual practices towards new-age technology-based procedures. This combination of AI and 3D printing is a revolutionary step forward for orthopedic bioengineering, ensuring improved surgical results and patient satisfaction through fewer complications and the ability to resume work sooner. While the promising applications of 3D print technology to orthopedic implants are of enormous potential, there are regulatory hurdles that must be addressed before such broad clinical application is possible. Regulatory bodies like the FDA and ISO play a fundamental role in ensuring the efficacy and safety of these new devices. The challenge lies in creating standardized validation procedures that are able to properly test the performance and biocompatibility of 3D-printed devices. Second, the uniqueness of bespoke implants raises ethical issues regarding production techniques and patient welfare long-term implications. As the industry evolves, it is paramount that researchers, engineers, and regulatory agencies collaborate, ensuring that innovations in 3D printing technology are not only beneficial but also compliant with safety regulations. This collaboration will ultimately pave the way for broad support of tailored orthopedic technologies as well as unravelling the complications of regulatory frameworks (Al-Zeregawe et al., 2025).

6.1.2. Dental Implants

The use of 3D printing technology in dental implant production is a paradigm shift in the efficiency and effectiveness of dental care. The majority of conventional methods involve lengthy production times and extensive manual labor, and because of this, they become difficult in accuracy and individualization. With the advent of 3D printing, however, dental implants are now produced in a fraction of the time, and with this, quick prototyping and spot treatment patient-specific interventions are achievable. This technology comes particularly handy in making anatomical models that enable enhanced pre-surgical planning to reduce the extent of complexity usually associated with implant placement. Enhanced surgical guides created through 3D printing further enhance accuracy in implantation, eventually leading to enhanced patient satisfaction and outcomes, thereby substantiating findings that show evidence of reduced surgery time and improved medical outcomes (Annemans et al., 2016). Moreover, the capacity to tailor 3D printing renders it particularly better suited to the dental implant process, which often has to be tailored to the individual anatomy of every single patient. Through the utilization of advanced imaging technologies, dental health care providers are able to create highly detailed models that replicate the exact dimensions required for proper implant integration. Such an approach not only enhances the precision of implant fitting but also lessens the risk of complications that might arise due to improperly fitting or improperly placed implants. I

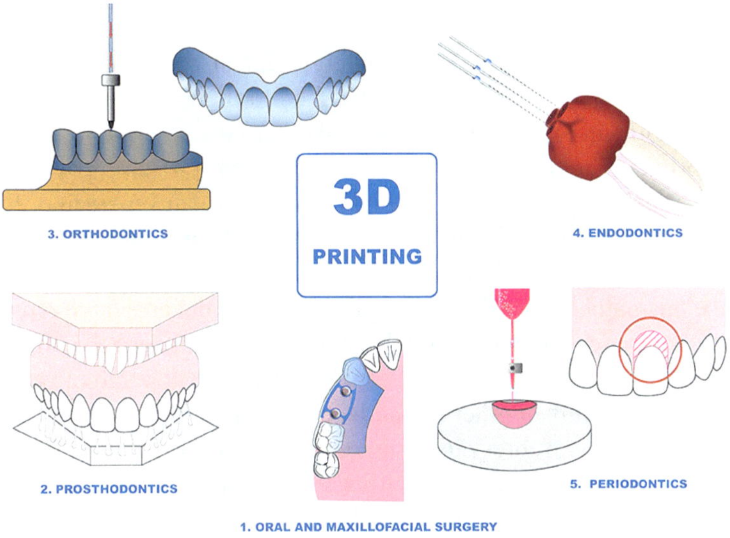

Figure 6.2. With the advent of 3D printing, dental implants can now be produced in a fraction of the time, allowing for rapid prototyping and immediate patient-specific solutions.

Source: https://www.frontiersin.org/files/Articles/420143/fbioe-06-00172-HTML/image_m/fbioe-06-00172-g002.jpg.

n addition, the potential for the development of bio-integrated implants that utilize biocompatible materials contributes to improved osseointegration, offering a smooth integration between the implant and bone tissue of the patient. With advancing technology in 3D printing, its role in dental practice for the future of personalized medicine is increasingly evident (Kasturi et al., 2016). Converting to 3D printing in the dental implant sector is not without its obstacles, however, particularly in terms of regulatory considerations and the expense. While the benefits of reduced surgical times and better outcomes are substantial, 3D printing technology is generally tied with higher upfront costs due to the cost of equipment and integration into digital workflows. This barrier requires more scrutiny into the cost-effectiveness of new technologies since clinicians will have to weigh the financial expense against the clinical value of

3D-printed implants. Further, navigating regulatory systems involves extensive awareness of organizational requirements set by the FDA and ISO to ensure patient safety and product efficacy. Keeping this in view, research has to be continuous to evaluate the long-term viability and acceptability of 3D printing of dental implants (Annemans et al., 2016; Kasturi et al., 2016) (Figure 6.2).

6.1.3. Craniofacial Reconstruction Implants

The process of surgical techniques in craniofacial reconstruction has been transformed by 3D printing technologies. Due to their ability to create highly customized implants, medical professionals can correct complex cranial and facial deformities more precisely. With this new process, patient-specific implants that are very similar to particular anatomy can be created. Research highlights the increasing use of 3D-printed craniofacial implants due to their potential to reduce the duration spent in surgery, improve the success of healing, and reduce mismatched prosthetic complications. Clinical research reports from several studies indicate that not only does 3D printing enhance the effectiveness of the surgical planning process but also improves postoperative recovery by providing a tighter fit than other methods. Hence, the application of 3D-printed craniofacial implants represents a pivotal shift in reconstructive surgery, which requires continued research on its long-term implications and efficacy (Annemans et al., 2016). Moreover, no larger role exists for rapid prototyping within craniofacial reconstruction. As it enables surgeons to create detailed anatomical models, they can better visualize and plan intricate procedures. Rapid prototyping techniques, as they are described in the literature, create individual prosthetic models that are not only aesthetically pleasing but also functional that have a direct impact on patient quality of life. This literature confirms that customized craniofacial prosthetics can effectively restore facial symmetry and enhance overall facial function, which is particularly important in reconstructive application after trauma or oncologic surgery. With the increased use of this technology, it makes it possible for a new model of surgical planning and action, ultimately transforming the way medical practitioners handle complicated craniofacial cases (Kasturi et al., 2016). Problems concerning regulation must be addressed in incorporating 3D-printed craniofacial reconstruction implants into practice. The transition to new manufacturing methods based on advanced technologies necessitates compliance with stringent safety standards established by agencies like the FDA and ISO. Regulatory guidelines are critical in determining the biocompatibility, efficiency, and general safety of 3D-printed implants. The production and approval process involves rigorous testing and validation to determine that such novel products pose no harm to patients. As 3D printing integration advances in the field of craniofacial reconstruction, it is increasingly important to resolve these regulatory challenges to ensure future applications not only enhance surgical outcomes but are also held to the highest quality of safety in patient care (Annemans et al., 2016) (Figure 6.3).

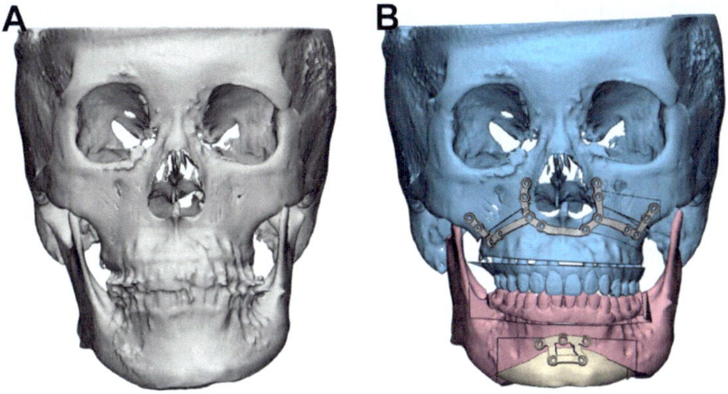

Figure 6.3. With the ability to create highly customizable implants, healthcare professionals can address complex cranial and facial abnormalities with greater precision.

*Source:*https://www.oralmaxsurgery.theclinics.com/cms/10.1016/j.coms.2022.06.004/asset/8128a3c5-da73-478d-9fe6-a8db4da9f573/main.assets/gr7_lrg.jpg.

6.2. PROSTHETIC LIMBS

Advancements in technology have ushered in a revolutionary era for prosthetic limbs, especially through the utilization of 3D printing technology. This new technology is superior because it has the unique capacity to build buildings in layers, and it is thus capable of carrying out intricate designs that are not possible using traditional manufacturing techniques. The flexibility of 3D printing enables the possibility of customized prosthesis for individual patients, enhancing comfort and fit. This customization has profound implications for patients since it can lead to increased functionality and quality of life. As is learned in some research, the application of 3D printing does not end at prosthetics but extends to many various medical situations, such as designing personalized implants that will integrate with the biological structures of the body. These technologies are an imaginary future in which prosthetic engineering is made increasingly integrated with the patient's anatomy and thus individual requirements are fulfilled in a better way. Incorporation of bio-integrated principles in the designing and manufacturing of prosthetic limbs is a developing field in biomedical engineering. By concentrating on osseointegration, which involves direct contact between living bone and implant material, researchers are discovering ways to enhance prosthetic stability and performance substantially. This natural process plays a critical role in delivering the endurance and functionality of both limb prosthetics and joint replacements and therefore provides an arena ready to be explored using 3D-printing technology. Current evaluations highlight the importance of design redesigns and new materials, such as bioactive coatings and titanium alloys, which are central to the efficacy of osseointegrated implants (Al-Zeregawe et al., 2025). With 3D printing allowing for rapid prototyping of such sophisticated features, prosthetic creation replicating natural movement of a limb becomes increasingly possible, providing better rehabilitation results for amputees. Despite the promise of 3D printing in prosthetics, regulatory challenges must be solved so that safety and efficacy are guaranteed. These institutions, the FDA and ISO, have a key role in overseeing approval processes for these new technologies, which often involve rigorous tests and verification to adhere to established safety standards. The shift from traditional techniques to cutting-edge manufacturing presents regulatory hurdles, particularly with patient-specific implants through the application of 3D printing. These regulatory barriers need to be addressed prudently in order to facilitate the introduction of new designs and materials into the clinic. As research fields evolve, there is going to have to be ongoing communication between researchers, clinicians, and regulatory agencies to map the direction of prosthetics so that the developments are turned into gains in practice by patients and healthcare systems alike.

6.2.1. Mechanical Prosthetics

Technological advancements have broad-reaching applications to the face of medical procedures, particularly in the field of prosthetics. As more patients seek alternatives with the capability of enhancing quality of life, mechanical prosthetics have become a vital part of the overall scope of 3D printing for implants and prosthetics. The use of 3D printing technology with mechanical prosthetics enables the use of personalized prosthetics that better fit the physiological needs of the patient, hence increasing functionality and comfort. Additionally, the quick capability to produce items enables iterative design procedures where medical doctors and engineers can collaborate better in producing prosthetic devices. These innovations not only enhance the performance of prosthetics but also resolve the complexities in orthopedic implants and craniofacial reconstruction, which are reflective of a growing trend towards customized medical care that exists in modern practices (Kasturi et al., 2016). The use of mechanical prosthetics is particularly relevant for patients who experience partial edentulism, which typically requires them to have some of their teeth replaced. Traditional substitutes, e.g., fixed partial dentures and removable partial dentures (RPDs), have been extensively utilized; nonetheless, these can be related to disadvantages affecting patient satisfaction. Recent research indicates trends towards improvements in materials and manufacturing technologies that might potentially overcome the disadvantages, offering a closer fit and greater comfort to users. Research indicates there is a significant need to enhance the manufacturing and designing of RPDs to counteract the discomfort associated with current prosthetic devices, including pain, esthetics, and long-term functionality.

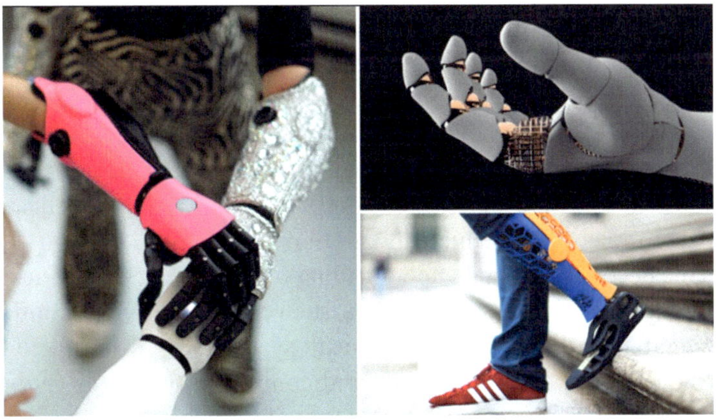

Figure 6.4. As patients increasingly seek solutions that enhance quality of life, mechanical prosthetics have emerged as a pivotal area within the broader domain of 3D printing for implants and prosthetics.

Source: https://www.mdpi.com/applsci/applsci-15-01350/article_deploy/html/images/applsci-15-01350-g006.png.

The innovation is vital because almost 40% of patients stop using their RPDs after five years, representing a critical shortage in prosthetic service that requires extensive attention and innovation (Abt et al., 2017). Regulatory matters are also of importance in the innovation of mechanical prosthetics through 3D printing technologies. Regulatory agencies such as the FDA and ISO play an important role in establishing safety and compliance standards for new materials and designs employed in prosthetics. Ensuring that mechanical prosthetics comply with these standards can have a considerable effect on the timeline of getting new innovations to market, as the intense testing and certification process is important in protecting patient health. In addition, compliance with these standards helps promote the credibility and efficiency of the prosthetics being produced. As researchers and producers work within these regulatory realms, they are frequently faced with the challenge of balancing fast innovation with ensuring adequate testing. Ultimately, coordination between technological innovations, regulatory bodies, and medical professionals will be critical in realizing the full potential of mechanical prosthetics in the broader framework of 3D printing technologies (Kasturi et al., 2016) (Figure 6.4).

6.2.2. Bio-Integrated Prosthetics

The latest development of prosthetics has put bio-integrated solutions at the forefront of orthopedic application, a far cry from traditional mechanical prosthetics. Through the implementation of techniques like 3D printing, which offers total levels of individualization and flexibility, researchers have begun exploring the possibility of combining biological tissue with synthetic material. This approach not only aims to regenerate function but also optimize the body-implant interaction. Unlike the conventional mechanical devices, which are likely to induce immune responses and complications, bio-integrated prosthetics are designed to maximize cellular integration and osseointegration. This shift highlights the necessity of total understanding of processing techniques and bio-material blends for addressing problems such as durability, biocompatibility, and functional behavior in biomechanical systems, as determined through continuous studies on titanium blends and composite structures (Ewart et al., 2019). With the progression of the subject matter, regulatory issues come into limelight, namely approval and standardization of bio-integrated prosthetics. The FDA and ISO regulations have a vital role of ensuring that these new medical devices are safe and effective prior to being made available to patients. Since the complexity in tissue-engineered medical products (TEMPs) is high, the regulatory system must change to accommodate the specificity of such biocomposite technologies. The process of manufacturing bio-integrated implants involves careful testing of manufacturing processes and material, especially where 3D printing is involved, which is constantly evolving. The regulatory standards must consider the newness of 3D printed tissues and their bioactivity, as highlighted in recent discussions on challenges in transforming such products to clinical use without compromising patient safety (Budharaju et al., 2021). Moreover, the application of bio-integrated prosthetics in medical practice is not merely functional progress; it also epitomizes the pursuit of patient-centered design concepts. This approach identifies the diversity in the needs of patients requiring orthopedic and dental implants, craniofacial reconstructive surgery, or prosthetic limbs. The possibility of customized solutions that better mimic the natural function of the limb underscores the necessary convergence of engineering, biology, and patient care. While bio-integrated solutions play catch-up, the nature of multidisciplinary teamwork will become all the more apparent, and thus a coalition of engineers, biologists, and clinicians will be called for. This cooperation will be required in solving the problems of clinical translation and overcoming the ethics of bioengineering so that bio-integrated implants not only meet the technical criteria but also truly improve the quality of life of the users (Figure 6.5).

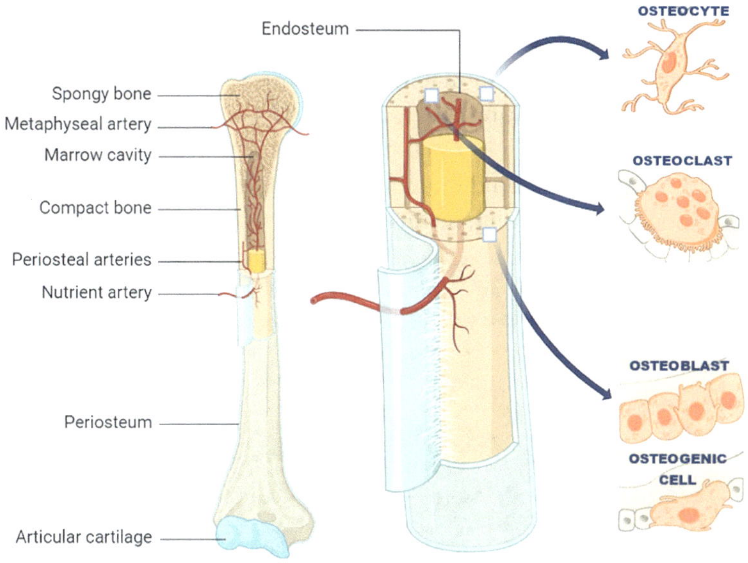

Figure 6.5. Bio-integrated solutions at the forefront of orthopedic applications, offering a significant advancement over traditional mechanical prosthetics.

Source: https://pub.mdpi-res.com/ijms/ijms-25-06012/article_deploy/html/images/ijms-25-06012-g001.png?1717062298.

6.2.3. Customization and Personalization in Prosthetics

Use of three-dimensional printing technology in the prosthetics industry is revolutionizing the process of customization and personalization required in order to deliver successful patient care. By offering a mechanism to create tailored implants as well as prosthetic devices that mirror the tailored anatomy of every patient, 3D printing enhances the functional efficiency of the medical solutions. This technology has particularly found widespread influence in orthopedic and dental implants, and craniofacial reconstructive surgeries. As demonstrated in literature, 3D printing not only aids surgical planning by way of delivery of patient-specific anatomical models but also facilitates the development of tailor-made implants that closely replicate individual patient needs, thereby ensuring maximized clinical results (Annemans et al., 2016). With their capability to reduce surgical time significantly and improve the precision of procedures, such bespoke solutions are becoming highly effective in meeting patients' variable requirements. Furthermore, developments in prosthetic limbs suggest a broad shift away from traditional mechanical ones towards more bio-interfaced ones due to advancements in 3D printing. This new technology supports prosthetic design not only meeting functional needs of the users but also offering personal aesthetics, helping in user satisfaction and self-image. Shape, weight, and material customization of prosthetic limbs can assure a smooth fit, mimicking the properties of human anatomy and motion. As seen in recent research into rapid prototyping application, the influence of this technology extends beyond mere functionality to include aspects of patient identity and social integration (Kasturi et al., 2016).

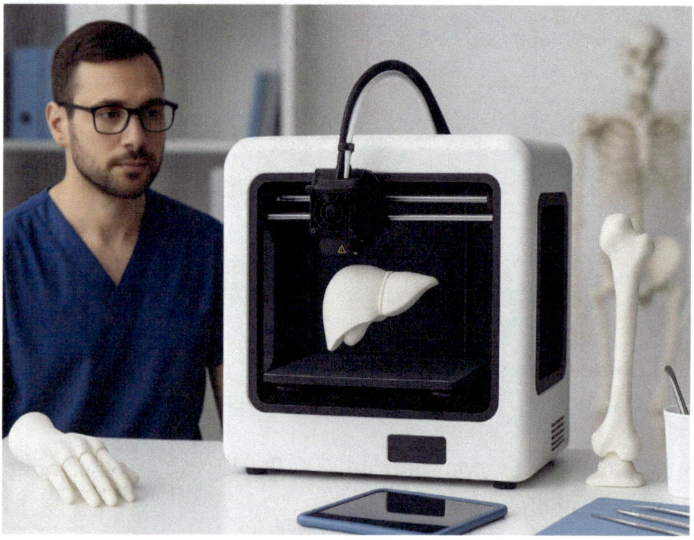

Figure 6.6. By allowing for the creation of tailored implants and prosthetic devices that mirror the unique anatomical features of each patient, 3D printing enhances the overall functional efficacy of these medical solutions.

Source: https://3dreality.in/wp-content/uploads/2025/08/3D-Printing-in-Health-care-1200x900.jpg.

Such technological advancement is symptomatic of the greater acknowledgment and acceptance of the need for personalized medicine, and it suggests that the future of prosthetics depends heavily on customized solutions facilitated by 3D printing. With the clinical advantages offered by customization come the regulatory benefits on behalf of 3D-printed prosthetics. The FDA and

ISO have established stringent requirements for safety and efficacy of custom medical devices. The regulations serve a critical role in guaranteeing that the intricacies related to the adoption of new technologies by mainstream medical practice are solved. Compliance with such policies ensures prosthetics are of high quality, dancing between innovation and patient safety. As the medical field embraces 3D printing in prosthetics, ongoing research and debate should be geared towards reconciling these issues in regulation with the tremendous capacity for customization, which requires intense interaction between medical doctors and engineers. Lastly, it is through this synergy that the full potential of individualized prosthetics can be optimized, optimizing patient benefits and the quality of life (Figure 6.6).

6.3. ADVANTAGES OF 3D PRINTING IN MEDICAL APPLICATIONS

Medical technology innovations have created unprecedented possibilities, and one of them is 3D printing, which holds tremendous promise for enhanced patient outcomes. One such example is how 3D printing can design customized orthopedic and dental implants tailored to the specific anatomy of the individual patient. By employing imaging data, surgeons are able to design implants that blend seamlessly with the complex geometry of a patient's anatomy, reducing the risk of complications and increasing interaction with surrounding tissues. The performance of such applications has been confirmed in various fields of surgery, including orthopedics and maxillofacial surgery. 3D-printed implants, as reported, not only increase the accuracy of surgery but also allow for fast surgical operations, thereby decreasing overall operative time as well as postoperative recovery times (Annemans et al., 2016). Such a combination of individualization and economy further clearly proves 3D printing's benefits in terms of applications in medicine including implants and prostheses. Additionally, 3D printing's rapid prototyping capability allows it to mimic and plan complex surgical procedures, and craniofacial reconstruction is particularly well suited for this. Surgeons can preview the patient's customized anatomy prior to surgery by means of the accurate anatomical models produced, thereby enhancing the surgical planning. This meticulous preparation minimizes intraoperative risk of complications and optimizes resource utilization, making surgery more efficient. Besides, they can also be employed as instructional guides for healthcare providers and learners, therefore making the dissemination of information within the healthcare fraternity much easier. Guides that have been established for surgery, as identified by recent studies, have proven capable of being able to augment surgical accuracy while reducing exposure to radiation when one takes images (Kasturi et al., 2016). Therefore, the use of 3D printing goes beyond the operational advantage and has a very significant contribution to the overall educational framework in medical science. Moreover, the use of bio-integrated prosthetic limbs is a significant breakthrough in patient care and rehabilitation. Having the ability to produce prosthetics with similar mimicry to natural limb functionality not only increases the esthetic acceptability but also the physiological interaction between the prosthetic device and the body. These developments give patients greater mobility and comfort, eventually leading to an improved quality of life. The trend towards personalized care by 3D printing techniques serves the diverse needs of patients, especially where the traditional prosthetics fail to deliver. Regulatory problems exist because the FDA and ISO are still actively involved in making sure these innovations are safe and effective, but the present contention over cost-effectiveness and net benefits says much for the future of 3D printing for medical applications (Annemans et al., 2016). The further these technologies improve, the more they will become part of medicine and rehabilitation.

6.3.1. Cost-Effectiveness

Progress in technology for 3D printing has transformed the area of medical implants and prosthetics, raising necessary questions regarding their cost-effectiveness. A strong argument expressed in recent literature is that while 3D printing maximizes customization and adaptability in orthopedic and dental implants, their expense can be an issue. The initial investment for scanning, printing material, and equipment is high, with most cases exceeding the traditional method. Also, other clinical requirements of the technology may entail additional unexpected financial expenses. As noted, the cost of printing and additional scans will add to the overall cost of the procedure (Annemans et al., 2016). Therefore, an accurate assessment of the economic results is required to guarantee that the improved precision of surgery and patient outcomes are justified with these additional costs. Its integration into craniofacial reconstruction and prosthetic limb manufacturing has been promising towards more patient-specific solutions but, economically speaking, is contentious. It has been established that there are dramatic improvements in surgical outcomes and reduced operation time, which indirectly lower postoperative treatment cost and recovery (Annemans et al., 2016). However, the problem at hand is to balance these clinical benefits against additional monetary investments to be incurred by 3D-printed solutions. Moreover, the comparative affordability of standard implants provokes further questions about the long-term viability of 3D printing technology for routine clinical practice. An official cost-effectiveness analysis is thus in order to address the long-term economic viability of this technology for use in surgery. As policymakers and healthcare providers navigate these budgetary concerns, use of computer-assisted orthopedic surgery (CAOS) systems also brings new opportunities for examining cost-effectiveness in 3D-printed implants and prosthetics. CAOS systems allow for precise surgical planning and execution, which in the long term reduces surgical complications and enhances patient outcomes. The complexity and assumed high cost of these systems necessitate an in-depth evaluation of their financial and clinical benefits. Studies on the implications of integrating CAOS in 3D printing technology can offer useful data on the decrease in overall cost in surgery, hence making it more cost-effective. Hence, achieving a balanced equilibrium between innovation and financial sustainability continues to be the highest priority as the medical sector guides 3D printing technologies.

6.3.2. Speed of Production

The revolutionizing impact of 3D printing on the medical sector extends far wider than that of its impact on manufacturing speed, a very important factor in designing and producing tailor-made implants and prosthetics. Compared to traditional manufacturing methods, which take time and involve a lot of manual input, 3D printing enables rapid prototyping and printing of patient-specific devices. 3D printing accelerates the design-to-delivery cycle, enabling clinicians to implement interventions in a timely manner. For example, when used in orthopedics and dental applications, the ability to make personalized implants quickly can enhance surgical planning and execution and ultimately result in improved patient outcomes and reduced recovery times. Evidence indicates that the speed at which the devices are produced is not only accountable for accelerating hospital medical processes but also facilitates early management of complex medical conditions requiring immediate intervention (Annemans et al., 2016). Furthermore, the rate of production enabled by 3D printing enhances the iterative design process, allowing for rapid accommodation to suit the specific anatomical needs of a patient. While clinicians utilize the rapid prototyping techniques, they can create multiple iterations of prosthetics or implants in significantly less time compared to alternative methods. The responsiveness in such applications as craniofacial reconstruction, where precise fit and alignment are most critical, is vital. The case studies illustrate that the quick turnaround time not only supports surgical planning but also trains medical practitioners with realistic anatomical models, boosting the educational value of this technology (Kasturi et al., 2016). Production speed thus powers an adaptive system of prosthetic design and application to support staying ahead of patient demand and clinical progress. In addition to the astounding increase in production rate, regulatory challenges remain, particularly with the clearing of 3D-printed prosthetics and implants by agencies like the FDA and ISO. With the technology becoming more widespread, compliance with efficacy and safety standards should be ensured. The acceleration of production enabled by 3D printing requires ongoing improvement of robust regulatory frameworks that are able to keep up with quick development in medical applications. Whereas the quick manufacture of customized devices has its unchallenged benefits, it raises questions of long-term performance and quality control. Future research must overcome these regulatory barriers while capitalizing on the speed and efficiency that 3D printing affords to healthcare innovation (Annemans et al., 2016). With increasing technology, the balance between rapid manufacturing and rigorous testing will be key to the successful integration of 3D printing into medicine (Figure 6.7).

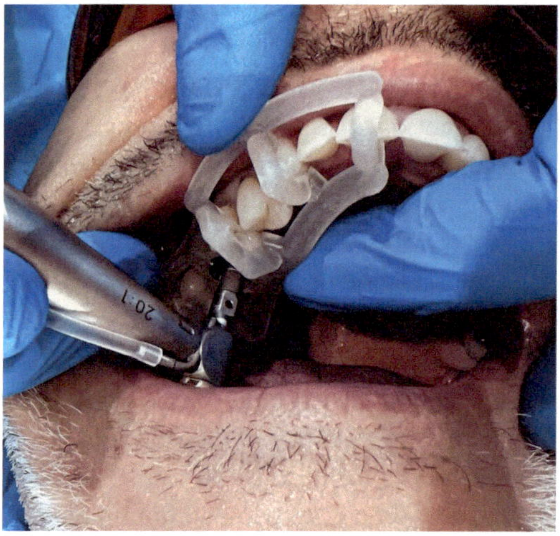

Figure 6.7. In orthopedic and dental applications, the ability to quickly produce customized implants can enhance surgical planning and execution, ultimately leading to improved patient outcomes and reduced recovery times.

Source: https://media.springernature.com/full/springer-static/image/art%3A10.1038%2Fs41415-024-7050-3/MediaObjects/41415_2024_7050_Fig2_HTML.jpg.

6.3.3. Enhanced Design Flexibility

The advancement in the manufacturing technologies has revolutionized medical device designing with great extent. Countries like the UK, Germany, and the US have used 3D printing technology, which has enabled medical practitioners to design complex and customized structures never before possible with conventional methods of manufacturing. This new manufacturing technique allows for accurate fabrication of orthopedic and dental implants with anatomical profiles of individual patients, enhancing overall function and comfort. Furthermore, the complex geometries available with additive manufacturing allow for improved osseointegration, which is critical to the longevity and functionality of implants. As imagined in existing research, the healthcare industry stands to benefit immensely from such advanced capabilities, progressing from off-the-shelf solutions to tailored treatments that respect the unique needs of patients (Akessa et al., 2021). That this progression itself emphasizes the incorporation of creativity into the design process is evidence of this. The capacity to provide enhanced design flexibility also opens into the area of prosthetics, where integration of bio-inspired design has made possible the development of mechanical as well as bio-integrated solutions. With the application of 3D printing technology, prosthetics can now also be designed with unique shapes, sizes, and functionalities suited to the specific needs of the individual user, leading to improved independence and quality of life.

Traditionally constrained production generally limited the possibilities of personalization, but the sequential deposition process involved in additive production allows for immediate prototyping and extensive personal adjustments. Not only does this accommodate physical dimensions, it also aesthetics, allowing individuals to engage with their prosthetic device as a part of their self. As technology advances, these technologies will continue to escalate user experience both practically and emotionally, underlining the synergistic collaboration of technology and human-centered design in healthcare (Syed et al., 2021). Despite high-profile capabilities available with 3D printing in providing added design flexibility, regulatory considerations remain the foremost priority in ensuring the safety and performance of prosthetics and implants. Regulatory agencies like the FDA and ISO have established guidelines that need to be complied with by manufacturers in the production of new medical devices, which present unique challenges given the innovative and heterogeneous designs that are facilitated by additive manufacturing. The intricate internal geometries of 3D printed devices necessitate rigorous testing and validation procedures to ascertain their biocompatibility and mechanical competence. As the industry matures, a balance has to be found in terms of encouraging innovation and meeting the strict requirements as required by the regulating bodies. In the long term, inclusion of greater flexibility in design through advanced manufacturing processes has the ability to revolutionize patient care, but this will have to be coupled with effective monitoring systems so that the benefits could be translated into safe and reliable health solutions for all (Akessa et al., 2021) (Figure 6.8).

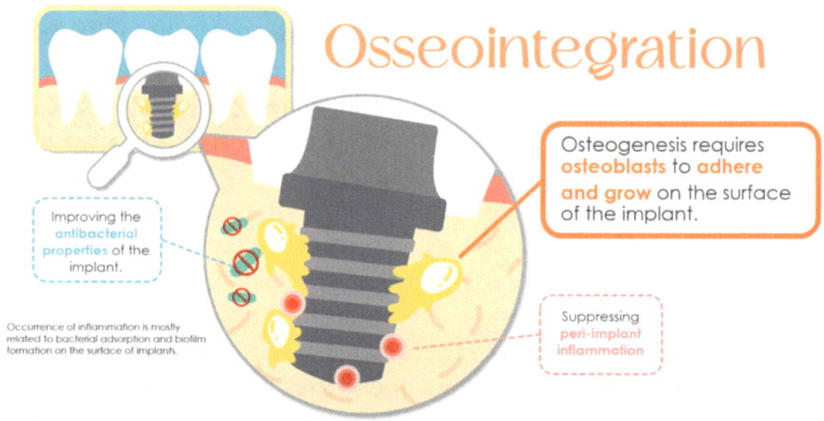

Figure 6.8. The intricate geometries that can be achieved through additive manufacturing facilitate improved osseointegration, which is crucial for the longevity and performance of implants.

Source: https://www.researchgate.net/publication/380186974/figure/fig1/AS:11431281387673697@1745130697928/Important-factors-for-the-successful-osseointegration-following-dental-implant-placement.tif.

6.4. CHALLENGES IN 3D PRINTING OF IMPLANTS AND PROSTHETICS

The technological advancement in 3D printing has transformed numerous fields in medicine, particularly prosthetic and implant manufacturing. Nonetheless, a few challenges still exist that hinder its use and performance on a large scale. Maintaining the mechanical performance of printed goods to meet the high standards for load-carrying functions, i.e., orthopedic implants, is one of the primary challenges. A majority of today's 3D printing materials lack the level of strength, durability, and biocompatibility necessary to be incorporated into the human body successfully. Specific attention must be paid to materials like poly(methylmethacrylate) (PMMA), which have been recognized as showing promise in biomanufacturing applications based on their biocompatibility and capacity to produce nanofibers, key characteristics for scaffolding within tissue engineering (Malshe et al., 2011). As such, continued research is imperative to enhance the properties of materials and processes to render 3D-printed implants more trustworthy. The regulatory framework that oversees the use of 3D-printed implants is another prime challenge. With advancing technology and complexity, it is imperative to set standards by bodies like the FDA and ISO to promote safety and effectiveness in such products. The current regulatory framework is often lagging behind technological evolution, leaving manufacturers in doubt. As a case point, prosthetic equipment—potentially with immovable and movable components—must be tested to ascertain that it can provide adequate stability and esthetic outcomes while subjecting the patient to minimal danger (Lazarova et al., 2018). This loophole in regulation will deter innovation and limit the capability of 3D printing in producing customized medical devices specifically designed to address the needs of individual patients. Thus, a coordinated effort by scientists, engineers, and regulators must come together to formulate comprehensive regulations that can keep pace with technological advancement. Additionally, the integration of 3D printing into the clinical workflow is also riddled with complications. Experts must adapt to new patterns of manufacturing and design that come with the application of additive manufacturing techniques. What this means is a transition from traditional manufacturing practices to 3D printing requires reframing the whole process, from design templates to digital fabrication processes. Additional training is also needed for medical professionals so that they know how to apply the 3D printing technology where practice is concerned. Second, maintaining hygiene and sterility during the printing and post-processing procedures must be achieved in order to eliminate infections, which is logistically demanding in clinical settings. Such challenges must be overcome in order to reach the full potential of 3D-printed prosthetics and implants, ultimately closing the gap between practicality and innovation.

6.4.1. Material Limitations

Increased utilization of 3D printing technology for the manufacture of implants and prosthetics has uncovered a variety of material shortcomings that can profoundly influence their function and lifespan. Various materials, such as polymers, metals, and ceramics, possess intrinsic mechanical properties that can be used to determine the implant function and lifespan. For instance, polymers, being lightweight and highly amendable, are generally weak mechanically for their application in high-load devices such as orthopedic implants. Metals, being stronger and less deformable, are generally susceptible to corrosion and issues of biocompatibility. Somewhere in between are ceramics that are capable of esthetic value and function in dental prostheses but are also brittle and therefore worry about their long-term behavior in load-bearing applications. Therefore, the choice of materials is a critical factor as it directly influences the overall success rate of 3D-printed implants and prosthetics. In addition, the complementary effect of these limitations in materials is augmented by the requirement for biointegration, particularly in the context of orthopedic and craniofacial applications. Biointegration is the capacity of an implant to biointegrate well with surrounding biological tissue, and this is essential to long-term implant and prosthetic survival. Optimal biointegration is required of materials to possess certain surface characteristics, mechanical response, and ideally bioactivity. While some of the 3D printing methods, such as selective laser sintering and stereolithography, allow intricate designs that are suitable for biointegration, none of the materials used in these methods are biocompatible. This disparity calls for ongoing research and development towards the identification of materials that can address the difference between mechanical stability and biological compatibility. A solution to this issue is essential for further enhancing the safety and efficacy of 3D-printed implants and prosthetics. Regulatory elements are also a key consideration when making material choice for 3D-printed medical devices, such as adherence to standards like the FDA and ISO. Introducing new materials or manufacturing methods typically requires a strict review process in the interest of safety, efficacy, and quality. Products which prove to lag in performance once examined by regulation have the ability not only to stall commercialization of emerging 3D printing technology but also to constrain potential for surgeons and practitioners to adopt cutting-edge solutions in the treatment of patients. Furthermore, ongoing competition in the market compels businesses to balance technological enhancement with affordability while adjusting to the regulatory landscape. This puts into focus the importance of selecting materials that not only meet clinical requirements but also meet regulatory requirements, ultimately affecting how seamlessly these 3D-printed implants and prosthetics can integrate into modern practice.

6.4.2. Technical Challenges in Printing

The technological revolution in 3D printing for the manufacturing of medical implants and prosthetics has opened very important doors to healthcare innovation. Nevertheless, the complexities surrounding this area provide insight into numerous technical issues that ought to be critically probed. Foremost among them is the accuracy needed in the production of orthopedic implants. For instance, the inclusion of CAOS systems is a growing tendency that aims to improve the success of musculoskeletal procedures.

These systems, utilizing advanced planning of surgery from volumetric images and real-time feedback, require absolute precision in 3D printing to enable correct fitting and function in the final implant products (Kalová et al., 2019). Material property changes, dimensional accuracy, and surface finish can significantly influence the performance of the implants and make highly rigorous testing and validation absolutely necessary before sale. Material selection is the biggest challenge in delving into technical issues of 3D printing. The development of suitable feedstocks that provide structural integrity under fluctuating loads is of utmost importance in prosthetic design. For instance, titanium alloys used in powder metallurgy are known to exhibit superior mechanical properties, but their hardness when fabricated via additive techniques tends to induce surface finish defects and part removal issues (Ewart et al., 2019). Such inherent issues need a multi-dimension solution taking into account the interaction between processing techniques and material properties. Moreover, by techniques that are both additive and subtractive in nature, like in the production of injection molds, performance of finished implants can be enhanced at lower costs of fabrication, thereby making 3D printed prosthetics more accessible. In addition to technological constraints in material behavior and fabrication, regulatory factors are important for the deployment of 3D printed implants and prosthetics. The tension between innovation and regulation is a compelling tale, with agencies such as the FDA and ISO developing challenging guidelines that must be thoroughly vetted for safety and effectiveness. As 3D printing technology advances, so must regulation keep pace to facilitate rapid development in tailored implant design and manufacturing processes. Such interaction is particularly important when considering bio-integrated rather than mechanical implants, as the former require separate regulatory clearances for ensuring patient safety and compliance with healthcare regulation. Hence, there must exist an active dialogue between engineers, medical specialists, and regulatory agencies to navigate the complex 3D printing application scenario in medicine (Figure 6.9).

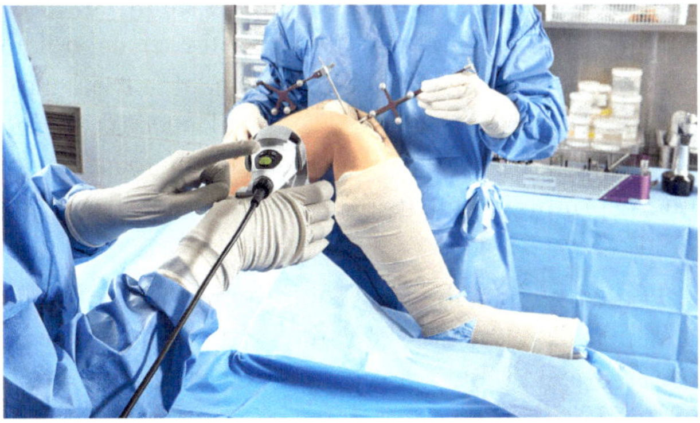

Figure 6.9. The integration of computer-assisted orthopedic surgery (CAOS) systems represents a growing trend aimed at enhancing the outcomes of musculoskeletal treatments.

Source: https://intellijointsurgical.com/wp-content/uploads/2020/03/Header-image.png.

6.4.3. Patient-Specific Considerations

In medical fields, patient-specific problems have gained even greater significance with the advent of technology bringing new solutions in the form of 3D printing. When used in orthopedic and dental fields, the facility to tailor implantation has the advantage of a more fitting implant that is both more functional and comfortable. The customized aspect of the technique not only maximizes clinical function but also minimizes the risk of complications that the off-the-shelf manufacture implants pose. For example, through the use of patient-specific anatomical information, medical professionals can design implants that adapt to unique patient morphologies, thereby enhancing integration and performance. Such benefits make way for an increasing evidence base in favor of incorporating 3D-printed implants into routine surgical procedures, as these are shown to shorten operative time, enhance immediate outcomes, and ultimately result in better long-term patient satisfaction (Annemans et al., 2016). Moreover, craniofacial reconstruction is one of the best examples of how patient-specificity in 3D printing can revolutionize classical procedures. The possibility of making custom implants from patients' own scans ensures that reconstructive surgery is performed with unforeseen accuracy.

Research has established that computer-designed cranioplasty implants, produced via additive manufacturing, are as accurate as or even more accurate than conventional methods that rely on hand-carved procedures (Burton et al., 2018). This push towards technological solutions emphasizes the significant advantages of embracing technology not only for visual rehabilitation but also for the development of functional dimensions of activities of daily living. Consequently, patients realize increased surgical success, reduced recovery time, and fewer complications, all of which greatly increase the quality of care in general. With 3D printing in the health context on the rise, regulatory factors cannot be ignored.

Regulatory bodies such as the FDA and ISO have significant roles to play in establishing standards to ensure the safety and efficacy of medical devices, especially those fabricated by additive processes. These are subjected to stringent testing and validation procedures, case-specific for patient-specific implants to check compliance and quality assurance. The problem is in balancing accelerating technological advancement with the need for systematic regulation. As health care continues to develop, it will be essential to have collaborative efforts between regulators and technology leaders like 3D printing in meeting the patient-specific needs efficiently while maintaining high safety standards. This equilibrium will ensure appropriate use of personalized prosthetics and implants without compromising patient safety (Annemans et al., 2016) (Figure 6.10).

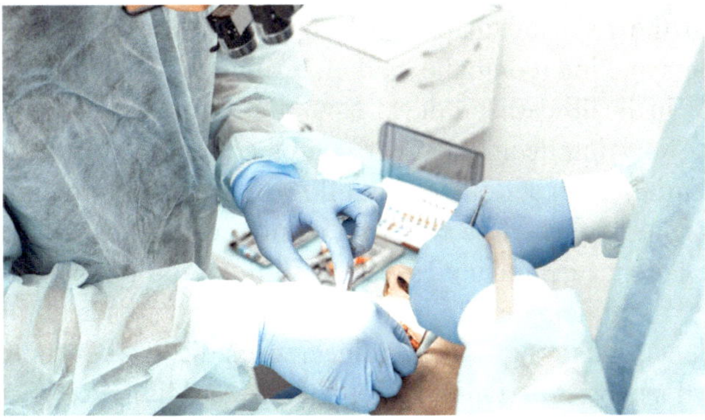

Figure 6.10. By utilizing patient-specific anatomical data, medical practitioners can create implants that accommodate individual patient morphologies, thus improving integration and performance.

Source: https://dgoavhl867cjd.cloudfront.net/0001/cd98f7d9/resize-crop(w=1920;h=1080):sharpen(level=0):output(format=jpeg)/up/dt/2024/04/Implant-placement-in-narrow-spaces%E2%80%94a-guided-approach_Shutterstock_1801190746.jpg.

6.5. REGULATORY CONSIDERATIONS

The 3D printing environment has redesigned the way numerous medical devices, such as orthopedic and dental implants, are manufactured. However, as this technology becomes increasingly integrated into medicine, it needs robust regulatory systems to ensure patient safety and quality of product. The unique characteristics of 3D-printed implants, such as the fact that they can be customized and new biomaterials can be used, present a challenge in understanding them through current regulatory frameworks. For instance, the FDA and ISO have made guidelines to gauge the safety and effectiveness of such products, but the advent of 3D printing technology poses challenges in conforming to accepted procedures for approval. As manufacturers innovate, they must work through a complex regulatory environment to remain compliant and keep their manufacturing processes open. Lastly, legitimate regulation is required to guarantee the minimization of risks and induce consumer trust in the safety of such newfangled medical procedures. Beyond matters of safety, the regulatory environment also has to make up for intellectual property rights concerns introduced by 3D printing technology. The potential to create duplicates of available implants or prosthetics using digital files poses burdensome issues of patent infringement and proprietary design protection. Such tension is a challenge for regulatory bodies, who must navigate on a tightrope to encourage innovation while protecting intellectual rights of inventors. With recent probes having placed the risks of unapproved copying at the forefront, the risk of quality products making it onto the market, leading to patient injury and erosion of confidence in healthcare products cannot be overstated. Clear regulatory guidelines on how intellectual property protections must be established are therefore essential. Such actions would allow manufacturers to invest freely in 3D printing technologies while fostering competitive practices that ultimately deliver better patient care and increase accessibility. Additionally, the regulatory system needs to anticipate the ethical implications related to 3D-printed medical products, including tissue-engineered medical products (TEMPs). As detailed, TEMPs consist of a mix of biomaterials and living cells, complicating the regulatory process due to their new therapeutic nature. The recent wave of bioprinting technologies holds much promise for individualized medicine; nonetheless, the advancements need customized regulatory guidelines. Regulations in place might not be fully equipped to manage the myriad concerns that arise due to 3D-printed tissues or organ architecture. It is imperative that these issues be addressed to effectively translate research from bench to bedside. Manufacturing complexities and the ethical imperative of extensive clinical trials underscore the importance of proper regulation to maintain these new health solutions patient-focused yet inclusive of scientific exploration and innovation in the practice of medicine, as emphasized by the literature citing the complexity of 3D bioprinted tissue and their regulatory needs (Budharaju et al., 2021; Pugliesi et al., 2020).

6.5.1. FDA Regulations for Medical Devices

Within the field of 3D printing technology for medical purposes, multidisciplinary regulatory frameworks govern the release of new devices and technologies, particularly for the development and design of orthopedic and dental implants. Because of the nature of such technologies that involve complex materials and processes, adherence to the FDA's guidelines is essential to ensure the safety of patients and efficacy. The FDA regulates medical devices by risk classification into Class I, II, or III, the most heavily scrutinized being III. The innovations with 3D printing present special challenges, particularly since they are most often printed with biocompatible materials with direct contact to living tissue. The importance of understanding and justifying these products and production methods is underscored by the increasing number of regulatory reports that critique the science underlying such devices and their potential impact on patient outcomes. Present developments in craniofacial reconstruction and prosthetic limb technology mirror the advanced regulatory challenges to manufacturers. 3D printing not only provides for personalization to fit rare anatomical variations but also presents a regulatory challenge with existing medical device regulations. Difficulty in merging biological material with technological components necessitates tissue-engineered medical products (TEMPs) to undergo serious testing to ensure their effectiveness and safety. The FDA has recognized the need for distinct regulatory pathways; therefore, TEMPs using new 3D printing technologies will often require tailor-made clinical trial protocols. Additionally, post-market surveillance approaches like adverse event reporting and long-term performance studies become the priority in monitoring these new devices continued safety and effectiveness throughout their lifecycle. Also, the ongoing updates in regulations of 3D-printed implants and prosthetics underscore the importance of a thorough knowledge of the science as well as the rules that regulate these advancements. Ongoing discoveries of new materials and technologies necessitate the updating of guidelines so that they remain effective and relevant in safeguarding public health. For instance, collaboration between industry players, regulatory bodies, and researchers can lead to the development of better standards that can capture the complexities of fabricating bio-integrated implants using 3D printing technology. The debate regarding regulations should also involve ethical considerations based on the societal impact of such innovations. Thus, regulating the regulatory environment is an ever-present challenge requiring coordination and adaptive understanding of innovation and patient care on which to establish more effective and safer medical solutions in the emerging universe of 3D bioprinting (Budharaju et al., 2021) (Figure 6.11).

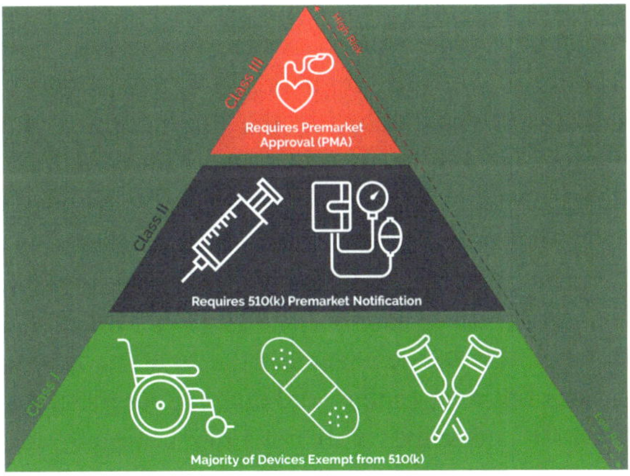

Figure 6.11. The FDA categorizes medical devices based on risk, assigning Class I, II, or III designations, which dictate the level of scrutiny required during the pre-market approval process.

Source: https://www.arenasolutions.com/wp-content/uploads/Medical-Device-Classification-Diagram-2.png.

6.5.2. ISO Standards for 3D Printed Implants

Incorporation of the 3D printing technologies in medicine also brought up the necessity to create solid standards for the development and production of implants. As the complexity of the 3D printed implants, particularly in orthopedic and dental surgeries, grows, it is necessary to provide assurance that the implants meet quality and safety criteria. The ISO standards form the critical framework to ensure that the manufacturing processes adhere to international safety and efficiency standards. Setting up standards such as ISO 13485, a quality management system standard, enables manufacturers to make dental and orthopedic implants that are safe and reliable for patients to use consistently. Besides, these standards also provide a platform to settle conflicts in products and processes, thus making healthcare practitioners confident of the implants they employ in surgeries.

In craniofacial reconstruction, ISO standards play an integral part in guaranteeing exactness and accuracy of custom implants. Various production techniques of cranioplasty implants have been contrasted on their clinical value, and it has been seen that digitally designed, additive-manufactured geometries possess precision levels comparable to traditional hand-crafted methods, according to recent studies (Burton et al., 2018). This not only solidifies the suitability of ISOs engagement but also positions 3D printing as a revolutionary technology capable of maximizing patient-specific solutions. But the lack of explicit guidelines for 3D printed medical implants remains an issue, and current practice must be supplemented in order to keep pace with technological advancements. Therefore, an entire regulatory framework must be put in place to provide for coherence and quality in the production of such life-altering implants. The regulatory climate for 3D printed implants has advanced, but significant problems remain in the area of remaining within ISO parameters. Research indicates that a large majority of NHS trusts in the UK have implemented 3D printing technology for many clinical applications, primarily utilizing them for preoperative planning and intraoperative navigation (Azeem et al., 2024). However, due to the absence of regulation-specific standards for 3D printing, questions regarding safety and efficacy for these devices have been raised. Having defined guidelines will not only be important for enhancing patient outcomes and safety but also to help medical professionals utilize 3D printed implants with optimal benefit. As the healthcare sector is shifting more towards technology, developing precise ISO standards will be crucial to addressing ethical as well as compliance issues, ultimately setting up a more responsible model for the integration of 3D printed prosthetics and implants within the clinical setup (Figure 6.12).

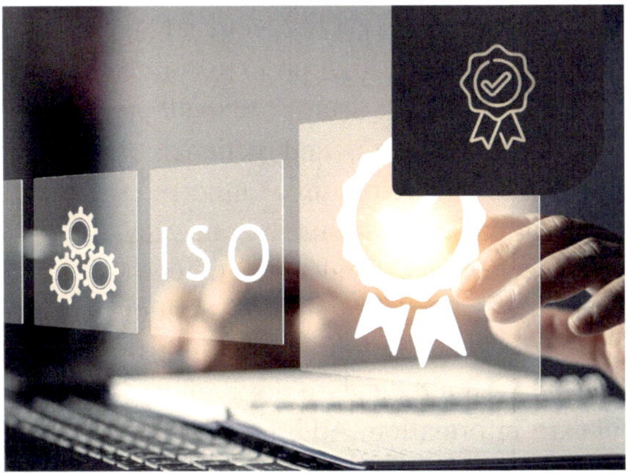

Figure 6.12. The ISO standards serve as a critical framework for ensuring that the manufacturing processes align with international safety and efficiency benchmarks.

Source: https://efor-group.com/wp-content/uploads/2025/02/QUALITE%CC%81.png.

6.5.3. Ethical Implications of 3D Printing in Medicine

The use of 3D printing technology in medicine also poses deep-rooted ethical issues, particularly with implants and prosthetics. Regular manufacturing methods prefer consistency, creating devices that need not necessarily suit individual patients' needs. However, 3D printing makes orthopedic implants and dental prosthetics more tailored to specifications, with enhanced fit and function. Such personalization, though, is questionable with its ethical dimensions on the quality control of such devices. There can be no uniform protocols, which may lead to variations in manufacturing and the risk of failure of the implants or reaction of the body. Patient safety being so important, there has to be a tight regulatory system to manage the manufacturing process and ensure the customized medical devices meet the needed standards of safety and efficacy (Pugliesi et al., 2020). These regulations are crucial to promoting trust between clients and healthcare providers and stimulating innovation in the industry. In addition, the intellectual property issue is highly critical in 3D printing, particularly in regard to medical devices and other health technologies. The ability to reproduce prosthetics and implants from existing designs gives rise to controversy on ownership and patent rights. As 3D models can be put on the internet, there is a strong possibility that copyrighted designs are illegally copied, which could harm the financial incentives required to keep research and development going. This might stifle innovation since companies will be reluctant to invest in new technology if there is a great possibility of losing their intellectual rights (Jena et al., 2024). The key to achieving the balance between stimulating innovation and intellectual property protection is in ensuring that the progress in 3D printing is made accessible to all parties involved, including manufacturers, health practitioners, and patients. Apart from this, as the application of 3D printing technology in healthcare continues to be entangled with the utilization of patient information, privacy and informed consent issues are compelling concerns. Production of customized medical devices involves collection of sensitive patient information, including anatomical data and medical histories. Protection of such information is important since unauthorized disclosure would lead to loss of patient trust and abuse of confidential healthcare information. Additionally, the complexity of informed consent in such cases cannot be overlooked. The patients must also be properly educated about the repercussions of being provided with 3D-printed implants, such as potential risk and uncertainty of these new options (Pugliesi et al., 2020). Medical practitioners must therefore exercise caution in communicating this information and applying strict consent procedures to allow the patients to make informed choices, making sure that there are ethical standards in place across all aspects of 3D printing for medical applications.

6.6. CONCLUSION

The promise of 3D printing in the field of prosthetics and implants is evidently becoming more evident with advancing technology. From orthopedic implants and dental implants to craniofacial reconstruction, the precision and flexibility offered by 3D printing methods hold immense advantages. As can be seen from the literature, advancements in this technology have been linked to improved patient outcomes, particularly when it comes to shorter operation times and improved surgical planning. Having the capability to create patient-specific models translates to improved surgical techniques, hence generally improved efficacy of medical interventions. While benefits like lessened surgery time and improved medical results are enticing, they are moderated by the complexities in implementation, including cost and regulatory considerations. Therefore, greater use of 3D printing in surgery needs to be carefully evaluated in terms of clinical and economic implications for effective integration into regular medicine. A more in-depth exploration reveals that the integration of 3D printing technology into medical practices, like prosthetics and surgery, has begun changing paradigms once dominated by conventional manufacturing. Literature reveals how 3D printing has been applied in medical settings ranging from tissue engineering to producing tailored implants specifically crafted to address precise anatomical needs. A review of case studies indicates that successful implementation of such technologies has the ability to enhance surgical accuracy and efficacy dramatically, transforming patient care by reducing recovery times and optimizing total satisfaction. The potential for increased intervention costs linked with new technology must be thoroughly researched, however. Future research needs to strive to produce a more balanced insight into the costs against which these advantages are gained through innovation in this field, moving toward making informed choices. Ultimately, while the advances in the 3D printing of implants and prosthetics present numerous possibilities for the enhancement of surgical procedures and patient results, they also pose the need for close examination and scrutiny of the accompanying challenges. The integration of new techniques in medicine is not without its challenges, particularly regulatory frameworks established by institutions like the FDA and ISO. According to the study, while there are certainly attractive applications of 3D printing, an official cost analysis will be needed to determine if and how the healthcare system can accommodate the expenses linked to such breakthrough technologies. As more research emerges, stakeholders will need to remain vigilant in assessing the clinical and economic impact of 3D printing so that progress in the field of medical science is not just sustainable but also to the advantage of all patients involved (Annemans et al., 2016; Kasturi et al., 2016).

6.6.1. Summary of Key Points

The face of medical technology is evolving, particularly around 3D printing, which is revolutionary for producing implants and prosthetics. One development is the production of cranioplasty implants tailored to patients' individual requirements. Studies have confirmed that both analog and digital methods are capable of delivering acceptable clinical results, with 3D-printed implants being as precise as more conventional methods. This finding highlights the growing feasibility of the use of digital design and additive manufacturing methods to fabricate patient-specific medical devices that fit the individual anatomical requirements of the patient. These advancements not only enhance surgical interventions but also give scope to a new generation of patient-specific medical interventions, facilitating the realignment toward customization in the medical field (Burton et al., 2018). In addition to cranioplasty, 3D printing has made significant strides in the areas of orthopedic and dental implants. By using additive manufacturing technologies, clinicians can design implants that interdigitate perfectly with the bone structure of the patient, increasing the likelihood of successful implantation and stability. Using advanced materials which promote biointegration, such implants are not just able to carry out mechanical functions but can interface with surrounding tissue more effectively, supporting healing and regeneration. The potential of these technologies is multidimensional and suggests an era where prosthetics and implants are engineered not just for fit, but also for biological compatibility. Thus, the addition of 3D printing to the manufacture of implants is a paradigm shift that combines mechanical engineering with biological knowledge (Ewart et al., 2019). Despite this, such technologies are replete with challenges, particularly in terms of regulatory methods for medical devices. Organizations such as the FDA and ISO have the mandate of establishing guidelines that safeguard the safety and efficacy of 3D-printed prosthetics and implants. The rapidly evolving technology of additive manufacturing demands close coordination between clinicians, engineers, and regulators to develop flexible standards that are poised for the unique risks and benefits of these technologies. As 3D printing re-engineers medicine, stakeholders need to work together in developing practices that promote patient safety without compromising innovation. This synergy will ultimately determine how effectively the technological innovation of 3D printing functions to become real in practical clinical application (Ewart et al., 2019).

6.6.2. The Impact of 3D Printing on Healthcare

Emerging technologies have revolutionized most sectors, with the healthcare sector being a prime area of benefit from the technological revolution. Among such emerging technologies, 3D printing has gained attraction owing to its transformative features, the most significant of which is in producing medical implants and prosthetics. Via patient-specific device printing, 3D printing reverses the limitations of traditional manufacturing methods, which produce mass products not designed to address individual anatomical variations. The ability to tailor implants, for instance, for orthopedic or dental procedures, offers better fit and functionality, allowing practitioners to diminish complications and enhance healing. With more advances in the technology, the growing integration of 3D printing into healthcare delivery sees a shift towards more tailored medicine that could substantially improve patients' outcomes while addressing individual health needs (Annemans et al., 2016). 3D printing is more than just prototyping and promises to unlock improved craniofacial reconstruction and prosthetic arm development. Using this technology, medical teams can create intricate models of the anatomy that can provide important insights in pre-surgical planning. The models raise the accuracy and efficiency of surgery by having a tangible representation, allowing surgeons to prepare for potential complications before they enter the operating room. Additionally, in prosthetics, 3D printing enables not just patient-specific designs to fit, but the construction of bio-integrated products that blend with human tissue. This has marked a departure from conventional mechanical prosthetics, which are typically unconformable to wearers and anatomically not aligned, promoting a paradigm in which patient-centered design is very desirable (Kasturi et al., 2016). Even with the potential benefits of 3D printing in medicine, regulatory issues are still a major stumbling block in its mass adoption. Ensuring the efficacy and safety of 3D-printed medical products requires intense scrutiny by regulatory agencies like the FDA and compliance with global standards like ISO. These organizations are faced with the daunting task of creating guidelines that will enable the innovative element of 3D printing so that the final devices are safe and reliable for patient use. Furthermore, the economic costs of employing 3D printing technology—e.g., the price of specialized equipment and training—must be weighed against the benefits. It is critical to balance the prospect of personalization by medical devices with regulatory paradigms compliance, as it ultimately defines the level to which 3D printing can be incorporated into mainstream healthcare practice (Annemans et al., 2016).

6.6.3. Future Outlook for 3D Printed Implants and Prosthetics

Technological improvements in 3D printing promise to revolutionize the manufacturing of medical implants and prosthetics, with significant repercussions for fields of practice such as orthopedics and dentistry. The ability to manufacture highly individualized implants tailored to a patient's specific needs addresses some conventional issues with surgical operations, particularly those relating to craniofacial reconstruction or total joint replacement. As demonstrated in most research, not only does this tailored solution provide enhanced patient comfort and function but also reduces surgical complication rates, making the healing process more effective. Ongoing research of these kinds of materials, such as biocompatible ceramics and metal alloys, further increases the performance functionality of these implants. Hence, in harmony with advancements in techniques, the landscape of implant manufacture will see a revolutionary change, with innovative but practical uses in clinics within the near future, suggesting a convergence of technology and medicine. The intricately organized structure of 3D printed limbs exposes the dual benefits of mechanical and bio-integrated models, which suggest a pivotal area of future study. Traditional mechanical prosthetics are less sophisticated in their response and function compared to bio-integrated prosthetics, which take advantage of advanced 3D printing to create prosthetics that are very close in limb mechanics. This trend towards bio-integration encourages rethinking material selection and complexity of design, favoring integration of smart technologies that are sensor-enabled for real-time feedback and adaption. The ability to produce such sophisticated prosthetic equipment using additive manufacturing not only improves performance but can also lead to a more personalized patient outcome. Encouragingly, the distinctiveness of 3D printed prosthetics could be an indication of a new direction in patient-centered treatment, positioning them firmly in medicine and stimulating further developments in biomechanical engineering. Despite the promising way for 3D-printed prosthetics and implants, regulatory matters remain the priority to their integration into clinical treatment. The FDA and ISO have established standards to ensure safety and effectiveness for medical devices, but the active nature of additive manufacturing provokes ongoing debate on standardization and conformity. With incorporation of stricter validation processes and overcoming unusual challenges inherent in the manufacturing process, as Ewart et al. (2019) puts forward, is responsible for the increase of 3D printed devices. With the healthcare industry embracing such innovations, the establishment of specific guidelines and regulations becomes more pressing in curbing safety issues while encouraging innovation. Thus, collective collaboration among stakeholders like producers, researchers, and regulatory bodies is paramount to overcome these limitations and achieve the full potential of 3D printed prosthetics and implants to solidify their position in modern medicine.

REFERENCES

1. Abt, A., Akaltan, A., Alla, K., Au, A., Becker, C., Benso, B., Bhola, R., et al. (2017). Removable partial dentures: The clinical need for innovation. https://core.ac.uk/download/74236409.pdf (accessed on 14th October 2025).
2. Akessa, A. D., Lemu, H. G., & Wakjira, Y. A. (2021). Overview study on challenges of additive manufacturing for a healthcare application. https://core.ac.uk/download/489823275.pdf (accessed on 14th October 2025).
3. Al-Zeregawe, A. H., Khalid, R., Al Mahmoud, M. A. M., Al-Hashimi, H., Sami Mahroq, O. A. M., Zwain, A. H., Abdulhasan Alaithi, N. A., et al. (2025). The role of osseointegration in orthopedics: The physiologic basis, new trends, and clinical implications. https://core.ac.uk/download/640071346.pdf (accessed on 14th October 2025).
4. Annemans, L., Gemmel, P., Tack, P., Victor, M., et al. (2016). 3D-printing techniques in a medical setting: A systematic literature review. https://core.ac.uk/download/84043719.pdf (accessed on 14th October 2025).
5. Azeem, R. U., Cheong, Y. K., Ilio, V. D., Kaye, J., et al. (2024). 3D printing adoption in NHS trusts within the United Kingdom. https://core.ac.uk/download/617962651.pdf (accessed on 14th October 2025).
6. Budharaju, H., Kalaskar, D. M., Sekar, M. P., Sethuraman, S., et al. (2021). Current standards and ethical landscape of engineered tissues—3D bioprinting perspective. https://core.ac.uk/download/477689723.pdf (accessed on 14th October 2025).
7. Burton, H., Eggbeer, D., Evans, P. L., Hanson, D., et al. (2018). Additively manufactured versus conventionally pressed cranioplasty implants: An accuracy comparison. https://core.ac.uk/download/161882301.pdf (accessed on 14th October 2025).
8. Clarke, A., Fink, A., Ayanniyi, A. A., Dyer, B., Raizada, D., McColl, E., Wu, G., et al. (2016). Questionnaire study to gain an insight into the manufacturing and fitting process of artificial eyes in children: An ocularist perspective. https://core.ac.uk/download/163076641.pdf (accessed on 14th October 2025).
9. Ewart, P. (2019). A comparison of processing techniques for producing prototype injection molding inserts. https://core.ac.uk/download/322841895.pdf (accessed on 14th October 2025).
10. Jena, M. C., Mishra, S. K., & Moharana, H. S. (2024). Application of 3D printing across various fields to enhance sustainable manufacturing. https://core.ac.uk/download/635776175.pdf (accessed on 14th October 2025).

11. Kalová, M., Kubíček, J., Oczka, D., Tomanec, M., et al. (2019). Recent trends, technical concepts and components of computer-assisted orthopedic surgery systems: A comprehensive review. https://core.ac.uk/download/287649034.pdf (accessed on 14th October 2025).
12. Kasturi, S. (S.), Nandi, P. (P.), Patil, A. N. (A.), Raikar, S., et al. (2016). Rapid prototyping assistance to medical science. https://media.neliti.com/media/publications/236937-rapid-prototyping-assistance-to-medical-a2067573.pdf (accessed on 14th October 2025).
13. Lazarova, L., Rogoleva Gjurovski, S., & Stoimenov, M. (2018). Application of combined fixed–mobile prosthetic allowances. https://core.ac.uk/download/154894189.pdf (accessed on 14th October 2025).
14. Malshe, H. (2011). Design, fabrication, and testing of an electrospinning apparatus for the deposition of PMMA polymer for biomedical applications. https://core.ac.uk/download/84120013.pdf (accessed on 14th October 2025).
15. Pugliesi, R. A. (2020). Ethical considerations in the advent of 3D printing technology in healthcare. https://core.ac.uk/download/578755760.pdf (accessed on 14th October 2025).
16. Syed, M. (2021). Designing for disability: Making activities of daily living more manageable through 3D printing. https://core.ac.uk/download/478749333.pdf (accessed on 14th October 2025).

CHAPTER 7

ORGAN AND SOFT TISSUE PRINTING

Contents

INTRODUCTION

The evolution of organ and soft tissue printing holds immense capability to revolutionize medical procedures and regenerative medicine. As research and technology are improving, the potential to engineer complex biological scaffolds has become much more efficient. The revolution is particularly evident in the fabrication of artificial skin, which is a critical answer for patients with burn injuries and chronic wounds. Through application of advanced bioprinting technologies, researchers are able to layer-print cells and bioinks to produce skin with properties close to natural tissue. Inclusion of stem cells into this process in effect enhances the potential of tissue regeneration by facilitating growth and repair of injured tissue. These technologies underscore the urgent need for further research into how bioprinting technology can address some of the medical challenges and thus provide a platform for a wide range of therapeutic applications. Bioprinting of cartilage and organs, such as liver and cardiac tissues, is also an encouraging field of regenerative medicine. The complexity of such tissues requires careful assessment of their structural and functional requirements, guided by the principles of tissue engineering. Through techniques like 3D Bioplotting, scientists are able to produce personalized scaffolds mimicking the extracellular matrix, promoting cell growth and differentiation. This method allows for the utilization of biopolymers and hybrid materials, which not only have the capability to induce soft tissue regeneration but can also be tailored to meet the mechanical demands for the hard tissues. As more experiments continue to advance, the potential of bioprinted organs as a viable option for transplantation becomes increasingly real, especially as more *in-vivo* experiments yield successful results, supporting the concept of personalized medicine. Besides, the uses of organ and soft tissue printing also reside in drug screening and disease modeling, and they represent a compelling milestone in pharmaceutical science. Traditional models never replicate the biological complexity of human tissues, warping the efficacy and safety test results of new drugs. However, bioprinted tissues can better reflect human biology, enabling the simulation of various drug interactions. This capacity not only confers vigor on the predictive role of preclinical research but can also potentially make drug development more efficient. Owing to technological progress, it is necessary to explore materials and methods applied in tissue engineering, more precisely including biodegradable materials that have the ability to sustain cell function and growth, as shown in recent publications (Abalymov et al., 2020; Carvalho et al., 2004). This continuing study has the potential to redefine our knowledge of human pathophysiology and physiology, leading eventually to better treatment options.

Definition of Organ and Soft Tissue Printing

The advancement in organ and soft tissue printing has significantly contributed to the practice of regenerative medicine, particularly in the development of artificial cartilages and skins. These bioprinted tissues contain multi-component bioinks composed of living cells, biomaterials, and growth factors that can replicate the intricate structures and functions of native tissues. For instance, artificial skin has been created using a combination of fibroblasts and keratinocytes to facilitate effective wound healing as well as potentially reducing the need for skin grafts. Bioprinting of cartilage has also shown promise in the treatment of joint and musculoskeletal disorders. By utilizing the physical attributes of hydrogel bioinks, researchers can achieve the desired mechanical and biological attributes necessary for cellular function support in order to create a scaffold that mimics the extracellular matrix in nature. These developments illuminate the possibility of organ and soft tissue printing as the key towards revolutionizing the management of numerous injuries and ailments. Aside from that, the capability of printing complex tissues like liver and heart tissues is a testament to the importance of bioprinting in organ replacement and drug testing. Liver tissues, for example, could be engineered to replicate metabolic functions, providing a platform for *in vitro* testing of hepatotoxicity and drug interactions.

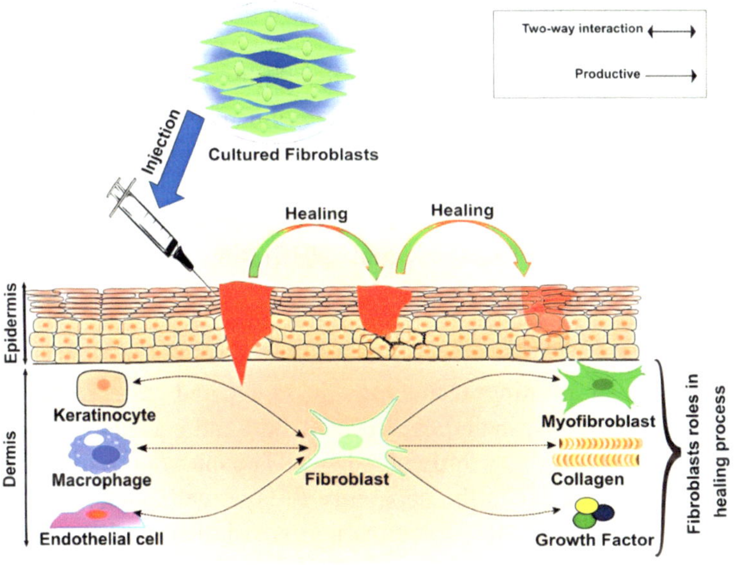

Figure 7.1. Artificial skin has been created using a combination of fibroblasts and keratinocytes, allowing for effective wound healing and potentially reducing the need for skin grafts.

Source: https://media.springernature.com/lw1200/springer-static/image/art%3A10.1186%2Fs13287-024-03892-0/MediaObjects/13287_2024_3892_Fig2_HTML.png.

This development is of utmost significance to the pharmaceutical industry because it makes more accurate predictions of drug action in humans and reduces reliance on animal models. Similarly, heart tissue printed from cardiomyocytes can simulate heart functions and rhythms and facilitate the study of cardiovascular diseases and therapy options. These tissue models not only enhance our understanding of disease mechanisms but also facilitate the planning of individualized medicine strategies as compared to conventional treatments, demonstrating a major shift towards more effective therapies. Central to the achievement of organ and soft tissue printing is the use of stem cells, which provide a versatile source for creating many cell types. Stem cells possess the capability to be converted into specialized cells needed for specific tissues, such as cardiomyocytes, hepatocytes, and chondrocytes, thereby making the challenge of obtaining cells for printing easier. The application of these stem cell-derived tissues in drug screening and disease modeling enhances understanding and treatment of various medical conditions also. For instance, tissue printed with bioprinting is capable of mimicking disease states, and scientists can investigate the effect of therapeutic compounds under controlled conditions. By and large, the combination of stem cells and organ and soft tissue printing significantly improve the ability to create functional tissue constructs and merging bioprinting with the aim of precision medicine. The ongoing progress in this field suggests the future in which bioprinted tissues would not only serve as experimental models but would also be at the forefront of advancing regenerative therapies in order to provide continuity to scientific growth (Barbetta et al., 2019; Blunk et al., 2016) (Figure 7.1).

7.1. THE TECHNOLOGY BEHIND ORGAN PRINTING

Advances in organ printing technology have created new possibilities to generate artificial organs, including artificial skin and cartilage, which are of extreme significance to regenerative medicine. The integration of the different bioprinting techniques offers the capability to layer cells and biomaterials in a controlled manner to create structures that are similar to the natural tissue architecture of human tissues. For example, researchers have been successful in printing artificial skin that has various cell types, such as keratinocytes and fibroblasts, creating functional properties that are akin to living skin. Furthermore, the ability to generate cartilage using such methods helps deal with shared issues in injury and degeneration, particularly in joints. The employment of bioinks that are diverse, with the majority being stem cells isolated from different sources, enhances the structural integrity and functional ability of these artificial tissues and positions them as future alternatives in regenerative therapies and tissue regeneration (Amrollahi et al., 2016). The liver is another organ of special interest under the organ printing system, mainly due to its intricate architecture and important functions in detoxification as well as metabolism. Current research in bioprinting has concentrated on replicating the livers microenvironment using advanced biomaterials and scaffolds that support hepatocyte growth and differentiation along with other cell types that support them. This has shown potential in creating liver models that are not just amenable to transplantation but also as a platform for drug screening and disease modeling. Integration of stem cells into these bioprinted structures has the capacity to enable scientists to generate liver tissue that is more physiological in behavior, enabling preclinical trials that are truer and reducing reliance on animal models.

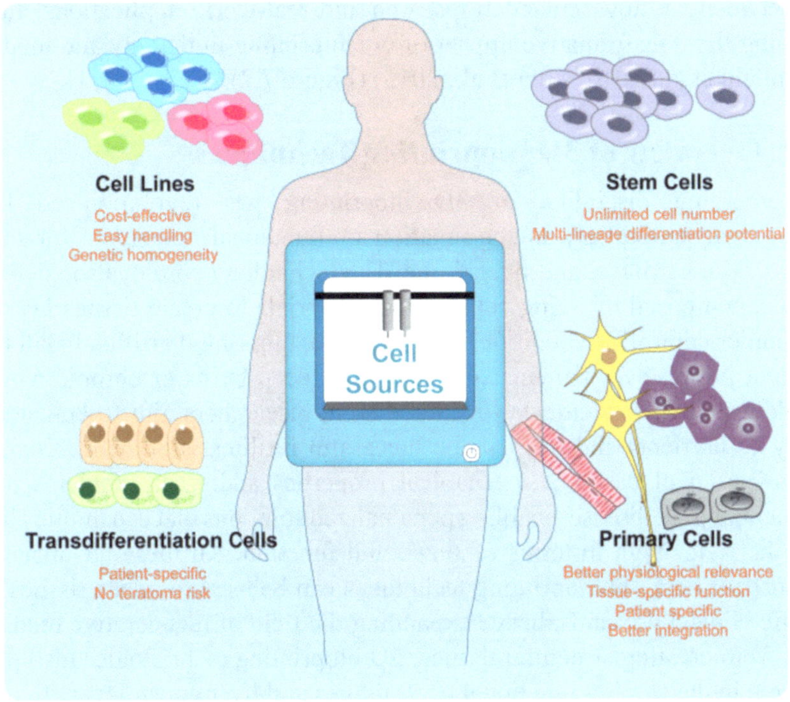

Figure 7.2. By incorporating stem cells into these bioprinted structures, researchers can yield liver tissues that more closely mimic physiological responses, thereby enabling more accurate preclinical trials and reducing reliance on animal models.

Source: https://ars.els-cdn.com/content/image/1-s2.0-S2405844024006248-gr3.jpg.

These advancements gesture towards the promise of revolutionizing drug discovery and disease information and making organ printing an essential focus area of biotechnology (Chia et al., 2015). Heart tissues are perhaps the most difficult targets in organ printing due to their complex structure and multi-functional demands. The ability of bioprinting cardiomyocytes with supporting vascular structures has deep implications for producing functional heart tissues. Progress in scaffold technology offers the platform to deliver bioactive factors and stem cell populations that are conducive to cardiac differentiation and maturation. This is all in pursuit of the final goal of not only repairing but also restoring damaged heart tissue in cardiovascular disease patients. Furthermore, bioprinted cardiac tissue usage extends beyond drug discovery, as it allows for testing of pharmaceutical drugs against human-like cardiac constructs. As scientists keep researching, these technologies will continue to bridge the gap between cardiovascular lab research and real-world applications, further affirming the transformative impact of organ printing in therapy and medicine (Amrollahi et al., 2016; Chia et al., 2015) (Figure 7.2).

7.1.1. Overview of 3D Bioprinting Techniques

The emerging discipline of 3D bioprinting has revolutionized tissue engineering, particularly in the creation of functional constructs for organs such as skin, cartilage, and liver tissue. The technology employs sophisticated bio-inks composed of living cells and biomaterials to create tissues layer-by-layer under controlled conditions. For instance, bioprinted artificial skin holds excellent promise for patients suffering from deep burns or chronic wounds. By adding vascular elements to printed skin, researchers aim to enhance the supply of nutrients and oxygen for successful healing. Moreover, bioprinted customization of cartilage mechanical properties addresses problems in the treatment of joint disease, enabling personalized solutions that can mimic natural tissue behavior both in terms of shape and function. All these advancements demonstrate how 3D bioprinting techniques can be used to create tissues with specific clinical demands, hence expanding the field of regenerative medicine. Apart from creating structural tissues, 3D bioprinting technologies also play a vital role in developing functional heart tissues and liver constructs with native organ-like characteristics. Establishment of cardiac tissues that are capable of rhythmic contractions is an impressive advancement in the direction of heart repair and cardiovascular regenerative therapy. Similarly, bioengineered liver tissues enable researchers to simulate vital metabolic processes and causative reactions to disease and produce appropriate drug-screening and disease models. This technology provides the pharmaceutical industry cost-efficient alternatives to animal use, enabling preliminary drug screening for efficacy and toxicity. Interestingly, the addition of stem cells within these bioprinted constructs has the potential to enhance regenerative capacities, allowing for the feasibility to heal damaged tissues or even completely replace failed organs. Such applications demonstrate the groundbreaking impact that 3D bioprinting technologies possess on the medical field. As the field has developed, several bioprinting techniques have been refined, each being utilized for different tissue engineering applications. For instance, techniques such as inkjet printing, extrusion-based printing, and laser-assisted bioprinting have emerged as leading methods, each employing a unique mechanism to deposit bio-ink with high accuracy. Among them, the choice of bio-ink plays an important role as it has a direct effect on cellular viability and functionality upon printing. Natural and synthetic polymers form the basis of most bio-inks, such as gelatin and polyethylene glycol used to retain desired properties for adhesion and cell growth. Cameron et al. (2017) highlights that selection of the appropriate bio-ink may affect structural stability and biological functionality of the printed structure. Furthermore, as researchers continue to develop better bioprinting methods and materials, there is a trend toward producing more complex, multi-cellular structures, and toward creating more functional capacities and clinical relevance in organ and soft tissue printing (Figure 7.3).

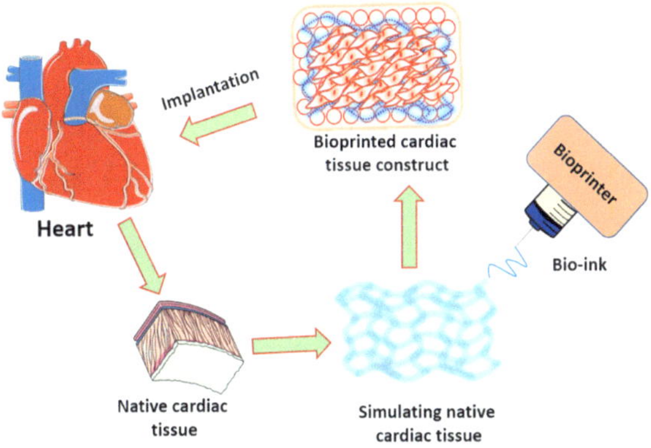

Figure 7.3. The creation of cardiac tissues capable of rhythmic contractions represents a significant leap towards heart repair and regeneration strategies for patients with cardiovascular diseases.

Source: https://media.springernature.com/lw1200/springer-static/image/art%3A10.1007%2Fs10856-021-06520-y/MediaObjects/10856_2021_6520_Figa_HTML.png.

7.1.2. Materials Used in Bioprinting

The significance of material selection in bioprinting cannot be overstated as it directly influences functioning and compatibility of printed constructs with native tissues. The hydrogels represent one of the most common materials applied in this novel technology due to their intrinsic resemblance to the extracellular matrix (ECM), which is pivotal in offering cell viability and function. For instance, the progress in using collagen and alginate has led the way towards the creation of artificial cartilage and skin so that biomimetic environments can be designed that facilitate cellular differentiation and growth. Moreover, these hydrogels can be loaded with stem cells, leading to greater regenerative capability. With the integration of such materials with bioprinting technology, researchers aim to design complex tissue architectures that replicate the mechanical and biological properties of human organs, bridging the gap between engineered tissues and actual physiological function in applications such as drug screening and disease modeling (Cho et al., 2018). In pursuing the bioengineering of organs such as the liver and heart, numerous other materials apart from hydrogels are explored.

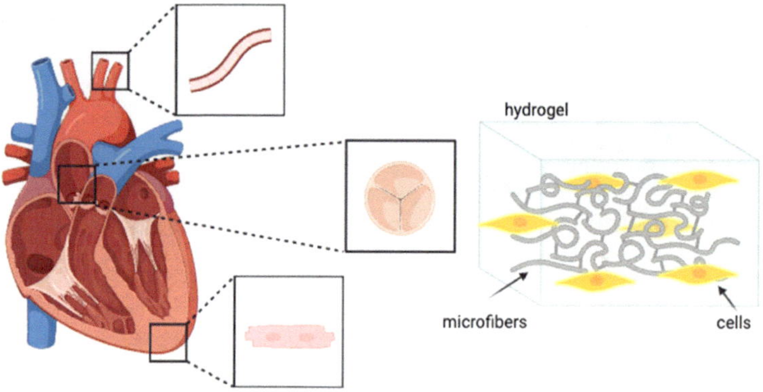

Figure 7.4. The use of polycaprolactone (PCL) and polyethylene glycol (PEG) provides a scaffold that supports the architecture of heart tissues, allowing for vascularization and electrical conductivity essential for cardiac function.

Source: https://pub.mdpi-res.com/bioengineering/bioengineering-11-00218/article_deploy/html/images/bioengineering-11-00218-g004.png?1709718817.

Synthetic and natural polymer bioinks are most instrumental in this endeavor because properties can be optimized to address the needs of mechanical strength as well as biocompatibility. For example, addition of polycaprolactone (PCL) and polyethylene glycol (PEG) bestows the scaffold that supports the heart tissue structure to facilitate vascularization and electrical conductivity which the heart needs. The intricacies involved in printing these tissues require new methods, such as coaxial extrusion, which enhance the resolution with which the printing is done and the incorporation of multiple cell types into the constructs. Targeting the specific properties that should be mimicked to match the functionality of such organs, scientists attempt to develop solutions that are physiologically acceptable in the human body (Cho et al., 2018). The adaptability of bioprinting materials makes them not only useful for the mere generation of tissue structures; they are also critical for disease modeling and drug testing. When stem cells are incorporated with tissue printed tissues, it is possible for researchers to produce patient-specific models that emulate unique disease stages, thus enabling personalized medicine strategies. For instance, liver tissue fabricated by bioprinting may be employed to assess drug metabolism and toxicity, providing a closer mimic of human reaction compared to existing techniques. This material-based strategy has been of special interest as it can potentially render preclinical research more accurate and reduce the application of animal models. As technology continues to evolve, the incorporation of advanced bioink formulations, such as nanogels with customized drug delivery characteristics, will increasingly extend the domain of bioprinting in medicine (Barbetta et al., 2019) (Figure 7.4).

7.1.3. Role of Computer-Aided Design in Organ Printing

CAD advancements have significantly revolutionized the technology of organ printing, particularly in the production of artificial tissues such as skin, cartilage, and complex organs like the liver and heart. CAD allows for intricate modeling, enabling accurate control and optimization of scaffolds to support cellular growth and functionality. The ability to tailor designs based on the individual patient anatomy ensures that such tissues are not only biocompatible but also exhibit properties much similar to that of native tissues. Customization is critical in achieving complete integration of printed tissues within the human body, which improves the prospects of restoring function in patients requiring organ transplant or tissue regrowth. Furthermore, incorporation of biocompatible material in scaffolds is critical for fostering cellular proliferation and adhesion, and CAD therefore takes a central position in organ printing successful strategies. Stem cells coupled with CAD strategies are a most powerful tool in regenerative medicine for organ printing, allowing for the development of tissue on an individual basis. With patient-specific data, CAD helps researchers design scaffolds that can provide the milieu for stem cell proliferation, which can develop into various tissue forms such as cardiac or hepatic cells. This technology can go a long way in addressing serious organ donor shortages, in addition to minimizing rejection hazards due to the employment of autologous cells. The combination of stem cell technology and CAD opens up new possibilities for the creation of very advanced structures that closely reproduce the native tissues architecture and thus result in improved outcomes in regenerative therapies. The influence of this amalgamation far exceeds transplantation, ushering in a new revolution in the treatment of degenerative disease and tissue injury. In addition, the use of CAD in organ printing has radical implications in drug testing and disease modeling, also demonstrating its biomedical research flexibility. Through the utilization of 3D printed tissue, researchers are able to create *in vitro* systems that model disease states, thus facilitating more precise identification of drug efficacy and toxicity. This capability not only accelerates the quest to find drugs but also optimizes the predictive value of preclinical models and reduces animal testing. Moreover, by printing tissues with specific patient-derived cells, researchers are able to model a patient's response to treatments, paving the way for personalized medicine approaches. Lastly, CAD is a fundamental foundation for continued development of bioprinting technologies that not only support organ replacement but also development of more effective therapeutic solutions to various diseases and states of health, as illustrated with the development of recent technologies in the field (Carvalho et al., 2004; Chia et al., 2015).

7.2. APPLICATIONS OF ORGAN PRINTING

The recent introduction of organ printing has significantly progressed the possibility of synthesizing artificial skin, cartilage, and other vital organs. These advancements draw on the capabilities of bioprinting technologies for producing three-dimensional structures that mimic the characteristics of biological tissue. With the application of a wide variety of biomaterials, researchers have had promising results in developing layers of skin capable of facilitating wound healing and preventing infection. Cartilage, being a major component of joints, is also one of the major uses of organ printing that address degenerative joint diseases through engineered tissues that have the ability to regenerate or replace damaged cartilage. With the expanding horizon of organ printing, scientists are also trying to engineer functional complex tissues, thereby opening doors for clinical application beyond the provision of mechanical support to the return of complete organ function in patients. One of the most hopeful applications of organ printing lies in the search for functional liver tissue. The livers important roles in metabolism, detoxification, and biosynthesis make it a prime candidate for bioprinting research. Newer organ printing technologies have been able to produce liver constructs with the capacity to replicate physiological behaviors, which holds promise in pharmacology and toxicology. These printed liver tissues are effective platforms for drug screening in which the scientists can investigate drug metabolism and interaction more accurately. The use of stem cells in organ printing also revolutionized the method of designing such hepatic constructs. Stem cells are involved in forming cellular diversity of the printed tissues, thus enhancing the functionality of the scaffolds and its applicability in regenerative medicine. In organ printing, the heart is of a very enticing frontier, both because of its complexity and because of the actual clinical need for treating cardiovascular disease. Present work includes bioprinting heart tissue with the goal of someday repairing or replacing a section of the heart to significantly improve treatment for heart failure patients. Such technology may set the stage for customized treatments that utilize patient-derived stem cells, addressing issues of compatibility and minimizing rejection rates. In addition, organ models produced using bioprinting also have immense potential as disease models. Organ models give researchers an indication of how disease progresses and how a therapeutic response can be seen, allowing them to explore conditions like myocardial infarctions in a controlled setting. The interdisciplinary collaboration mentioned in other reviews signifies the significant role that bioengineers and materials scientists have played in attaining such advancements and introducing significant innovations in regenerative medicine (Figure 7.5).

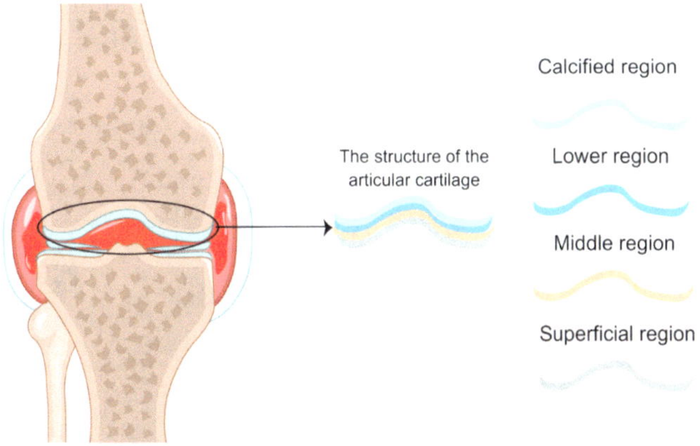

Figure 7.5. Cartilage, being a crucial component in joints, is now also an important application of organ printing, addressing joint degenerative diseases through engineered tissues that can regenerate or replace damaged cartilage.

Source: https://media.springernature.com/lw1200/springer-static/image/art%3A10.1186%2Fs12938-024-01260-w/MediaObjects/12938_2024_1260_Fig1_HTML.png.

7.2.1. Development of Artificial Skin for Burn Victims

The technological advancement in bioprinting has stimulated vast growth in the production of artificial skin, which is aimed at patients suffering from burns. Traditional skin grafting methods are painful, as the skin is obtained from healthy regions on the patient, which might lead to extended recuperation time and complications. Using 3D bioprinting techniques, researchers can create skin substitutes that have the same natural structure and physiology as human skin.

These artificial constructs can be engineered from a combination of stem cells and tissue-compatible biomaterials that provide a matrix for cell growth and incorporation into host tissue. This novel approach is not only faster to heal but also reduces the risk of rejection and infection. The uses of such advancements extend beyond the healing of burns in the present context, but can also serve as a model for more broad applications in tissue engineering, including repairing liver, cartilage, and heart tissue, as proof of the revolutionary potential of organ and soft tissue printing for medical application. Lastly, the creation of organ printing technologies is inextricably linked to the creation of stem cells, which have the fundamental role of generating new tissue to be used in regeneration. Stem cells possess the capacity to differentiate into a wide range of cell types and hence are ideal for use in bioprinting. Isolation and manipulation of stem cell populations provide researchers with the ability to pursue means of constructing complex tissues and even functional organs whose anatomy will mimic that of the original human body.

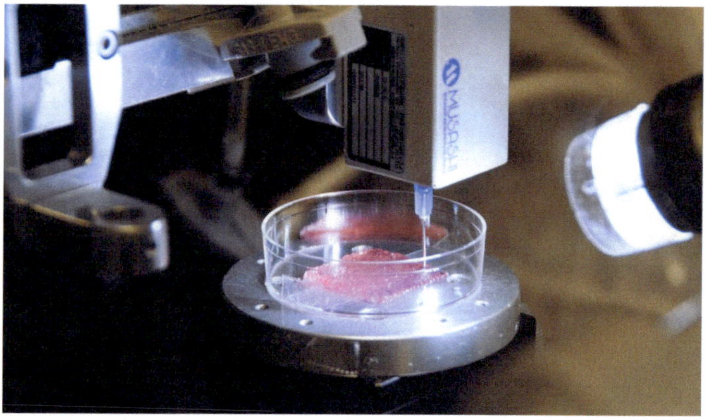

Figure 7.6. By employing 3D bioprinting techniques, researchers can create skin substitutes that replicate the natural structure and function of human skin.

Source: https://i.all3dp.com/workers/images/fit=scale-down,w=1200,h=675,gravity=0.5x0.5,format=auto/wp-content/uploads/2022/05/10174219/3d-bioprinting-involves-the-creation-of-biological-ny-times-220419.jpg.

This promise not only affords possible future organ transplantation but also makes it a powerful tool for personalized medicine through tailor-made tissue constructs. Furthermore, these constructs will be amenable to drug screening and disease modeling, providing rich information on the pathophysiology of the conditions. This two-fisted application of bioprinting technologies underscores the need for continued research and development in the field, in keeping with the rising demand for novel solutions for primary healthcare challenges. Lastly, the addition of organ and soft tissue printing into practice will revolutionize how we treat tissue regeneration and burn patients. With ongoing research and emerging technology like what is seen here, being able to print living tissue within a lab environment is a very appealing option compared to conventional surgery. The ongoing manufacture of artificial skin and other tissue types is indicative of the cooperative synergy of materials science, stem cell technology, and bioprinting. With scientists working relentlessly to render engineered tissues more functional, viable, and complex, remarkable strides are being made in making fully functional organs an attainable reality. This interdisciplinary approach not only guarantees to enrich the lives of burn patients but also presents a broader vision for addressing systemic deficits in organ transplantation and even overall enhancing the quality of patient care in an increasingly strained healthcare setting, as proposed by the challenges raised by Elmahjub (2025) and Parikh et al. (2024) (Figure 7.6).

7.2.2. Creation of Cartilage for Joint Repair

The intricate process of bioprinting revolutionized the field of regenerative medicine, offering groundbreaking methods for the production of various tissues, including cartilage for joint repair. When age wears us down or trauma hits us, the cartilage that cushions joints is compromised, causing significant pain and limited movement. Recent advances in bioprinting cartilage utilize the novelty of stem cells, which can differentiate into various cell types. This use of stem cells is in line with the goals of tissue engineering, wherein the creation of a biological replacement for damaged cartilage not only needs scaffolds but also an appropriate microenvironment that may promote chondrogenesis, or the development of cartilage. By combining cellular components and biomaterials, researchers aim to create functional cartilage constructs that not only restore joint function but also circumvent the complications associated with traditional surgical methods (Almeida et al., 2017). Hybrid bioprinting is a highly promising technique in cartilage engineering for joint repair. Such an approach effectively combines concepts of developmental biology and biomaterials science with 3D bioprinting technologies to produce better cartilage constructs. With the use of scaffold-free cartilage microtissues as a building block, researchers have been able to incorporate human bone marrow-derived mesenchymal stem cells into bioprinted constructs. The hybrid constructs not only exhibit enhanced biological function but also maintain their viability and chondrogenic phenotype following printing. The use of specialized hydrogels is shown to facilitate microtissue assembly with an organized spatial layout to mimic that of natural cartilage. Consequently, the development of these complex systems enhances the promise of effective joint repair, ultimately providing an improved quality of life for those suffering from cartilage disorders (Asadian et al., 2020). Besides joint repair, the application of bioprinted cartilage extends beyond the avenues of production of other necessary tissues such as skin, liver, and heart tissue. The development of bioprinting technologies holds the promise of generating complex, multi-layered tissues that replicate the natural cellular structure and function. This opens up new avenues in drug testing and disease modeling, with the potential to study the efficacy and toxicity of drugs in a closer resemblance to the biological environment. With organ printing using stem cells, scientists can generate patient-specific models that offer individual response to treatment, significantly improving personalized medicine. Combined, these technologies show the potential of organ and soft tissue printing to not only solve the problem of cartilage repair but also revolutionize more widespread medical applications, revolutionizing therapeutic strategies for a wide variety of diseases and conditions (Almeida et al., 2017) (Figure 7.7).

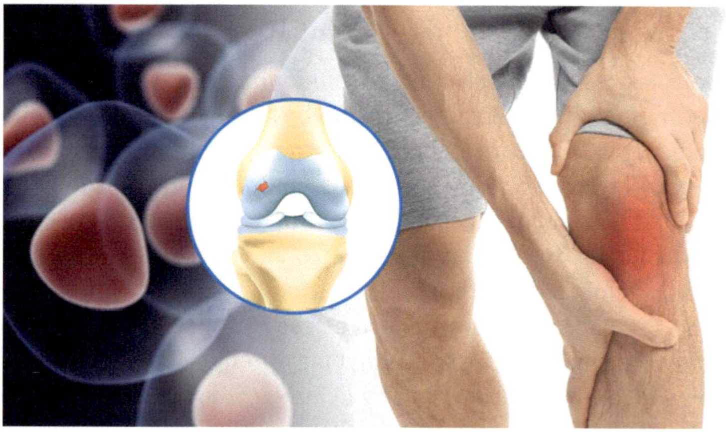

Figure 7.7. As the body ages or experiences injury, the cartilage that cushions joints can deteriorate, leading to significant pain and mobility issues.

Source: https://www.stemcellcareindia.com/wp-content/uploads/2024/07/Stem-Cell-Treatment-for-Cartilage-Repair.jpg.

7.2.3. Printing of Liver Tissues for Drug Testing

Advancements in bioprinting technologies have opened up new opportunities for the development of human tissue models, significantly transforming the preclinical drug testing scenario. Among all these models, liver tissues are critical structures since they have important functions to perform in drug metabolism and detoxification processes. The ability to print liver tissues precisely means scientists are able to create more lifelike *in vitro* systems that can mimic human liver function, thereby providing insight into drug pharmacokinetics and toxicity. These systems incorporate various cell types, including hepatocytes, endothelial cells, and fibroblasts, in a configuration that mimics the natural microenvironment of the liver. Moreover, the application of bio-inks composed of synthetic and biological polymers enables the preservation of cellular function and viability, enhancing drug response analysis precision in liver tissue bioprinted, which is critical for successful drug development (Cameron et al., 2017). The ongoing research on stem cells has also contributed to the promise of organ printing, particularly for liver tissue engineering. Stem cells possess excellent regenerative and differentiative potential, enabling them to create hepatocyte-like cells, which are required for replicating liver function in bioprinted tissue. With the help of techniques such as directed differentiation, researchers can create liver tissues that not just retain liver-specific functions but also exhibit required metabolic functions of very close proximity to native tissue of the liver. Application of the technology extends beyond pharmacological study, such as disease modeling, in which the bioprinted liver tissue may serve as a platform to investigate hepatic pathologies like hepatitis and cirrhosis. This gives insight into disease mechanisms with new therapeutic options and opportunities for drug testing (Badi et al., 2015). Integration of bioprinted liver tissue into drug testing pipelines also provides several benefits in safety and efficacy assessments. Standard drug screening procedures rely on animal models that can produce results not fully translatable to human physiology. Bioprinted liver tissues, on the other hand, offer a human-relevant solution that significantly increases the value of preclinical information. The potential for high-throughput screening of drug candidates in such model systems can speed drug discovery with reduced reliance on animal testing. As organ printing advances, application of advanced technologies, such as 3D printing and microfluidics, enhances the functionality and complexity of printed tissues. This convergence of technologies is opening up new paradigms for personalized medicine, where liver models can be tailored to replicate individual patient profiles, thus revolutionizing the paradigm of drug testing and development (Cameron et al., 2017).

7.3. HEART TISSUE ENGINEERING

The recent advances in tissue engineering have brought much enthusiasm to the possibility of bioprinting for most of the organs, even heart tissue. Bioprinting takes advantage of stem cells' potency, which can form bioengineered tissues with regard to functional morphology of native organs. By using bioinks derived from natural and synthetic polymers, scientists have managed to create scaffolds that enable cellular development and permit the establishment of extracellular matrices—of equal value to tissue functionality and survival. Beyond the simple restoration of damaged tissues, applications include being delivery vehicles for drug discovery and disease modeling, with possible new avenues for the investigation of pathophysiological processes and responses to therapy. This purpose dualism highlights the increased pertinence of using heart tissue engineering methods in the fast-growing area of organ and soft tissue printing. Hybrid materials have been particularly promising within the context of heart tissue engineering since these composites can precisely emulate the mechanical and biochemical properties of hard and soft tissues, respectively. The ability to tailor the makeup of such materials allows for applications of defined nature among varying tissue types, an emphasis emphasized by the idea of a one-matches-all model presented in modern literature. Viscous polymers of various inorganic composition in bioprinting not only allow for cell proliferation but also promote the intricate formation of the extracellular matrix, a key to effective tissue engineering. Additionally, the integration of drug delivery systems into these scaffolds expands their role so that they can be used to deliver growth factors and therapeutic molecules locally and control their release to enhance healing and tissue regeneration. These developments offer a more sophisticated and efficient approach to heart tissue building, further cementing its role in revolutionizing regenerative medicine (Abalymov et al., 2020). The study of co-axial wet-spinning extrusion methods is an example of the establishment of new bioprinting strategies with the potential to revolutionarily optimize heart tissue construction. One such strategy revealed improved printing resolution and shape fidelity, vital parameters in the fabrication of anatomically relevant tissue constructs. By allowing the decoupling of printing accuracy from bioink rheological response, this process allows simple design of complex bioinks for cardiac applications. Furthermore, the ability to produce heterogeneous multi-material constructs expands the potential for producing tissues that reflect the intricate architecture and function of natural heart and embraces the intricacies of cellular interactions. With the research continuing to define the challenges and expanding the scope of these technologies, it is clearer than ever that heart tissue engineering is the cornerstone to overcome critical deficiencies in current therapeutic approaches (Barbetta et al., 2019).

7.3.1. Challenges in Printing Functional Heart Tissues

The intricacy of bioprinting heart tissues puts enormous challenges that identify the limitations of current methods. Among various tissues, cardiac tissue is most complex due to its unique structure composed of highly organized cardiomyocyte, endothelial cell, and extracellular matrix component arrangements. The degree of mimicking such organization is decisive for the mechanical and electrical functions characteristic of native heart tissue. Materials science breakthroughs have provided polymer-based and hybrid biomaterials that are conducive to tailoring towards cardiac cell proliferation as well as tissue repair. Their employment in bioprinting, as encouraging as it might seem, calls into question their possible integration with existing cardiovascular architectures and functional efficacy *in vivo* in general, hence the need for further studies to further tailor their properties towards cardiac tissue engineering (Abalymov et al., 2020).

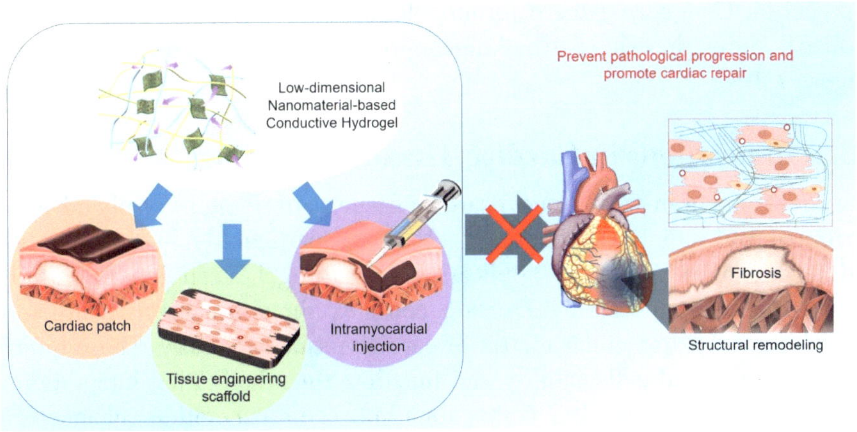

Figure 7.8. Innovations in materials science have led to the development of polymer-based and hybrid biomaterials that can be tailored to promote cardiac cell growth and tissue repair.

Source: https://www.dovepress.com/file/img/graphical_abstract/386763/xlarge.

The second prominent field of challenge for heart tissue biofabrication lies in choosing and preparing bioinks. The rheology, mode of gelation, and cytocompatibility of the bioink all significantly contribute to successful bioprinting outcomes. In the case of cardiac tissue, not only must the bioink support cell viability, but also mimic the elastic character of heart tissue to enable matching functionality when under physiological conditions. Traditional types of bioink formulations fail to achieve this delicate balance. New methods like co-axial wet-spinning extrusion present a potential solution to reduce the challenges, with a better resolution in printing and the capability to create heterogeneous and multicellular structures resembling the natural tissue architecture. Constant development in the technology of bioink can surmount the limitations of achieving the structural and functional fidelity during the printing of heart tissues (Barbetta et al., 2019). Besides, the new field of organ printing transcends mere structural duplication; it involves the new use of stem cells in the aim of enhanced tissue regeneration and versatility of application in fields such as drug screening and disease modeling. Stem cells used within the bioprinting process can provide the cell diversity necessary for functional heart tissues because they can differentiate into various cell types necessary for the aim of enhanced tissue complexity. But the challenge is to control the pathways of differentiation with high cell fidelity in printing. Further, printing tissue application to drug testing and disease modeling is future breakthroughs in personalized medicine with the potential to define patient-specific therapeutic approaches. Conquering these formidable challenges is critical to advancing cardiac tissue engineering and making bioprinted constructs clinically applicable (Figure 7.8).

7.3.2. Innovations in Cardiac Tissue Scaffolding

The development in creating new cardiac tissue scaffolding has truly advanced the organ and soft tissue printing technology, particularly in cardiac repair and regeneration. With the application of hydrogel-based bioinks' ability, it is theoretically possible to create complex three-dimensional structures mimicking the extracellular matrix of cardiac tissues naturally. These bioinks allow for enhanced cell viability and function, thus facilitating integration of stem cells, which form a key cornerstone in tissue regeneration enhancement. As emphasized by recent studies, the fast growth in patenting applications on hydrogel formulations is a reflection of an ever-evolving reality of cardiac tissue engineering solutions (Afridi et al., 2024). The integration of these technologies not only increases the survivability of printed tissues but also places emphasis on sustainability in regenerative medicine as such technologies might in the long run translate to improved therapy for heart disease, a widespread killer around the world. Concurrent with cardiac scaffolding, multi-functional intelligent materials are now starting to take their place in the rapidly expanding arena of 4D printing, presenting intriguing avenues for dynamic tissue engineering approaches. Smart materials that are capable of responding to various stimuli—such as temperature change, pH change, or mechanical stress—hold immense promise for creating responsive and dynamic heart tissues (Akrami et al., 2022). This technology has been employed to augment traditional bioprinting techniques to allow scientists to print scaffolds whose structural properties can dynamically change over time, thus presenting a supportive microenvironment that favors cell integration and tissue maturation. The development of such smart scaffolds is particularly important in cardiac tissue engineering because it can enhance implantation outcomes and tissue repair and integration after implantation. This convergence of material science and biomedical engineering not only fuels innovation but also promotes further research into the potential of 4D bioprinting in regenerative strategies. In view of the advances in organ printing, detailed understanding of diverse applications like artificial skin, cartilage, and liver tissue engineering becomes imperative. The technical innovations gained from cardiac tissue scaffolding offer valuable insights that can be transferred to other organ systems, greatly enhancing the manufacturing of functional tissue constructs needed for drug screening and disease modeling. For instance, bioprinted tissue derived from cardiac scaffolds can provide valuable platforms for therapeutic testing, allowing the accurate forecast of human responses compared to traditional preclinical models (Afridi et al., 2024). Besides, these advances position tissue engineering at the focal point in personalized medicine, where scaffolds tailored to one's biological pattern would be developed. In total, the trajectory of innovations towards cardiac scaffolding not only promotes the creation of living organ tissues but also enhances the fusion of engineering and medical sciences in addressing the growing public health challenge in organ failure.

7.3.3. Potential for Heart Disease Treatment Through Bioprinting

With the advent of newer bioprinting technologies, the applications of their use in heart disease therapy have become clearer. The new three-dimensional (3D) bioprinting technique integrates a variety of fields such as developmental biology and materials science to engineer the structures of bio-hybrid that can mimic human tissues. With the use of decellularized extracellular matrix (dECM) scaffolds derived from human donor organs, researchers have been able to develop organ and tissue models that are similar to normal human physiology. Specifically, with the addition of human pluripotent stem cells (hPSCs), researchers can recellularize the scaffolds to enable functional heart tissue growth. This parallel development of stem cell technology and bioprinting not only provides a model for engineering heart tissues but also offers a platform to develop further advances in regenerative medicine for the treatment of heart disease (Plana et al., 2017). The therapeutic applications of tissue created by bioprinting go beyond individual organ anatomy, such as use in artificial cartilage and skin, which would transform patient outcome in the treatment of cardiovascular disease. For instance, bioprinted skin grafts can facilitate wound healing and cosmetic improvement in cardiac surgery patients, while cartilage printing will correct related musculoskeletal deformities. The intricate role of the liver in drug metabolism and detoxification has also led to the need for bioprinted liver tissues that can mimic drug action. When scientists design complex tissue architectures in stacks of bio-inks with different kinds of stem cells, the precision of 3D bioprinting not only enables the reproduction of functional tissues but also the simulation of the pathophysiology of disease, giving valuable insight into mechanisms of heart disease (Cameron et al., 2017). In addition, integration of bioprinting in drug screening and disease modeling represents a revolution in biomedical science. Traditional *in vitro* models are not likely to exactly replicate the complexity of human tissue, which can be debilitating for drug performance. Cardiac tissues printed using bioprinting, designed to reflect the specific physiological properties of human myocardium, have been developed as a durable platform to measure cardiac response to novel therapeutics. Scientists can track interactions between drugs and bioengineered tissues in real time using bioprinting technologies, thus opening the door to more customized treatment strategies for heart disease. This interaction between drug screening and bioprinting not only accelerates biomedical innovation speed but also opens up novel avenues for the elucidation of pathophysiological mechanisms yet again highlighting organ and soft tissue printing as a pillar of modern regenerative medicine (Ameron et al., 2017; Plana et al., 2017) (Figure 7.9).

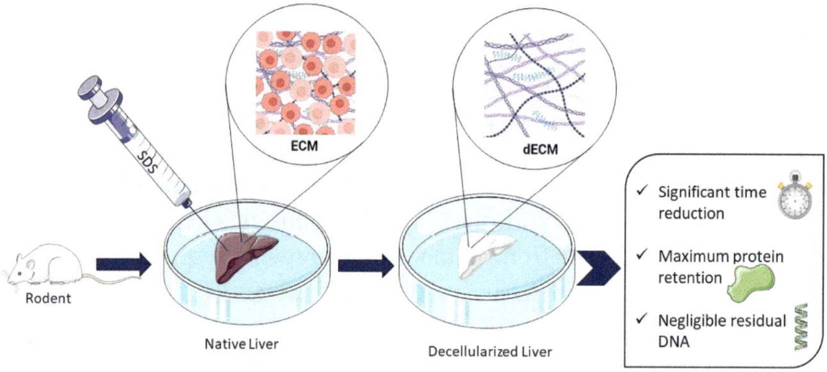

Figure 7.9. By utilizing decellularized extracellular matrix (dECM) scaffolds derived from human donor organs, researchers have been able to develop organ and tissue models that closely replicate natural human physiology.

Source: https://www.tandfonline.com/action/showGraphicalAbstractImage?doi=10.1080%2F21691401.2024.2319893&id=ianb_a_2319893_uf0001_c.jpg.

7.4. STEM CELLS IN ORGAN PRINTING

The intricate relationship between organ printing and stem cells is transforming the branch of regenerative medicine, particularly the construction of intricate tissues such as artificial cartilage, skin, and vital organs such as the heart and liver. Stem cells have the extraordinary ability to differentiate into specialized cells, therefore becoming a vital element in the creation of tissues that bear features close to what occurs naturally. By employing bioprinting, researchers can precisely layer these stem cells so that they create scaffolds upon which cells grow and become ordered into tissue. Not only can this facilitate the creation of functional tissue, but it has a basis for mass-scale application in drug testing and disease modeling as well. The incorporation of stem cells in organ printing is a revolution that can possibly resolve the shortage of donor organs and enhance therapeutic treatments in patients with chronic diseases. Furthermore, the potential of stem cells is not only the manufacturing of tissues but encompasses the delicacy of generating biocompatible scaffolds that promote integration within the human body. Recent advances in materials science have introduced innovations in hybrid polymer-based biomaterials, which may be designed to replicate the properties of various tissues. These biomaterials can support cellular growth and stimulate the deposition of extracellular matrix, playing a significant role in functional organ formation. For instance, biodegradable scaffold generation allows for the controlled delivery of growth factors, resulting in enhanced tissue regeneration. This is also supplemented by the integrated work of bioengineers, material scientists, and clinicians in attempting to develop ideal milieus for specific kinds of tissues to enhance the utilization of stem cells in organ printing and addressing a variety of medical complications associated with tissue regeneration and repair (Abalymov et al., 2020). The consequences of incorporating stem cells into organ and soft tissue printing extend beyond simple sonic engineering; they have the potential to revolutionize treatment interventions. For instance, in maxillofacial reconstructive surgery, the application of stem cells with very sophisticated scaffolding technology has been of considerable promise in restoring tissues of cartilage and bone to near-optimal levels. Preclinical testing has demonstrated the reconstitution of various tissue types, which indicates the potential of such bioprinted tissues in meeting the needs of individuals with severe trauma or congenital conditions (Almeida et al., 2017). Furthermore, drug testing through stem cell-derived tissues poses a new paradigm for modeling disease effectively and allowing researchers to test therapeutic response at the cellular level. This union of biology and technology not only encourages innovation in regenerative medicine but also provides an entry point to ethical considerations in the use of biodegradable products and living tissues for enhancing patient outcomes in the clinic.

7.4.1. Types of Stem Cells Used in Bioprinting

Bioprinting advancements have resulted in new methods of functional tissue production, and a variety of stem cell types of benefit with different advantages, particularly for skin, cartilage, and organ constructs. Pluripotent stem cells, such as induced pluripotent stem cells (iPSCs), are increasingly employed due to the ability to differentiate into nearly any cell type and thus act as a substrate for bioprinting. For instance, iPSCs can be engineered to make specialized skin cells that replicate the epidermal and dermal layers, providing a potential solution for the repair of burns and other skin wounds. Further, MSCs are employed to print cartilage, which helps with the treatment of degenerative joint diseases and enhancing the regenerative potential of cartilage by their ability to secrete trophic factors that promote tissue healing. In exploring organ constructs, liver tissue and heart tissue have been significant focus points in the study of bioprinting.

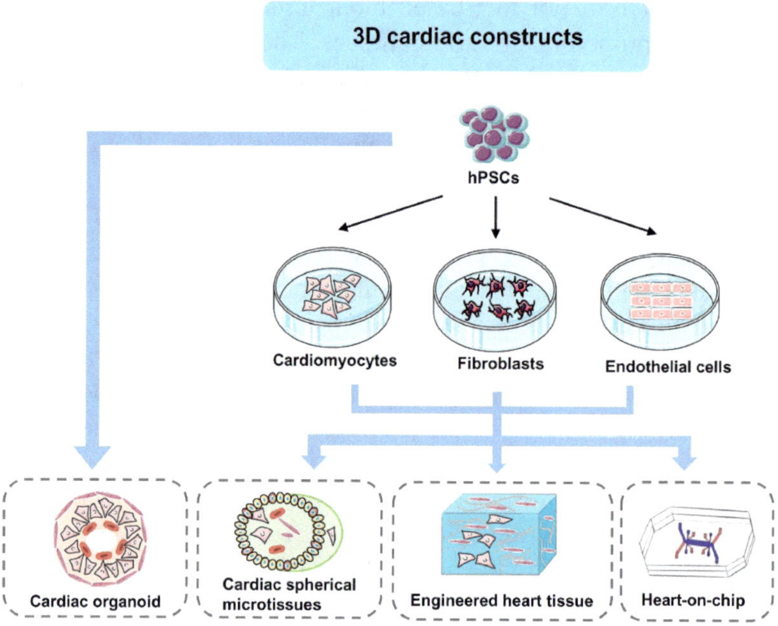

Figure 7.10. Pluripotent stem cells, such as induced pluripotent stem cells (iPSCs), are increasingly favored for their ability to differentiate into nearly any cell type, making them a cornerstone for bioprinting applications.

Source: https://www.thelancet.com/cms/10.1016/j.ebiom.2022.103813/asset/b503e059-dba3-4e2e-ae07-8f64222d4ec8/main.assets/gr2_lrg.jpg.

The use of hepatic stem cells in the construction of liver tissue permits the exploration of drug metabolism and disease progression *in vitro*, providing a highly sophisticated platform for drug testing and development. Cardiac stem cells, conversely, are of primary importance in bioprinting heart tissue, permitting scientists to examine the effect of varying conditions on the cardiac system. This kind of application has the potential to make significant contributions towards heart disease knowledge and drug intervention evaluation, thereby bridging the gap between clinical practice and *in vitro* research. Advances in bioprinting technologies are enabling the synthesis of these complex tissues and, in turn, offering new insights into organ function and pathology, eventually improving the treatment methodologies of cardiovascular and liver-related pathologies. Heterogeneity at the cellular level is critical in the replication of native tissues in close simulation, an aspect that informs the selection of appropriate stem cells to apply in the construction of functional constructs. For example, the introduction of additional cell types can provide strength and functionality to the resultant bioprinted product, providing opportunities for enhanced efficient modeling of disease. In addition, the co-axial wet-spinning extrusion technology has been regarded as an advanced method for achieving this complexity without compromising fidelity and print resolution (Barbetta et al., 2019). Integration of various bioinks, such as natural or synthetic polymeric components supported by stem cells, can also play a significant role in the mechanical properties and biological function of the printed tissue (Cameron et al., 2017). With such sophisticated methods, bioprinting is set to revolutionize the field of organ and soft tissue printing towards successful transplantation and regenerative medicine (Figure 7.10).

7.4.2. Advantages of Using Stem Cells for Tissue Regeneration

Stem cell use in tissue regeneration has a revolutionary potential in several fields of medicine, particularly organ and soft tissue printing. Employing stem cells to construct artificial skin, for instance, allows one to create grafts that can be used to heal and repair burns. This ability stems from the inherent ability of stem cells to differentiate into numerous different cell types, thereby mimicking the dermal natural condition. Consequently, not only do these tissue-engineered tissues show enhanced incorporation with host tissues but also reduce the risk of rejection and complications related to traditional grafts. Through the creation of techniques such as bioprinting, in which three-dimensional scaffolds are seeded in precise configurations, researchers find new avenues through which to replicate not only skin but also more complex tissues such as cartilage and organ shapes towards better outcomes in regenerative medicine (Abalymov et al., 2020). Cartilage and liver tissue studies through the use of stem cell techniques are another area of their regenerative ability. Cartilage, being an avascular tissue, is a difficult tissue to be repaired, but stem cells have proved capable of regenerating this critical structure, especially in patients with degenerative joint disorders. At the same time, advances made in liver tissue engineering confirm the promise of stem cells in regenerating functional hepatic tissues, which are crucial in most metabolic processes. This capability not only offers the potential for the treatment of liver injuries but also the creation of platforms for drug testing and disease modeling. With the integration of stem cells and bioprinting, microenvironments can be designed that are precisely controlled with the ability to replicate the native structure and function of these tissues, thereby facilitating more effective therapies and models (Chia et al., 2015). The incorporation of stem cells into organ printing technology represents a step towards personalized medicine, offering tailor-made therapeutic strategies that closely match the individual patient's specific requirements. The same strategy is also used in the fabrication of heart tissue, which plays a vital role in heart disease, one of the leading causes of mortality worldwide. The potential to print vascularized heart structures through bioprinting technology, not only raises hope for transplant patients but also offers invaluable resources for drug development and disease modeling. Patient-specific stem cell utilization enhances the authenticity of these models such that how responses to pharmacologic therapy can be better comprehensively understood and optimized. With continued advances in research, the rewards of using stem cells not only pave the way to functional organ regeneration but also open the door to revolutionary progress in disease research and treatment (Abalymov et al., 2020) (Figure 7.11).

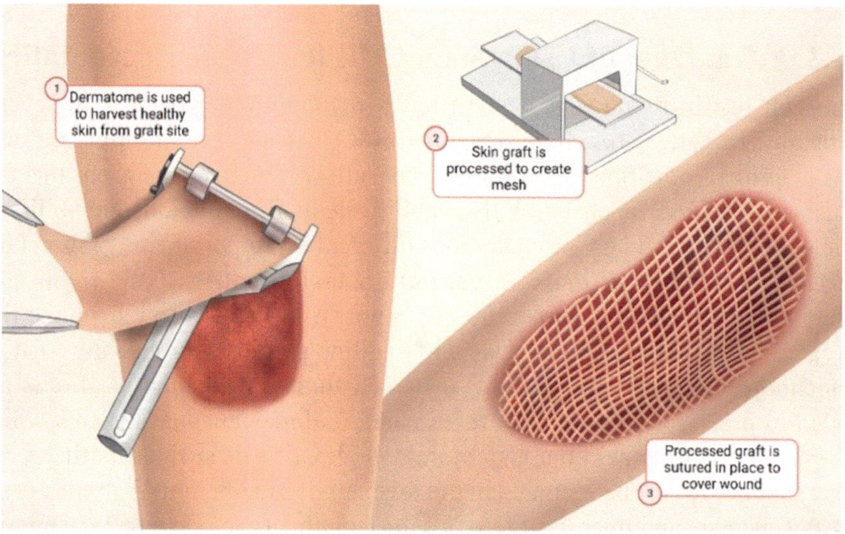

Figure 7.11. Utilizing stem cells to create artificial skin, for instance, allows for the development of grafts that can aid in wound healing and repair post-burn injuries.

Source: https://pub.mdpi-res.com/bioengineering/bioengineering-10-01378/article_deploy/html/images/bioengineering-10-01378-g002.png?1701327881.

7.4.3. Ethical Considerations Surrounding Stem Cell Use

The research into stem cell use in the context of organ and soft tissue printing raises a complicated debate about ethical issues that must be addressed. As bioprinting technology advances to enable the growth of artificial skin, cartilage, liver, and heart tissues, where stem cells are obtained becomes a priority concern. The ethical implications of employing embryonic stem cells, commonly derived from human embryos, elicit strong emotions and public debate. It is held by some that the potential to rescue lives in tissue engineering should be shouted from the rooftops, while others express ethical reservations based on the belief that life begins at conception. Such contradictory opinions necessitate a serious examination of the benefits of regenerative medicine and also the ethical issues of stem cell procurement, particularly in the context of organ replacements that would fundamentally transform the treatment of several degenerative diseases.

Moreover, the utilization of stem cells in organ printing raises matters of consent and commodification of human biological material. Instances of bioprinting technologies used for drug testing and disease modeling highlight the need for open policies regarding purchase and use of stem cells. Bioengineered tissue commercialization, even as it has the potential to lead to great improvements in medicine, can lead to unequal access to such technology. This has a tendency of deepening inequalities since the affluent have a greater opportunity to access sophisticated treatments and thus diminish the principle of universal access to healthcare.

It is important to address these ethical challenges to establish confidence in regenerative medicine technologies so that they serve the common good while being morally developed and sourced, supporting human dignity. In addition to individual rights and access disparities, long-term social implications of mass application of stem cells in organ and tissue printing must be considered. With the prospect of creating such highly intricate tissues as heart valves and liver cells, there is an implied responsibility to investigate and mitigate resultant harms from their use. Ensuring biocompatibility and avoiding harms are paramount in the clinic. The moral implications entail the risk of unforeseen consequences in human health and ecological equilibrium, following the increased manipulation of biological material. Further, as new 3D bioprinting technologies evolve, the discussion has to involve the scientists' ethical responsibility to prioritize safety and efficacy above any other factor, so that scientific progress stays in harmony with ethics and societal values, and establishes public trust in such cutting-edge applications of stem cells (Aebi et al., 2017; Birchall et al., 2016).

7.5. BIOPRINTING FOR DRUG TESTING

Bioprinting innovations have contributed significantly to the drug testing arena, particularly by the creation of artificial tissues that closely mimic human biological environments. Engineered tissues such as artificial skin and cartilage offer valuable platforms for testing the efficacy and safety of pharmacological drugs. Bioprinted constructs have the ability to replicate complex tissue architecture and function, thus allowing for more accurate drug responses than traditional 2D cell cultures. In addition, through the use of stem cells in tissue production, scientists are able to produce various cell types that mimic patient-specific biology. This diversity is important in determining individual drug responses and refining personalized medicine strategies. The build-up of such bioprinted models improves not only the reproducibility of drug testing but also facilitates the establishment of strategies against deleterious drug reactions, thus having a profound influence on improved patient safety and therapeutic outcomes (Cameron et al., 2017). The integration of 3D bioprinting into pharmaceutical research allows new *in vitro* models for better disease modeling and drug screening.

The generation of multilayered tissues from bioprinted structures, i.e., liver and heart tissue, is the promise of replicating organ-specific drug response. Techniques to create microscale tissue structures, as observed in work on developing integrated microfluidic devices, enable real-time pharmacokinetic evaluation. Bioprinted liver models, for instance, can disentangle metabolic profiles and toxicological reactions, enabling quick evaluation of drug candidates. These models enable researchers to examine the impact of drug interactions on cellular metabolism, and this leads to opportunities for the discovery of novel therapeutic approaches. By utilizing bioprinting technology, drug testing procedures can be enhanced in terms of efficacy and accuracy, leading to improved treatment eventually (Chang et al., 2006). In addition to the enhancement of drug testing processes, bioprinting presents opportunities in comprehensive disease modeling, particularly for those diseases that necessitate tissue-specific responses.

Structures from various stem cell sources can lead to the generation of complex heterogenous tissue that mimics cell signaling networks as in organs of nature. Some examples include the use of bioprinted cardiac tissues, where scientists would examine the effect of drugs on heart activity and learn about cardiotoxicity. The ability to produce these focused constructs not only accelerates drug discovery but also allows dissecting disease mechanisms so that targeted therapies can follow. Furthermore, as the technologies get better, the potential to harness cells from individual patients will increase the relevance of drug test models by enabling more realistic models of disease states. Thus, bioprinting is an essential tool in maximizing both therapeutic approaches and our understanding of a number of diseases (Cameron et al., 2017).

7.5.1. Advantages of Using Printed Tissues for Pharmacological Studies

The study of artificial skin and other tissues in the course of pharmacological research is the ultimate example of the modern advancement possible through organ and soft tissue printing. With the use of bioprinting techniques, researchers are able to create intricate structures that closely mirror human tissues, simplifying the process of creating more precise *in vitro* models. Artificial skin, for instance, allows researchers to assess topical drugs and the healing process, thus providing them with information two-dimensional cultures do not. In addition, tailoring of artificial tissues also enables strategies for personalized medicine, where drug effects can be evaluated in terms of individual patient-derived cellular mixtures. These advances in reproducibility and pharmaceutical relevance of pharmacological studies show tremendous advantages of printed tissues towards further integration into future medical research and drug development. Another potential application lies in liver and cartilage tissue bioprinting, which is significant for physiological and pharmacological functions. Cartilage models present a previously unexplored opportunity to explore joint-associated diseases and the efficacy of anti-inflammatory drugs and enable accurate prediction of therapeutic efficacy. Similarly, printed liver tissue is capable of replicating drug metabolism in the liver, thus enabling scientists to analyze the pharmacokinetics and toxicity of chemicals under a controlled environment. This aspect bridges the gap between *in vivo* and *in vitro* studies, which hitherto has been difficult to link. The construction of bioprinted tissues therefore not only enhances the drug interaction knowledge but also the reduction of animal models usage, thereby aligning with the international standards in present research. The use of stem cells in organ printing further enhances the advantages of printed tissues for pharmacological studies. Stem cells possess the unique characteristic of differentiation and have the potential to develop into various cell types required to form functional tissues, such as cardiac or hepatic cells. Such a possibility of generating patient-specific tissues by this approach can lead to more targeted drug testing and disease modeling and eventually to precision medicine. Further, cell entrapment in hydrogels also offers controlled microenvironmental conditions specific to cellular function, supporting tissue viability and functionality. As elaborated in the literature, Abalymov et al. (2020) stresses that molecular delivery systems incorporated into biomaterials support drug delivery and bioactivity. Use of these advanced methods in drug research will most likely open up breakthroughs in disease mechanisms and drug treatments, further solidifying the place of printed tissues in modern medical science (Figure 7.12).

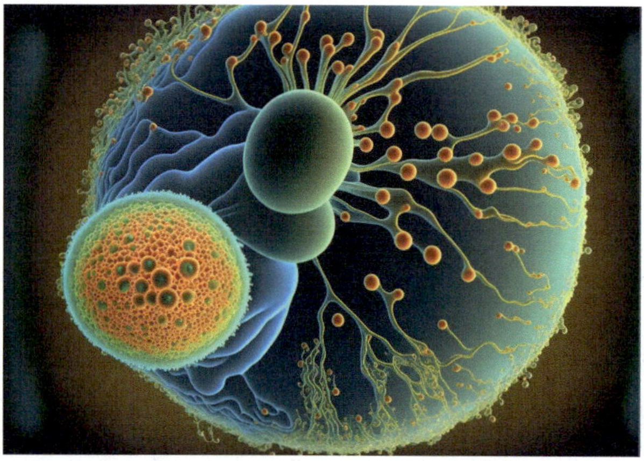

Figure 7.12. Stem cells possess the unique characteristic of differentiation, allowing them to develop into various cell types necessary for creating functional tissues, such as cardiac or hepatic cells.

Source: https://cdn.prod.website-files.com/5d9667bad4a41e222995e15b/63d44713a930ee51916600e4_embryonic%20stem%20cell%202%20copy.webp.

7.5.2. Case Studies Demonstrating Successful Drug Testing

The convergence of organ and soft tissue printing has created major breakthroughs in drug testing methods, especially with the creation of artificial skin and other tissue types. Most significant of all is the development of bioengineered skin that has dramatically changed preclinical testing by offering a more human environment than animal models have to offer. Scientists have demonstrated that these skin models can accurately mimic *in vivo* conditions, thus enabling it to measure drug absorption, toxicity, and efficacy accurately. Such advancements not only enhance drug testing predictability but are also in line with ethical considerations by reducing animal testing. Additionally, these artificial skin models are valuable platforms for the evaluation of dermatologic treatments and suggest serious ramifications for pharmaceutical use and the treatment of patients. In parallel with skin models, cartilage and organ tissue bioprinting of liver and heart has also been found to be positive in drug testing models. Various works of research have pointed to stem cell application in the engineering of these tissues, which are found to have better functional qualities than those engineered in 2D culture. For instance, drug-treatable cartilage tissue engineered from human stem cells can be used to assess the effectiveness of osteoarthritis drugs therapeutically. Liver tissue constructs can also be used to model metabolic processes, providing valuable information on drug metabolism and hepatotoxicity. The application of these advanced tissue models not only strengthens the pipeline of drug testing but also opens the way for new breakthroughs in the area of personalized medicine, where therapy can be formulated based on differential responses *in vitro*. Besides, the application of cardiac tissues from bioprinting technology has transformed drug testing and disease modeling. Stem cells that are used to prepare myocardial constructs allow researchers to investigate drug response in conditions that are extremely similar to human cardiac physiology. These tissue-engineered constructs enable the exploration of new treatments for cardiac disease while providing useful information on arrhythmias and other heart diseases. The flexibility of these models serves to explain disease mechanisms and facilitate candidate drug screening in a controlled environment. As technology advances, the integration of sophisticated fabrication techniques, such as optofluidic fabrication and microfluidics-based hydrogels, as outlined by Chung et al. (2015) and Bae et al. (2012), is likely to enhance organ printing processes' quality and effectiveness, eventually culminating in a new revolution in drug testing that is not only ethical but scientifically sound.

7.5.3. Future Prospects for Bioprinting in Pharmaceutical Development

Bioprinting technology development is going to significantly change the pharmaceutical development process, particularly in artificial tissue manufacturing such as skin, cartilage, and other organ constructs. The intricate layering of living cells embedded into the bioinks allows for the manufacturing of tissues that will be able to mimic the natural form and function of human organs. For instance, advances in bioprinting have allowed scientists to design artificial skin that can be utilized for drug efficacy and toxicity screening and thus reduce the application of animal models in pharmaceutical research. With the advancement in regenerative medicine, the integration of stem cells into bioprinting programs also holds great promise in creating functional cardiac and hepatic tissues, hence making way for new avenues of disease modeling and therapeutic applications. These advances will ultimately lead to the enhanced understanding of physiological responses and drug screening techniques, ensuring a faster and more efficient path to drug discovery (Kumar et al., 2023). In addition, the utility of bioprinting for drug screening also includes the potential to create organ-specific models, enabling researchers to screen drug interactions in target tissues. Development of functional cardiac and liver tissues through bioprinting can be used as critical testing platforms to predict metabolic responses and cardiac effects of new drugs. Pharmaceutical companies, using such bioprinted models, are likely to conduct more accurate *in vitro* screening, thereby enhancing the predictability of clinical response. The ability to print complex tissue architectures that closely replicate the natural organ microenvironment also provides new opportunities in personalized medicine, where therapies can be tailored to individual patient profiles. Lastly, these developments emphasize the promise of bioprinting technologies not only in advancing drug testing paradigms but also shortening the gap between research in the lab and clinical practice (Fernandes et al., 2017). The application of bioprinting in drug development also creates challenges to be overcome to realize its full potential. Maintaining viability and function of printed tissues poses technical challenges, given that cells need to perform their physiological functions within the engineered tissues. Additionally, regulatory aspects concerning the application of bioprinted tissues for drug testing and clinical use need to be addressed to guarantee safety and efficacy. Ethical concerns over the use of stem cells and the implications of bioprinting human organ tissue will also come into focus as the technology advances. Nonetheless, continued research and collaboration between scientists, ethicists, and regulatory bodies will be essential to overcome these obstacles. With these issues solved in an orderly manner, the prospects for bioprinting in drug development appear brighter still, holding out the promise of a new morning both in drug development and regenerative medicine (Kumar et al., 2023) (Figure 7.13).

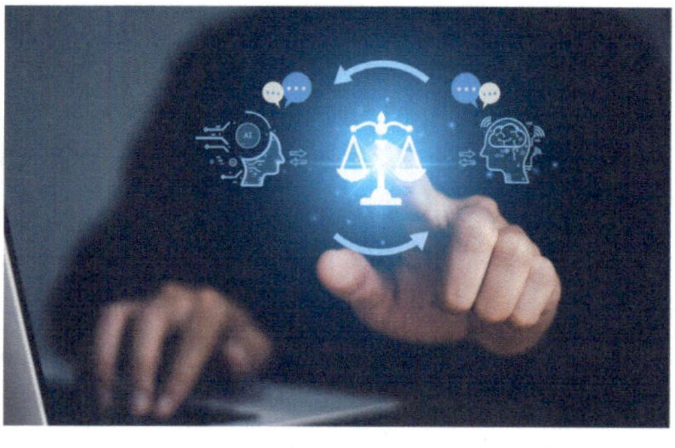

Figure 7.13. Ethical considerations surrounding the use of stem cells and the implications of bioprinting human organ tissues will also garner attention as this technology advances.

Source: https://images.squarespace-cdn.com/content/v1/56a042fb25981d9326c9bbdb/0858ce4b-8054-49b0-9d28-7f815d32fbe7/Ethical+Considerations+in+Clinical+Trials+blog+image.png.

7.6. DISEASE MODELING WITH BIOPRINTED TISSUES

Advances in bioprinting technology have made it possible to fabricate intricate tissue structures with high accuracy in relation to human organ physiological attributes. Of particular note is the fabrication of artificial skin, which is of relevance when studying wound healing and the effects of various dermatological treatments. Utilization of various cell types such as keratinocytes and fibroblasts makes it possible for researchers to create layered structures that can mimic epidermis and dermis. This new technique not only is used as a testing site for drugs but also serves to clarify disease formation and therapeutic responses in skin diseases. Furthermore, the use of stem cells within these scaffolds makes them more regenerative competent, allowing one to examine cellular differentiation processes as well as the effects of external influences upon skin status and disease (Plana et al., 2017).

On a wider scale, bioprinting of organs such as cartilage, liver, and heart has revolutionized disease modeling studies, offering information on pathologies such as osteoarthritis, liver fibrosis, and heart disease that was not earlier accessible. Engineered tissues, which commonly consist of various cell types and biomaterials, can be employed to model disease states *in vitro*. For instance, cartilage bioprinted might be subjected to mechanical stress to study the process of degradation with respect to arthritis, while liver tissues might be employed to study drug-induced liver injury (Aleman et al., 2016). Stem cells that are derived from sources varying from one to another can be employed to build patient-specific models improving the accuracy of disease research and therapeutic response, ultimately resulting in personalized medicine approaches formulated based on individual patient requirements.

Furthermore, the potential of bioprinted tissues does not stop at modeling; these constructs are drug-testing platforms, and therapeutic agents can be tested in a controlled environment. Traditional drug testing methods are riddled with human predictability of response issues. Engineered tissue models, like liver replication, offer a more accurate simulation of drug metabolism and toxicity. This innovative application not only streamlines the drug development pipeline but also reduces the reliance on animal testing, which aligns with ethical research considerations. As there is progress in organ and soft tissue printing technology, the use of bioprinted tissues for disease modeling and drug screening has the potential to strongly affect preclinical drug discovery and therapeutic development in regenerative medicine (Aleman et al., 2016; Plana et al., 2017).

7.6.1. Importance of Disease Models in Research

The success of organ and soft tissue printing relies heavily on the development of accurate disease models that can mimic human physiological status. The work has been motivated by the need to investigate intricate diseases due to the ineffectiveness of traditional *in vitro* and *in vivo* models to replicate the precise biochemical and mechanical interactions of human tissues. For instance, bioprinting processes involving artificial skin, cartilage, and heart tissue can significantly enhance our ability to study the pathophysiology of diseases like diabetes, heart disease, and arthritis. Such engineered tissues can also serve as platforms for drug testing so that investigators are able to observe how therapy could interact with living cells and thus have information about the efficacy and safety of the therapy before clinical trials. Moreover, organ printing with stem cells also promises the development of patient-specific tissues, planned not only for studying disease mechanisms but also for facilitating tailored therapies. With continuous advancements in bioprinting technologies, disease modeling has emerged as a key aspect of organ printing. By printing three-dimensional structures closely approximating native tissue, researchers are able to explore the mechanisms of disease at a previously unimaginable degree of detail. For example, drug toxicity and metabolism can be studied using liver tissue models printed with bioprinting, contributing to the knowledge of liver disease and drug interaction. Similarly, bioprinted heart tissues can be used to explore arrhythmia and heart failure and develop new therapies. The employment of bio-inks constituted of cells, polymers, and extracellular matrix proteins increases the functionality of such models to develop a yet tighter integration between fundamental research and clinical application. Disciplinary convergence in this instance underscores the importance of disease models in the sense that not only do they provide information on disease mechanisms but also allow for the testing and verification of bioprinted tissues as reliable testing platforms. The uses of disease models extend beyond basic research; they are also of utmost importance in the field of regenerative medicine. As has been noted in recent studies, the integration of 3D bioprinting with next-generation biomaterials enables the ability to fabricate multifunctional scaffolds that possess the mechanical properties of native tissues, thereby promoting cell growth and function (Abalymov et al., 2020). In addition, disease models generated via bioprinting allow for drug screening in a more physiologically relevant setting, increasing the predictive value of preclinical studies (Cameron et al., 2017). This process not only speeds up the drug development process but also minimizes the use of animal models, encouraging ethical research protocols. As organ and soft tissue printing continues to develop, the ability to make and utilize disease models will be central to revolutionizing how we approach addressing the treatment of complex health conditions, providing a more efficient and customized medicine environment (Figure 7.14).

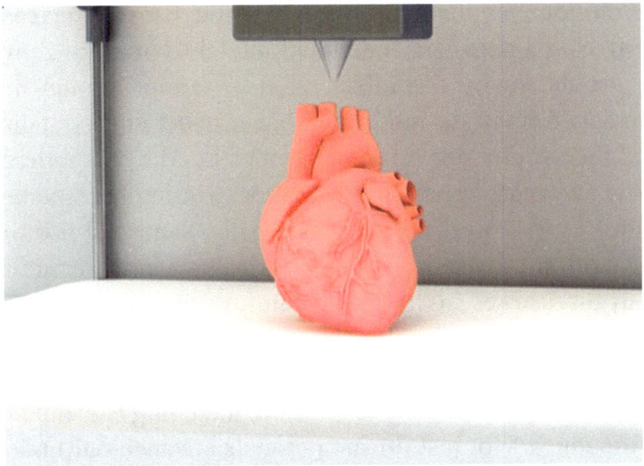

Figure 7.14. Bioprinting techniques that incorporate artificial skin, cartilage, and heart tissues can significantly enhance our ability to study the pathophysiology of conditions like diabetes, heart disease, and arthritis.

Source: https://www.labiotech.eu/wp-content/uploads/2019/04/tissue-bioprinting-heart-israel-1200x900.jpg.

7.6.2. Examples of Diseases Modeled Using Bioprinted Tissues

Recent technological developments in bioprinting have greatly expanded the range to model numerous diseases by printing bioprinted tissues. One of the major uses is the construction of artificial skin, which provides a critical platform for the study of skin-associated diseases such as psoriasis and dermatitis. Using three-dimensional printing techniques, researchers can mimic the complex architecture of human skin, including elements like dermal fibroblasts and epidermal keratinocytes. It allows for more advanced understanding of disease pathophysiology and treatment response. Moreover, drug-testing platforms can be deployed using bioprinted skin tissues, allowing one to assess the efficacy and toxicity of drugs without the ethical conundrum of animal use. These new technologies promise a future with a more efficient, personalized, and more humane process of developing drugs, attesting to the high stakes of organ and soft tissue printing in modern medicine. The usefulness of bioprinted tissues extends to other major uses, including cartilage regeneration and simulation of liver disease. For instance, bioprinted cartilage has been shown to model conditions like osteoarthritis, which affects millions of individuals globally. Using scaffolds with the same biomechanical properties as native cartilage, scientists are more likely to explore the onset and treatment of disease. Similarly, bioprinted liver tissues are revolutionizing the treatment of hepatic diseases such as cirrhosis or hepatitis by offering a real-like, functional model to investigate liver function and toxicity. As shown by the intersection of computational modeling and bioink design, data from tissue models enable a deeper understanding of disease pathology and therapeutic response, as demonstrated by Laporte et al. (2020). With these new methods, organ and soft tissue printing become key players in the fight against long-term disease. Additionally, stem cell use in bioprinting creates a new path in disease modeling, particularly in the creation of cardiac tissue for heart disease research. The dynamics of cardiovascular disease call for a model that is capable of replicating the dynamic personality of the heart. By using stem cells to create bioprinted cardiac tissues, scientists can study the cellular response towards various pathologies, including ischemic heart disease and cardiomyopathies. Not just do such models advance our understanding of cardiac functions but also give rise to the development of personalized medicine approaches where patient-specific tissues can be created for the screening of drugs and therapy evaluation. The ability of bioprinted systems to demonstrate their strength is proven through their ability to offer flow conditions that mimic blood circulation, therefore optimizing drug delivery strategies as shown in studies based on engineered hydrogel formats, according to Parodi et al. (2025). The marriage between stem cell technology and organ printing strategies is instrumental in advancing preclinical studies and therapy plans.

7.6.3. Impact of Disease Modeling on Personalized Medicine

The synergy between disease modeling and personalized medicine is increasingly key, particularly organ and tissue printing. Advances in stem cell technology have pushed the development of artificial cartilage, skin, liver, and heart tissues, which have made it possible for an era when patient-specific treatment can become the new standard in the not-so-distant future. The constructed tissues are not only regenerative medicine tools but also valuable platforms for disease modeling. By the recreation of human organ cellular makeup and microenvironment, researchers can now research disease processes, drug action, and treatment within a controlled setting. It supports more effective treatment strategies tailored to specific needs of individual patients, thereby underlining the significance of personalized medicine in contemporary healthcare. Lastly, the coming together of these technologies has the promise to further enhance patient outcomes as well as widen the gap between bench and clinical translation immensely. Building on the foundation established by advances in bioprinting technologies, the engineering of functional organ constructs plays a dual role in understanding human diseases and charting the map toward personalized treatment options. The employment of decellularized extracellular matrix (dECM) scaffolds that are obtained from human donor organs and human pluripotent stem cells (hPSCs) allows the recellularization of scaffolds with diverse cell types needed for organ function. This enhances not only the physiological applicability of the printed tissue but also allows research into how a certain disease affects cellular response within such constructs. The ability to print a patient's own individual biological environment with 3D bioprinting effectively transforms traditional drug testing paradigms since drug efficacy can be assessed with respect to patient-derived tissues to optimize the translational value of research in personalized medicine (Plana et al., 2017). Organ printing also has applications in the modeling of disease, advancing our understanding of drug efficacy and safety. Bioprinted tissues provide a more sophisticated platform for drug response testing, allowing for higher fidelity determinations that can reduce the need for animal testing and offer more suitable data for human therapeutics. By integrating patient-specific characteristics into these models, personalized medicine is significantly enhanced, allowing for tailored therapeutics that are closer to the varied genetic and phenotypic context within the patient population. Thus, as organ and soft tissue printing advances, the knowledge obtained through disease modeling will certainly shed light on the routes to better, personalized treatment approaches that have the potential to transform patient care (Azouna et al., 2016).

7.7. CONCLUSION

The advances in soft tissue and organ printing announce a new era in regenerative medicine when traditional limits in medicine might be overstepped. At the top of the most promising opportunities are the creation of replacement skin, cartilage, liver, and heart tissues, which showcase the capability of bioprinting techniques to replicate the complexity of human organs. Interestingly, the use of stem cells within this procedure provides an increased possibility for these bioprinted tissues to be more biocompatible and functionally incorporated upon implantation. This incorporation is key, in that the ultimate goal is not only to create tissue but to create tissue capable of sustaining function within an organism and therefore fill the pressing need for organ transplantation and disease treatment through degenerative disease. Lessons learned from challenges faced in developments of organ printing technology unlock the door to innovation. Nanogels-based tissue development—a top area of 3D printing—has unlocked a variety of biomedical applications, including tissue regeneration and drug delivery systems (Cho et al., 2018). Nanogel application extends to their inclusion in bioprinting, which advances precision in creating patient-specific constructs that cater to their individual biological needs. With increasing demand for personalized medicine, the role of 3D printing technology becomes more important with each passing day, hinting that with these technologies advancing, these will change the way we approach organ replacement and rehabilitation. In addition, the promise of organ and soft tissue printing extends beyond transplantation; drug development and disease modeling are given a new window of opportunity with the technology. Through the application of bioprinted tissues, researchers are in a position to design more accurate *in vitro* models that replicate human physiological responses and hence improve the process of drug discovery. The models allow for the assessment of drug efficacy and safety through mechanisms closely mimicking patient responses, thereby avoiding the use of the traditional animal models. Furthermore, technological advances in interfacing microtechnologies have made feasible the recording of high-resolution nerves, permitting an insight into disease mechanisms and treatment outcomes (Alice et al., 2019). The synergy of such advanced technologies, thus, facilitates a holistic approach to health beyond the traditional paradigms, a new frontier in medical science and patient therapy.

7.7.1. Summary of Key Points Discussed

Advances in the field of organ and soft tissue printing have facilitated overwhelming progress in developing functional tissues such as artificial skin, cartilage, liver, and heart tissue. The application of three-dimensional (3D) bioprinting methods allows for the serial layering of biomaterials and cells, resulting in constructs that virtually mirror the complex structure and function of native tissues. This capability can be observed most prominently in the development of artificial skin, which may serve as a protective and functional barrier in severely burned or chronically wounded patients. Bioprinted cartilage also holds the potential to minimize joint injuries through the replacement of the intricate architecture of this load-bearing tissue. These advancements are a testament to the promising future of regenerative medicine, with not only alternatives to organ transplant but also aiding patients in recovering and enhancing their well-being. Stem cells have been the focal point in the recellularization of human donor organ-derived decellularized extracellular matrix (dECM) scaffolds that retain the original natural structure for proper tissue integration and regeneration. Specifically, human pluripotent stem cells (hPSCs) have proven to be a cell source with versatility to seed these scaffolds with all the required cell types that are capable of facilitating the development of functional organs. Through this new approach, researchers can generate personalized tissue grafts for individual patients, which is a critical step towards the end of the organ shortage crisis. Moreover, the employment of patients own cells for recellularization of organs reduces the risk of rejection and facilitates compatible integration with host tissue, which has been a major contribution of organ printing. Besides regenerative medicine, bioprinting technology has been highly beneficial in drug screening and disease modeling, which gives an opportunity for high-throughput drug analysis in regard to pharmaceutical-pharmacology or the manner in which a drug will respond to human tissues. By creating 3D tissue constructs that mimic disease states, researchers can observe cellular response to compounds within a representative and controlled system. Not only is this more predictive of drug safety and efficacy, but it also decreases reliance on traditional animal models, which themselves are limited in their ability to accurately represent human biology. The potential of these developments is realized in the development of therapeutics specifically designed to treat specific conditions, highlighting the multidimensional value of organ and soft tissue printing. As research into the subject area continues, it holds the potential to transform not just transplant medicine but the whole landscape of drug development and individualized healthcare.

7.7.2. Future Directions for Organ and Soft Tissue Printing

The landscape of organ and soft tissue printing is about to see revolutionary innovations, with the power of advanced techniques of bioprinting that are capable of enabling the fabrication of complex tissues. Among the developments is the growing focus on artificial skin, which has immense possibilities not only for treating burn patients but also for cosmetic purposes. Stem cell integration into the printing process is most promising in that stem cells are able to enhance printed tissue regenerative capabilities. Moreover, the techniques employed for culturing stem cells are becoming increasingly enhanced, and scientists anticipate that the printed construct will better reflect the natural tissues, which will enhance biocompatibility and function. Besides, artificial skin printed through bioprinting could also serve as a platform for drug testing for pharmaceuticals, enabling drugs to be tested more efficiently in a controlled setting closely mimicking human skin, hence eliminating further use of animal testing, and enhancing preclinical analysis accuracy. Technologies for printing complex structures such as cartilage emphasize another promising area for soft tissue printing. This is particularly crucial for patients with joint disease because traditional treatments fail to restore function to any significant degree. Tissue engineers have been exploring hybrid materials made of biodegradable polymers and inorganic components, enabling them to design scaffolds that can closely replicate the mechanical properties of natural cartilage (Abalymov et al., 2020). This approach not only facilitates cell proliferation and growth but also supports the development of extracellular matrix (ECM), an essential element in tissue engineering. With innovative technology, the capability to create tailor-made cartilage grafts will be facilitated, offering personalized treatment to patients. This can conveniently alleviate the influence of joint diseases and improve the life of patients. In parallel, the objective of bioprinting complicated organ geometries like the heart and liver is gaining popularity with researchers in the past few years. Liver tissues, which control numerous body functions, are being researched extensively to develop viable hepatic constructs with the capability of metabolizing drugs and disease modeling. Additionally, efforts toward the creation of heart tissue aim to develop cellularized constructs that mimic cardiac function and assist in research related to cardiovascular disease (Barbetta et al., 2019). Additionally, studies on enhanced methods of bioprinting, particularly co-axial wet-spinning extrusion, offer new possibilities in overcoming challenges associated with printing fidelity and material variability. Such technology is applicable for the layering of various cell types and biomaterials to form multicellular constructs that closely resemble native organ structures. The future of organ and soft tissue printing therefore has much potential to provide unprecedented methods of drug testing and the observation of complex disease processes.

7.7.3. Final Thoughts on the Implications for Healthcare and Research

Recent organ and soft tissue printing technology has illuminated the path to ground-breaking health applications, particularly through the development of artificial skin, cartilage, and multi-layered organ architecture such as liver and heart tissues. Bioprinting with stem cells presents unprecedented regenerative medicine potential. This feature allows for tailor-made arrangements of tissue that mimic the original biological characteristics of the patient and hence enhance compatibility and reduce the risk of rejection. Secondly, the use of such bioprinted structures in implantation can be combined to develop tailor-made treatment regimens to overcome the personalized demands of every patient. As technology continues to improve techniques of tissue engineering and bioprinting, the ability to create living tissues that can be employed to cover injured or degenerating areas of the body becomes increasingly viable, marking the dawn of a new era in personalized medicine that may transform patient outcomes in revolutionary means. The promise of such technology does not end at drug screening and disease modeling, either. Bioprinted tissue is also applied as a precise model, simulating human response to drugs, eliminating altogether the traditional approach of animal testing. Such advancements rationalize drug development, avoiding time and cost while maximizing predictive value of drug response. Specific applications, for example, printed liver tissue allow not just an enhanced insight into metabolic function but more effective screening for hepatotoxicity, significantly avoiding side effects in clinical use. Further, advancements in microfluidic systems further enhance these models by allowing for more intricate cellular interactions that accurately reflect true physiological conditions. This union of research and real-world use reflects the revolutionary scope of organ and soft tissue printing in both the pharmaceutical and healthcare sectors, offering new frontiers for exploration and discovery. In summary, the way of organ and soft tissue printing is clearly leading to a future where medicine is becoming more defined by innovations derived from bioprinting technologies. With methods changing, the potential for 3D-printed organs could make the lack of organ donors become a norm, offering not only substitutes for failing organs but also personalized solutions according to the disease states of individuals. Enhanced regenerative capacity, coupled with personalized therapies based on such technologies, represents a paradigm shift toward treating medical conditions and managing patients. There is a need to meet the ethical, regulatory, and technical challenges underlying such advances. Continued research, coupled with reflective consideration of the societal implications, will ensure that the potential for such technologies to be actualized is so done in a responsible and effective manner, paving the way for extensive advancement in healthcare and research contexts (Bechthold et al., 2015; Casanova et al., 2024).

REFERENCES

1. Abalymov, A., Parakhonskiy, B., & Skirtach, A. (2020). Polymer- and hybrid-based biomaterials for interstitial, connective, vascular, nerve, visceral and musculoskeletal tissue engineering. https://core.ac.uk/download/299792280.pdf (accessed on 14th October 2025).
2. Aebi, M., Ahmed, A., Ahn, J., Aho, T., Aibe, N., Akmal, M., Alan, B., et al. (2017). 3D bioactive composite scaffolds for bone tissue engineering. https://core.ac.uk/download/141194116.pdf (accessed on 14th October 2025).
3. Afridi, F., Alaoui, C. H., Chigr, M., Fatimi, A., et al. (2024). Recent progress in hydrogel-based bioinks for 3D bioprinting: A patent landscape analysis and technology updates. https://core.ac.uk/download/620924710.pdf (accessed on 14th October 2025).
4. Akrami, M., Bodaghi, M., Karamimoghadam, M., Sahafnejad-Mohammadi, S., et al. (2022). 4D printing technology in medical engineering: A narrative review. https://core.ac.uk/download/519709208.pdf (accessed on 14th October 2025).
5. Aleman, J., Assawes, P., Bakht, S. M., Dell'Erba, A., et al. (2016). 3D bioprinting for tissue and organ fabrication. https://core.ac.uk/download/78071761.pdf (accessed on 14th October 2025).
6. Almeida, L. E., Dashtimoghadam, E., Fahimipour, F., Jazayeri, A., et al. (2017). A current overview of materials and strategies for potential use in maxillofacial tissue regeneration. https://core.ac.uk/download/213072267.pdf (accessed on 14th October 2025).
7. Amrollahi, P., Seifi, A., Shah, B., Tayebi, L., et al. (2016). Recent advancements in regenerative dentistry: A review. https://core.ac.uk/download/213080485.pdf (accessed on 14th October 2025).
8. Asadian, M., De Geyter, N., De Moor, L., Declercq, H., et al. (2020). Hybrid bioprinting of chondrogenically induced human mesenchymal stem cell spheroids. https://core.ac.uk/download/323232718.pdf (accessed on 14th October 2025).
9. Azouna, N. B., Goncalves, A. I., Introna, M., Khoshbin, A., Kim, J. Y., Leferink, A. M., Popa, E. G., et al. (2016). Current approaches and future perspectives on strategies for the development of personalized tissue engineering therapies. https://core.ac.uk/download/55640855.pdf (accessed on 14th October 2025).
10. Badi, L., Berrera, M., Bishop, R., Certa, A., et al. (2015). Functional analysis and transcriptional output of the Göttingen minipig genome.

https://core.ac.uk/download/33303086.pdf (accessed on 14th October 2025).

11. Bae, H., Dokmeci, M., Khademhosseini, A., Oh, J., et al. (2012). Microscale strategies for generating cell-encapsulating hydrogels. https://core.ac.uk/download/78053361.pdf (accessed on 14th October 2025).
12. Barbetta, A., Colosi, C., Costantini, M., Święszkowski, W., et al. (2019). Co-axial wet-spinning in 3D bioprinting: State of the art and future perspective of microfluidic integration. https://core.ac.uk/download/188825522.pdf (accessed on 14th October 2025).
13. Bechthold, L., Fischer, V., Hainzlmaier, A., Hugenroth, H., et al. (2015). 3D printing: A qualitative assessment of applications, recent trends and the technology's future potential. http://hdl.handle.net/10419/156627 (accessed on 14th October 2025).
14. Birchall, M. A., Mehrban, N., & Teoh, G. Z. (2016). 3D bioprinting for tissue engineering: Stem cells in hydrogels. https://core.ac.uk/download/79497944.pdf (accessed on 14th October 2025).
15. Blunk, T., Boland, T., Burdick, J. A., Cho, D. W., et al. (2016). Bio fabrication: Reappraising the definition of an evolving field. https://core.ac.uk/download/77034391.pdf (accessed on 14th October 2025).
16. Cameron, N. R., Donderwinkel, I., & van Hest, J. C. M. (2017). Bio-inks for 3D bioprinting: Recent advances and future prospects. https://core.ac.uk/download/110168777.pdf (accessed on 14th October 2025).
17. Campistol Plana, J. M., Fernández Avilés, F., Garreta, E., Montserrat, N., et al. (2017). Tissue engineering by decellularization and 3D bioprinting. https://core.ac.uk/download/83830377.pdf (accessed on 14th October 2025).
18. Carvalho, C., Landers, R., & Mülhaupt, R. (2004). Soft and hard implant fabrication using 3D-Bioplotting TM. https://core.ac.uk/download/287648471.pdf (accessed on 14th October 2025).
19. Casanova, C. R., Casanova, M. A. R., Oliveira, J. M., Reis, R. L., et al. (2024). Advancing diagnostics and disease modeling: Current concepts in bio fabrication of soft microfluidic systems. https://core.ac.uk/download/619582162.pdf (accessed on 14th October 2025).
20. Chang, R., Culbertson, C., Gonda, S., Holtorf, D., et al. (2006). Freeform bioprinting of liver encapsulated in alginate hydrogels tissue constructs for pharmacokinetic study. https://core.ac.uk/download/287648502.pdf (accessed on 14th October 2025).

21. Chia, H. N., & Wu, B. M. (2015). Recent advances in 3D printing of biomaterials. https://core.ac.uk/download/323078409.pdf (accessed on 14th October 2025).
22. Cho, H., Jammalamadaka, U., & Tappa, K. (2018). Nanogels for pharmaceutical and biomedical applications and their fabrication using 3D printing technologies. https://core.ac.uk/download/212859248.pdf (accessed on 14th October 2025).
23. Chung, A. J., Di Carlo, D., & Paulsen, K. S. (2015). Optofluidic fabrication for 3D-shaped particles. https://core.ac.uk/download/323076965.pdf (accessed on 14th October 2025).
24. De Laporte, L., & Duarte Campos, D. F. (2020). Digitally fabricated and naturally augmented *in vitro* tissues. https://core.ac.uk/download/525035337.pdf (accessed on 14th October 2025).
25. Elmahjub, N. A. (2025). Bioengineering advances in tissue regeneration: Current trends and future prospects. https://core.ac.uk/download/663684355.pdf (accessed on 14th October 2025).
26. Fernandes, E. M., Oliveira, J. M., Pina, S. C. A., Reis, R. L., et al. (2017). Natural-origin materials for tissue engineering and regenerative medicine. https://core.ac.uk/download/132797692.pdf (accessed on 14th October 2025).
27. Parikh, D., & Shah, M. (2024). 3D bioprinting–Recent advances in tissue regeneration. https://core.ac.uk/download/658783618.pdf (accessed on 14th October 2025).
28. Parodi, I. (2025). Engineering 3D *in vitro* tissue models through integrated computational and experimental approaches. https://core.ac.uk/download/661555116.pdf (accessed on 14th October 2025).
29. White, A. E., Lee, B., Holinski, B. J., Michas, C., Chew, D. J., Semu, D., Gleick, J., et al. (2019). Printable microscale interfaces for long-term peripheral nerve mapping and precision control. https://core.ac.uk/download/322973176.pdf (accessed on 14th October 2025).

CHAPTER 8

MEDICAL DEVICES AND SURGICAL PLANNING

Contents

INTRODUCTION

Progress in surgery has been significantly influenced by the arrival of medical devices that facilitate complex procedural planning. The technologies enable doctors to transition from traditional techniques to precision-based methods that enhance the safety and efficiency of operations. Personalized surgical guides and instruments are a breakthrough in this area, providing surgeons with customized instruments that perfectly align with a patient's anatomy. This individualization improves the outcome of surgery and minimizes recovery time because interventions can be done with increased accuracy. Advances in imaging modalities such as CT and MRI also support these advances by enabling accurate visualization of the area to be operated on, thereby facilitating precise pre-operative planning and techniques specific to each patient's requirements. Thus, the integration of sophisticated medical devices in surgical planning forms a critical foundation for modern surgical practice. The application of three-dimensional anatomical models in surgical planning reflects the revolutionary impact of technology on surgical practice. The models enable surgeons to appreciate better complex anatomy and plan procedures before stepping into the operating room. With the simulation and training models, medical personnel can refine their approaches, improve performance and outcome under actual operating conditions. Virtual reality and augmented reality software application use in surgical training is also on the rise, supplementing an immersive learning experience that mediates theoretical and practical skills. With the adoption of these innovations by surgical societies, the capacity to mitigate the risks of novel procedures is evident. The application of such advanced technology is not only beneficial to the operating crew, but it ultimately enhances patient safety and recovery, justifying pre-operative investment in innovation. As the medical device world continues to evolve, surgical planning increasingly relies on automation and self-operating systems to maximize and accelerate procedures. The introduction of computer-aided orthopedic surgery (CAOS) systems is an example of the emerging trend towards advanced technological integration, where procedure precision is significantly augmented by real-time feedback and biomechanics (Kalová et al., 2019). Moreover, the future possibility of robotic assistance for surgery represents a new paradigm, enabling sub-millimeter precision and potential for conducting surgeries beyond human hand abilities (Das et al., 2017). This shift towards automation not only peaks operating effectiveness but poses pertinent ethical and practical concerns regarding the prospective position of human surgeons. By exploring these technological developments and the implications they bring, deeper insight into how medical devices recast surgical planning will be gained, giving rise to further developments within the medical sector.

Definition of Medical Devices

Medical device innovation has left a profound impact on surgical planning, with improved accuracy and efficiency of operations in the various specializations. Computer-assisted orthopedic surgery (CAOS) systems are among the most exemplary developments of the ongoing revolution in the surgical instrument department. They rely on advanced imaging tools such as computed tomography

(CT) and magnetic resonance imaging (MRI) to construct accurate anatomical models. Integration of these volumetric images into surgical planning allows individualized methods, hence maximizing patient outcomes. Furthermore, various types of CAOS systems—from those that utilize kinetic data on joints and morphological data on target bones—are revolutionizing traditional methods by providing more accurate surgical guides and personalized devices. Lastly, CAOS not only establishes the definition of medical devices but also illustrates their importance in modern surgical procedures (Kalová et al., 2019). Secondarily, the overlap of robotics and automation in the operating room illustrates another dimension in the definition of medical devices. Autonomous surgical systems enhance the precision of surgery through sub-millimeter control to facilitate improved execution of complex tasks that might be beyond human capability.

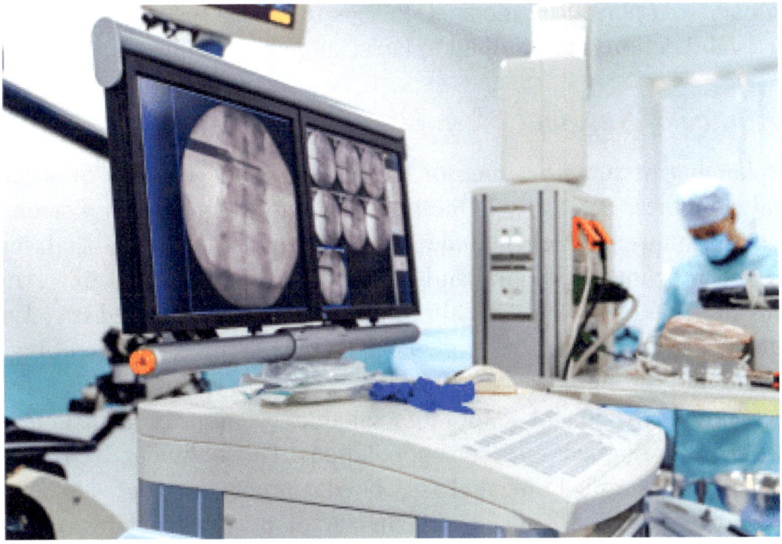

Figure 8.1. Computer-assisted orthopedic surgery (CAOS) systems exemplify the ongoing transformation in the realm of surgical instruments.

Source: https://acf.com.tr/wp-content/uploads/2021/05/admin-ajax-1-min.png.

These technologies can be calibrated to real-time biosignals, speeding interventions and minimizing the likelihood of human error. By reconceiving the surgeon's role, these technologies also create ethical and operational concerns, in this instance, trust in robotic performance and effects on surgical teams. With these stand-alone machines entering commercial use, they create the need for clear definition of what a medical device is. As such, the union of automation and robotics not only raises compliance standards but also redefines surgical planning itself, with improved accuracy and patient-friendliness (Das et al., 2017). In broadening the meaning of medical devices in the realm of surgical planning, then, one cannot help but consider how patient-specific instrumentation and simulation become valuable. Preoperative planning is also increasingly on an individualized basis considering the anatomical differences specific to each patient, and thus they present the entry point for custom surgical guides and instruments. Personalized care represents the essence of new-fangled medical devices, emphasizing the significance of putting together the latest imaging with surgical skill. Simulation models and simulators provide new surgeons valuable experience in a risk-free environment, underlining the value of careful planning prior to actual application. Thus, these new devices not only enhance surgical outcomes but also enhance anatomical information and surgical techniques. Synoptic outcome of all these developments highlights the primary role played by medical devices to obtain successful surgeries, to derive a valid definition according to latest surgical techniques (Figure 8.1).

Importance of Surgical Planning

Good planning of surgery is one of the distinguishing features of successful surgical outcomes, especially in the field of complex operations. Personalized surgical techniques, which include the production of personalized surgical guides and instruments, significantly contribute to the success of operations in terms of accuracy. The personalized instruments are designed based on the individual anatomical features of patients, thereby facilitating better alignment and positioning of surgical tools. The use of patient-specific instrumentation allows surgeons to see and adapt more suitable techniques for the anatomical variations present in heterogeneous populations. This individualized technique not only reduces surgical time and associated complications but also optimizes postoperative recovery. Thus, the inclusion of personalized instruments in planning the surgery reiterates its pivotal role in achieving enhanced accuracy and overall patient satisfaction in surgery. In addition to the adjustment of surgical equipment, pre-operative planning with anatomic models is particularly helpful with the tailoring of the surgery. From virtual modifications that mimic human anatomy to 3D printed replicas, the models enable surgeons to make extensive studies of the surgery site prior to entering the operating theater. By allowing visualization of the complex anatomical relationships, these models give the experts an opportunity to develop strategic plans that include likely challenges. Remarkably, such sophisticated planning leads to a more significant understanding of spatial relationships that pertain to surgical procedures. As pointed out by recent literature, this pre-operative phase not only enhances the surgeon's preparedness but also optimizes the potential for achieving optimal surgical results, thus ensuring the importance of extensive surgical planning (Kalová et al., 2019). Besides, training and simulation models enhance the surgical planning process by providing a safe platform for procedure mastery and skill enhancement. These models serve as valuable learning devices for residents and practicing surgeons alike to hone skills and test new methods of surgery. Enhanced with virtual reality and haptic feedback systems, simulations provide life-like experiences replicating real surgical contexts. These practice exercises allow muscle memory and decision-making to be established, which then convert into more competent surgery when performed in actual patients. The application of the use of these models illustrates the significant role surgical planning serves not only in individual surgeries but in the continuous evolution of surgical training, adapting to increased levels of accuracy and more concern for the patient (Das et al., 2017).

8.1. TYPES OF MEDICAL DEVICES

In the constantly evolving environment of surgical planning, individualized surgical guides and instruments occupy a prime position in promoting procedural achievement. Carefully crafted to complement the unique anatomy of each patient, these instruments provide surgeons with the precision they need for procedures. Through the use of advanced imaging techniques such as CT or MRI scans, guides facilitate interventions optimized for precision and reduced risk of complications. Guides can also make real-time adjustments as they are able to adapt and accommodate variations in anatomy to ensure the approach is optimized for the specific needs of the individual patient. In addition, the development of custom tools is another significant move towards personalized medicine that has led to enhanced postoperative recovery and worldwide patient satisfaction. Incorporation of custom devices and surgical planning is one of the best examples of moving towards more personal healthcare practices. The use of pre-operative planning aided by anatomical models has also revolutionized the surgical fraternity. Surgeons can now visualize detailed anatomical structures preoperatively, enabling them to devise more ideal operative strategies. The three-dimensional models from imaging scans are a physical and visual model of the surgery site, enabling an enhanced understanding of the patient's individual anatomy. Such sophisticated planning not only enhances the accuracy of the procedure but also serves as a valuable teaching tool, allowing surgical teams to rehearse complex procedures in a simulated setting. By allowing surgical staff to communicate and coordinate more effectively, pre-operative models significantly enhance team efficiency and morale, as each member becomes well-prepared for the real procedure. Thus, emphasis on such meticulous planning underlines the importance of innovation in surgical techniques. The adoption of training models and simulation in teaching surgery is indicative of ongoing advancement in medical equipment. Training models allow for realistic simulation of training settings, with surgeons able to practice skills through various techniques and scenarios without putting patients at risk. By simulating real operative situations, these devices increase the skill and confidence of operating surgeons, ultimately leading to improved patient care. Furthermore, the application of patient-specific instrumentation, inherently related to these simulation models, enhances the operation by allowing instruments specifically tailored to the patient's anatomical structures. This integration of training and specialized instrumentation creates new possibility in surgical planning, bridging the gap between theoretical and clinical use. As surgeons learn to work with these newer instruments, the possibility for patient outcome and surgical success is vast and expansive, portending a rosy future for surgical development (Figure 8.2).

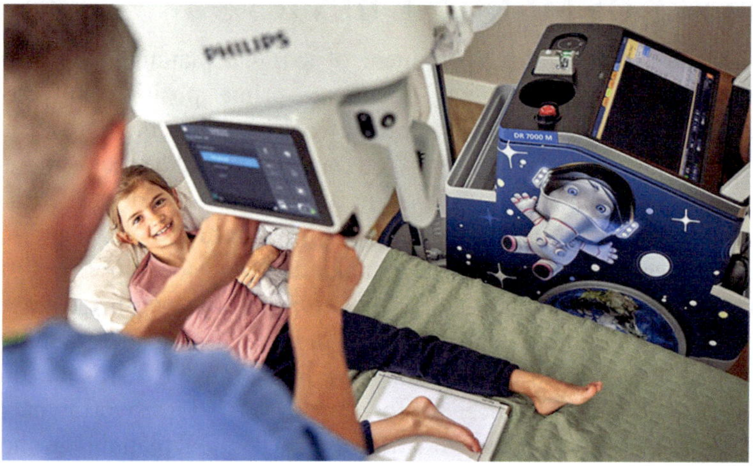

Figure 8.2. By utilizing advanced imaging techniques such as CT or MRI scans, these guides facilitate targeted interventions that can improve accuracy and reduce the risk of complications.

Source: https://www.philips.com/c-dam/corporate/newscenter/global/standard/resources/healthcare/2024/q-and-a-with-atul-gupta-md/dr-7000-m-application-tech-pediatric-eth.jpg.

8.1.1. Surgical Instruments

Technological innovation in surgical instruments has transformed the landscape of medical treatment, both in efficiency and safety. One of the major advances is the development of customized surgical guides and instruments, exactly adapted to suit the anatomy of each patient. Personalization makes surgeries more accurate, reducing the potential for complications and improving results. By the use of pre-operative planning involving anatomical models, surgeons can visualize the field of operation in real terms. The technique not only helps one to identify important structures but also enables one to develop custom instrumentation to adapt to one's anatomical subtleties. These customization solutions are the interface of technology and medicine where a more concentrated and methodical application of surgical performance is made possible. In addition, the integration of simulation and training models into surgical procedures has revolutionized how surgeons hone their skills and prepare for complex operations. The models provide a platform where surgical instruments can be utilized in simulated settings, bridging the gap between practice and theory.

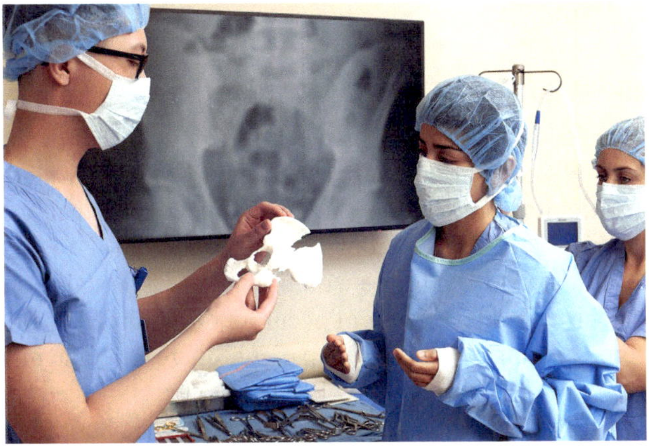

Figure 8.3. By leveraging pre-operative planning that incorporates anatomical models, surgeons can visualize the surgical field accurately.

Source: https://formlabs-media.formlabs.com/filer_public_thumbnails/filer_public/27/7c/277c2953-0591-4a09-a4b5-00a88cca4bb6/11092017_medical_pelvis_354_flat.jpg__1184x0_q85_subsampling-2.jpg.

Through the use of advanced simulation technology, trainees can practice with virtual simulations of surgical situations, honing their skills with various instruments without putting patients at risk. By this process, the surgical teams get proficient in utilizing their instruments properly, building up confidence and competency prior to performing actual surgical procedures. This step is very important because it prepares the surgical team for the time they spend in the operating theatre, ensuring that they use the instruments to their maximum capability. Patient-specific instrumentation is fast emerging as a vital component of modern surgical procedures, holding specific advantages that strongly appeal to the domain of surgical planning. The method individualizes surgical instruments according to the anatomical and procedural requirements of individual patients, leading to better surgical outcomes and recovery rates. As indicated in new publications on computer-assisted orthopedic surgery (CAOS) systems, three-dimensional imaging and accurate anatomical data have facilitated the introduction to more accurate surgical planning. The systems give a greater awareness of the operating environment to allow instruments to be created to meet specific requirements. These developments underscore the importance of blending the latest surgical instruments with careful planning so that operations not only meet the clinical requirement but also integrate the unique aspects of patients anatomy, resulting in tailored care that upholds the highest achievable standards of medical practice (Das et al., 2017; Kalová et al., 2019) (Figure 8.3).

8.1.2. Diagnostic Equipment

The integration of advanced diagnostic technology into the clinical environment has revolutionized surgical planning, particularly through the production of patient-specific instrumentation and customized surgical guides. These technologies enable surgeons to tailor their approach on the basis of detailed anatomical data obtained from high-resolution imaging modalities such as MRI and CT scans. Through the creation of accurate three-dimensional images that reflect the unique anatomy of a specific patient, diagnostic machinery not only supports pre-operative planning but also facilitates enhanced surgical team communication. Personalized instruments with such technology reduce both surgical time and complication risk significantly because they allow for cautious and well-informed decisions during surgery. Such technological advancement indicates the necessity of new regulatory frameworks, as existing EU directives may not necessarily adapt to such quick developments, illustrating the complex interrelation between technology and regulatory practice in healthcare systems (Altenstetter et al., 1995). The role of simulation and training models, propelled by diagnostic equipment, cannot be overestimated in surgical planning. By exposing healthcare professionals to real-world situations and challenges, these models provide greater surgical competence and preparedness, which ultimately benefit patient outcomes. The combination of virtual reality and augmented reality in surgical education is an exemplary demonstration of diagnostic tools moving beyond the bounds of traditional methodology, allowing surgeons to practice and refine their skills under well-controlled circumstances. Apart from this, these simulations can be programmed to simulate individual patient conditions, contributing to learning in young surgeons. As new technology advances, there is a learning curve to adapt to using it, but what is learned through these simulations provides a strong basis for competent and confident surgery (Fortina et al., 2015). Apart from direct impact of diagnostic devices on operations, the implications of patient safety and device performance are most critical. Ensuring that medical devices, including diagnostic devices, adhere to high standards of safety and performance presents a challenge ever-present to regulatory bodies. The intersection of the ability of institutions to implement new regulations and the precedents in medical practice history forms the terrain of diagnostic device uptake. It is crucial that such devices not only comply with current regulations but also with the prevailing medical practices and conventions of the region. Thus, continuous evaluation and adaptation of the regulatory framework are vital to ensure a setting under which innovation may flourish without victimizing patient safety and the reliability of devices. Such equilibrium is essential as the medical devices sector continues to grow, shaping the future of surgical planning and treatment of patients (Altenstetter et al., 1995).

8.1.3. Implantable Devices

In the past few years, technology has revolutionized the planning of surgery, particularly where implantable devices are involved. Enhanced pre-operative planning has become increasingly significant as surgeons strive to make procedures more individualized for patients. For instance, creation of precision surgical guides and instruments allows for correct implant placement, improving outcomes while reducing intraoperative complications. These tailor-made tools, created using accurate models of anatomy, ensure that the technique of surgery is ideally aligned with a patient's specific anatomy. Thus, application of technology in surgery planning not only enhances the effectiveness of surgery but also spurs better patient satisfaction because procedures are more predictable and aligned with specific needs. The landscape of medical devices, i.e., implantable devices, also comprises sophisticated features such as telemetry systems. These technologies are primarily responsible for monitoring patients' post-surgery. Implantable telemetry systems, for example, monitor significant physiological alterations that may signal complications, such as the onset of rejection in transplanted tissues. This type of technology best demonstrates where medical science and engineering converge, and how specialized devices work to monitor health in real time. These advancements ensure that surgeons can respond swiftly in case of any complications, thereby improving patient care and postoperative outcomes better, ultimately leading to a paradigm shift in what constitutes successful surgery in contemporary medicine (Culclasure et al., 2025). Also, patient-specific instrumentation has been a key driver to enhance the effectiveness of surgeries using implantable devices. By employing models that reproduce the patient's individual anatomy, surgeons can create detailed pre-operative planning which directs their technique. This level of preparation reduces surgical times and reduces trauma while also facilitating simulations and training that can assist both beginner and experienced surgeons. For instance, incorporation of aerospace science technologies, such as those from NASAs Biomedical Application Team, has led to tremendous progress in device form and function to ensure reliability in sophisticated surgery. This is proof of ongoing diligence toward improved patient outcomes using precision medicine-based approaches, thus demonstrating the critical position of implantable devices in the dynamic field of surgical planning (Culclasure et al., 2025) (Figure 8.4).

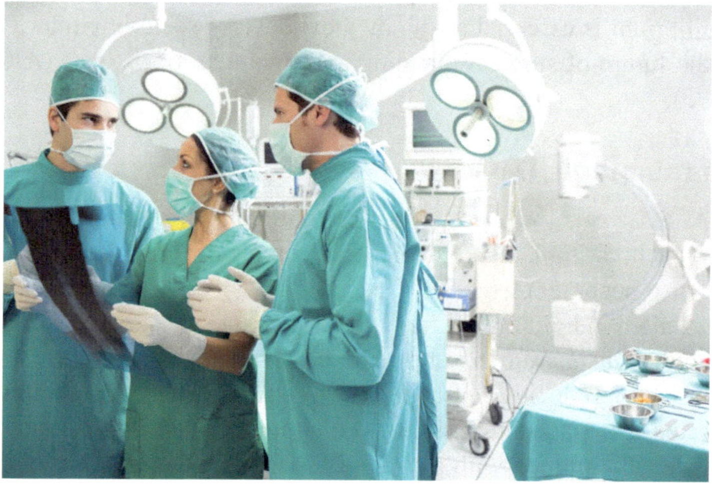

Figure 8.4. Enhanced pre-operative planning has become increasingly critical as surgeons aim to customize procedures for individual patients.

Source: https://cdn.prod.website-files.com/651c14815121543d83a69af8/67dacb27da71e47be8d2468e_BLOG%202021-05-20%20Preoperative%20Planning%20Can%20Help%20Improve%20Patient%20Recovery.webp.

8.2. ROLE OF TECHNOLOGY IN SURGICAL PLANNING

With technology seeping into various areas of healthcare, the surgery practice has embraced innovative solutions that ensure enhanced pre-operative planning and implementation. Among the key advances is the use of custom-designed surgical guides and instruments, through which surgeons are able to perform operations with more accuracy than ever before. Such instruments are designed based on the individual anatomy of every patient and hence ensure decreased chances of complications and improved outcomes of surgery. For instance, in complex surgeries such as orthopedic surgeries, patient-specific implants can be designed using the assistance of 3D printing technology, which facilitates appropriate alignment and fixation of the implants. Such personalization not only leads to reduced surgery time but also enhanced patient recovery, symbolizing the core role of technology in contemporary surgeries. In addition to specialized instruments, pre-operative planning is also dependent on advanced anatomical models offering essential visual data about a patient's individual requirements.

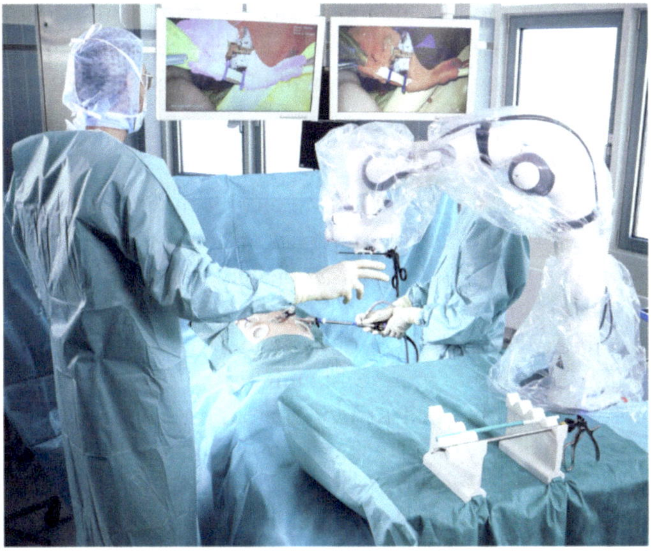

Figure 8.5. By employing anatomical models, surgeons can simulate surgical interventions, enabling them to anticipate challenges and identify potential complications before entering the operating room.

Source: https://media.springernature.com/lw685/springer-static/image/art%3A10.1038%2Fs43856-024-00581-0/MediaObjects/43856_2024_581_Fig2_HTML.png.

By utilizing advanced imaging methodologies like MRI and CT scans, anatomical structures can be reconstructed in 3D by surgeons, and the spatial relationships involved in intricate operations are better comprehended. This careful planning is most essential in surgical specializations like cardiac surgery, where anatomical complexity calls for attention to detail. Using these anatomical models, surgeons can practice surgeries, which enables them to anticipate complications and identify potential problems before attending the operating room. For the most part, the integration of these technologies in surgical planning mirrors their groundbreaking impact on patient safety and operative success. Besides, the use of simulation and training models in surgical training cannot be overstated. These technology-oriented tools enable medical practitioners to enhance their competence in actual practice, therefore overall capacity. Examples of these technologies include computer-assisted orthopedic surgery (CAOS) systems that enable trainees to practice on both virtual and augmented reality platforms. Such simulator training aids the learning curve to surgical procedures, allowing trainees to better learn anatomical subtleties and procedural specifics without the direct stresses of real-time surgery. Such integration of training models aids not only safer operating routines but the confidence of newly qualified surgeons, thereby representing the broader implications of technology for both surgical planning and training (Figure 8.5).

8.2.1. Imaging Technologies

In the midst of the swift progression of medical technology, the importance of imaging technologies in surgical planning has grown even more crucial. Imaging technologies make it possible to generate accurate anatomical representations that allow surgeons to see complex structures ahead of time before doing anything about them. Through three-dimensional imaging modalities, surgeons can perform thorough pre-operative planning, and they can then tailor their methods according to individual patient anatomies. The use of virtual reality (VR) and augmented reality (AR) technologies in this field has further enhanced the pre-operative phase. By allowing medical professionals to be immersed within a digital simulation mimicking actual conditions, such technologies help improve surgical skill and overall outcomes. The combination of these imaging technologies highlights their underlying use in personalized and effective surgical planning, ultimately resulting in enhanced patient safety and operating room effectiveness (Dellavalle et al., 2020). Advances in imaging technologies have also led to the creation of patient-specific surgical instruments and guides, which are customized based on a patient's anatomy. These technologies greatly improve the accuracy of surgical procedures by enabling instruments to be accurately aligned with the unique geometry of the surgical environment. Preoperative imaging enables the creation of these tailored guides, which are usually developed using advanced 3D printing techniques. This process not only provides the utmost precision but also reduces procedure time, thereby reducing patients' recovery time. As more of these custom solutions are employed by surgeons, the potential for improved surgical results is obvious. Furthermore, having the ability to see and manipulate anatomic models in real time not only enhances surgical planning, but also confidence, allowing practitioners to handle difficult cases with greater assurance (Kupelian et al., 2011). In addition to enhancing surgical precision, imaging technologies have transformed simulation and training models for healthcare professionals. High-fidelity simulation offers a method for surgeons to practice complex operations in a controlled environment, ultimately augmenting their ability and judgment skills when performing operations. These modules utilize advanced imaging to simulate patient-specific cases, which present the learner with a variety of anatomical challenges. Thus, the introduction of improved imaging technologies in training curricula builds a generation of more skilled surgeons who can manage the complexities of surgeries better. With the consistent incorporation of these advances in education as well as in practice, the medical profession can expect a future to be even more competent, leading to better patient outcomes in the long run as well as an improved quality of care (Dellavalle et al., 2020) (Figure 8.6).

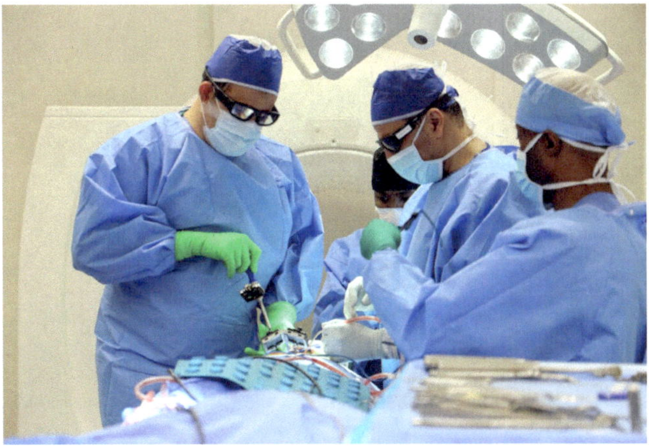

Figure 8.6. By allowing healthcare professionals to immerse themselves in a digital environment that mirrors real-world conditions, these technologies aid in refining surgical techniques and improving overall outcomes.

Source: https://media.springernature.com/lw1200/springer-static/image/art%3A10.1038%2Fs41746-025-01575-5/MediaObjects/41746_2025_1575_Fig4_HTML.png.

8.2.2. Software for Surgical Simulations

Within the ever-changing field of surgical planning, sophisticated surgical simulation software has emerged as key components that have assisted in enhancing the precision of medical procedures. The sophisticated systems allow for the creation of tailored surgical guides and instruments that are directed by patient-specific data derived from imaging equipment. Through the utilization of software for importing DICOM images from CT scans and MRI scans, surgeons can create accurate anatomical models for pre-operative planning. This personalized approach not only aids in the visualization of complex anatomical relationships but also allows simulation of various surgical conditions, thereby preparing surgical teams for complications that could occur during actual surgeries.

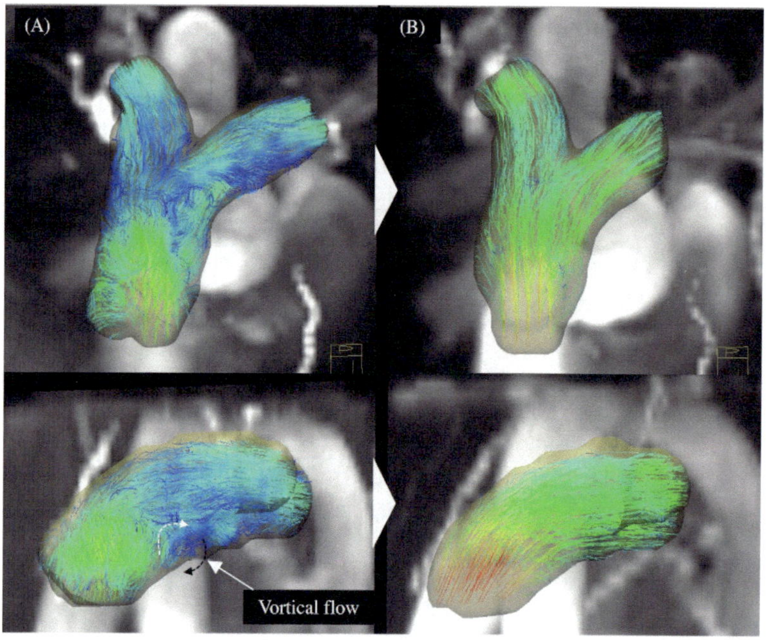

Figure 8.7. The ability to model hemodynamic alterations through computational fluid dynamics (CFD) enables surgeons to evaluate the impacts of various surgical approaches on blood flow and wall shear stress, essential parameters that influence patient morbidity.

Source: https://www.journal-of-cardiology.com/cms/10.1016/j.jjcc.2022.05.007/asset/501574ec-2963-4379-94c0-89c5bca0fb77/main.assets/gr4_lrg.jpg.

Overall, the application of this technology increases effectiveness while lowering risks associated with surgical interventions. Besides, software simulation is not only used for visualization; it is also an essential training instrument for surgeons of all levels. Enhanced simulation models enable realistic environments wherein surgeons can practice their skills without compromising patient safety. Learners train in a controlled environment using realistic surgical simulations, enhancing proficiency and confidence before actual procedures. The equipment developed using simulation software, in addition to what is learned from rehearsing complex maneuvers, assists surgeons in honing their craft, ultimately bringing surgical results closer in line with pre-operative predictions. This element of surgical training highlights the key role played by new software in getting healthcare professionals ready for what is encountered in the operating room. In more clinical specific settings, surgical simulation software has been shown to improve procedural skill significantly, particularly in dynamic clinical situations such as coarctation of the aorta (CoA). The ability to simulate hemodynamic alterations with computational fluid dynamics (CFD) enables surgeons to evaluate the impact of various surgical methods upon blood flow and wall shear stress, important parameters that influence patient morbidity. Using this technology, the surgical teams have the possibility to go through the effects of different stent geometries and surgical methods on patient outcomes and thereby evidence-based choices during surgery. Moreover, advances in haptic feedback systems, as shown in new techniques of bone manipulation, allow for adaptation during real-time simulation, further enhancing the surgical planning process as a whole (Arnez et al., 2012). This type of fusion of planning and simulation software is evolving beyond that, with potential for even more personalized and effective patient-specific instrumentation for modern medicine (Feinstein et al., 2010) (Figure 8.7).

8.2.3. Integration of AI in Planning

The application of modern technology for surgical planning has revolutionized the practice of patient care, particularly through the integration of artificial intelligence (AI) in various areas of medical devices. Surgeons are now relying more on AI-based algorithms to create custom-made surgical guides and instruments based on individual patient anatomies. The guides not only increase accuracy for surgical procedures but also minimize the likelihood of complications, hence improving patient outcomes. Apart from this, AI is also capable of reviewing extensive databases of past surgeries and predict potential problems which may arise in a specific surgery so that it may be prepared for better. Such seamless integration of technology into planning procedures is essential to incorporate greater levels of care into surgical practice and provide every patient with the most personalized and optimal care. Preoperative planning, as well, has been significantly improved with the use of AI, most notably through the generation of detailed anatomical models that reflect the complexity of human physiology. Through the generation of these models, which can be generated using AI algorithms working with medical imaging, surgeons can view and play with patient-specific anatomy long before any procedure is ever done in the operating room. This level of preparedness allows for higher situational awareness and decision-making during procedure. As the literature has noted, these anatomy models not only support surgical interventions directly but also improve the learning environment for surgical teams generally, promoting a culture of safety and quality improvement. This move towards better educated planning can eventually translate into reduced operative times and improved clinical outcomes, processes which are always supported by evidence from medical research (Annemans et al., 2016). Moreover, improvements in simulation and training models with artificial intelligence have drastically changed the learning landscape for surgical experts. These models offer life-like training conditions under which surgeons are able to hone their skills in a risk-free environment and practice repeatedly without compromising real patients' lives. The analytical power of AI allows these training models to respond to the individual trainees' level of proficiency and deliver customized feedback and focused skill development. As has been emphasized in comparative studies, the techniques so utilized lead to an enhanced level of surgical competence and greater practitioner confidence. The integration of AI within such teaching methods not only helps to train future surgeons but also reinforces the need for continued surgical planning methodology adjustment with an ever-evolving changing healthcare landscape (Figure 8.8).

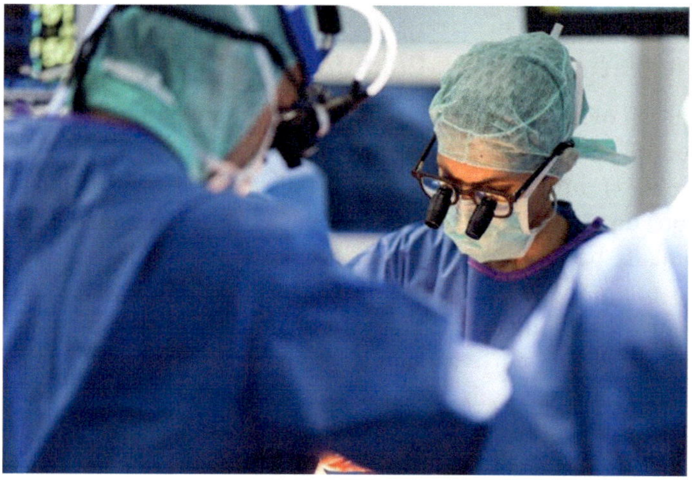

Figure 8.8. Surgeons increasingly rely on AI-driven algorithms to create custom surgical guides and tools tailored to individual patient anatomies.

Source: https://imageio.forbes.com/specials-images/imageserve/67200dc48f7355f56031cdd1/two-cardiovascular-surgeons-operate-on-a-patient/960x0.jpg?height=473&width=711&fit=bounds.

8.3. CUSTOM SURGICAL GUIDES AND TOOLS

The use of technological innovation in medicine has revolutionized the manner in which surgical procedures are planned and executed. The transformation has led to a remarkable increase in the application of customized surgical guides and instruments, which have become vital tools for enhancing the accuracy of surgical operations. By facilitating enhanced flexibility in patient handling, the tools contribute extensively to the effectiveness of surgeries. They not only fit the particular anatomical configurations of patients but also enable pre-operative planning, so that surgeons can see steps of procedure beforehand. Such meticulous preparation is crucial as it contributes to surgeons' confidence and general efficiency of surgical teams intra-operatively. Therefore, custom surgical guides enhance patient safety as well as surgical outcomes. Together with customized surgical tools, anatomical models produced with high-resolution imaging modalities also provide surgeons with useful visual references during pre-operative planning.

The models facilitate precise assessments and enable complete familiarity with the operating field. The resulting detailed models help with the identification of important anatomical structures, thereby increasing familiarity before the procedure. Furthermore, technologies such as three-dimensional printing have progressed the production of low-cost, patient-specific devices that support surgical planning. Particularly in complex specialties such as spinal surgery, patient-specific guides and instruments can assist with enhancing precision of intervention, for instance, pedicle screw placement. This capability for tailored anatomical modeling encourages a paradigm shift towards patient individualized treatment, making it possible for tailored strategies that are specific to the unique challenge presented in each case (Kalaskar et al., 2017). Additionally, models for simulation and training are most suitable with regard to the need for continuous surgical skill and technique improvement. They provide a state-of-the-art platform for practicing, allowing surgeons to rehearse intricate procedures in a risk-free environment. By integrating patient-specific guides along with these training devices, clinicians are able to obtain a greater understanding of the unique challenges each case of patients poses. The integration of such tailored guides and simulation technologies not only enhances surgical skills but also significantly helps minimize operative time and enhanced patient satisfaction. As the medical fraternity embraces these techniques increasingly, emphasis on teamwork dynamics in surgery even more underlines the importance of bridging individualized tools and planning methods with routine practice, ultimately contributing to improved patient outcomes and working efficiencies within the surgical setup (Burity et al., 2014) (Figure 8.9).

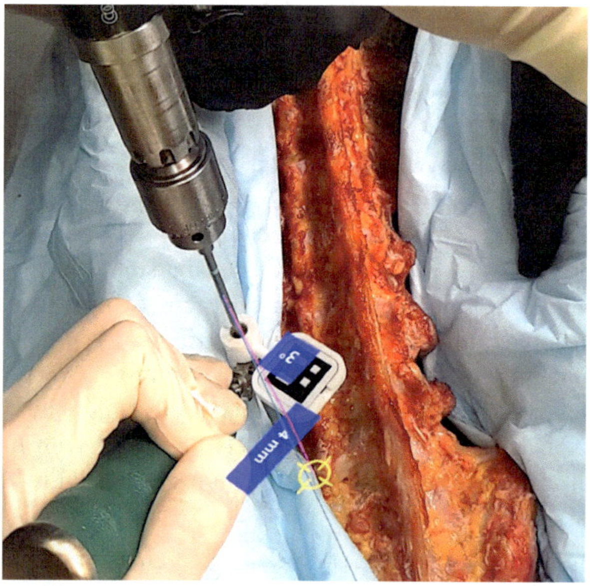

Figure 8.9. Particularly in complex fields like spinal surgery, custom guides and tools can assist in increasing the accuracy of interventions, such as pedicle screw placement.

*Source:*https://www.nassopenaccess.org/cms/10.1016/j.xnsj.2021.100084/asset/17e0c2e9-efe1-4521-bc9f-911755f843f7/main.assets/gr2_lrg.jpg.

8.3.1. Definition and Purpose

The use of sophisticated technology in surgical environments has altered the definition and the function of surgical devices in surgical planning. Surgical planning is a lengthy process for the optimization of surgical outcomes by carefully resolving all the pre-operative concerns. At the center of this is also the use of individually tailored surgical guides and patient-specific instrumentation, developed from high-definition imaging information that follow the unique anatomy of a patient. This uniqueness enhances the precision of surgery, thereby limiting risks that can accompany one-size-fits-all solutions that are not aligned with individual variation. As highlighted in the literature, volumetric image-based systems, i.e., CT and MRI, have emerged as essential tools in this regard, enabling accurate visualization of the anatomical structures to be transcended in the management of musculoskeletal disease (Kalová et al., 2019). The use of training and simulation models also highlights the necessity of incorporating technology in surgical planning. These models provide a safe environment where surgeons can hone and refine their skills, becoming familiar with the precise problems they may encounter when operating on actual patients. Through haptic interfaces and virtual spaces, surgeons can engage with realistic replicas of patient anatomy, thereby skillfully performing delicate maneuvers such as bone cuts or joint reconstructions (Arnez et al., 2012). This form of training not only enhances surgical proficiency but also serves to improve decision-making under real-time conditions and adaptability. This new pre-operative planning model is a shift from the traditional method of training towards an exciting and more efficient system of training that more adequately prepares surgeons for the intricacies of modern surgical procedures. Ultimately, the aim of these sophisticated surgical instruments transcends the optimization of surgical accuracy; they also aim to improve patient outcomes through the creation of an individualized sense of each patient's surgical requirements. Pre-operative planning with anatomic models allows meticulous inspection and consideration of patient-specific variations in morphology, which is crucial in developing tailor-made surgical plans. In addition, as computer-aided orthopedic surgical systems increase, they offer promising methods of integrating dynamic and kinetic information about bones and joints into educational surgery (Kalová et al., 2019). Consequently, the role of medical devices in surgery becomes a multilateral approach which not only enables precision but also promotes a patient-centered ideology in medicine, bridging the gap between the latest technology and clinical requirements.

8.3.2. Benefits of Customization

In the field of surgical planning, the use of custom-made surgical guides and instruments has revolutionized the field of patient care by enhancing the accuracy and efficiency of procedures. By utilizing patient-specific instrumentation, surgeons can carry out operations with a greater degree of conformity to the unique anatomical features of each patient, thus drastically reducing the risk of error. This is a personalized process that has the advantage of guaranteeing that the instruments used are suited to the individual characteristics of the patient's anatomy, thus leading to improved surgical outcomes. Therefore, the development and implementation of such personalized devices aid not just in efficacy in the process of surgery but also alleviates anxiety in the patient through provision of a more predictable experience. The drift toward specialized surgical equipment points to the need for customizing medical devices for patients' unique needs in order to enhance overall surgical performance in the practice of medicine. Preoperative planning with anatomical models is an invaluable tool for the reinforcement of surgical success. Surgeons are able to undertake careful preparatory procedures by making precise replicas of a patient's anatomy so they can see and plan beforehand before interventions are carried out. These models not only allow them to plan effectively for different methods of intervention but also help them have a comprehensive understanding of the problems that are likely to be encountered during intervention. Moreover, such use is useful in providing communication between patients and surgical teams, which enhances a spirit of cooperation where expectations are effectively defined.

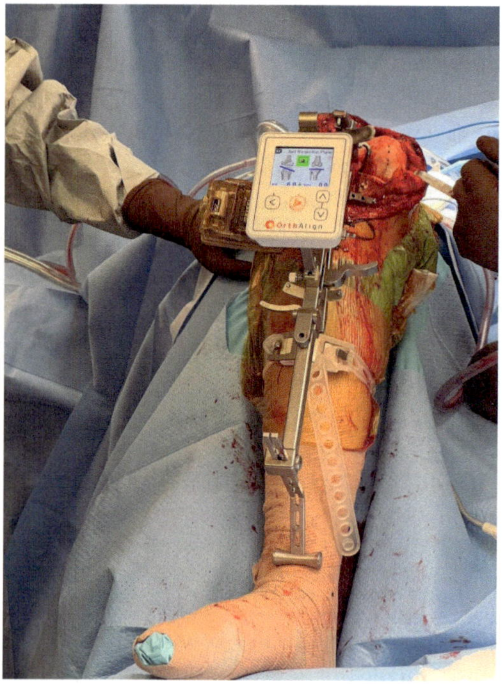

Figure 8.10. By utilizing patient-specific instrumentation, surgeons can operate with a greater alignment to the unique anatomical features of each individual, substantially reducing the risk of error.

Source:https://www.arthroplastytoday.org/article/S2352-3441%2823%2900177-2/fulltext

Such interaction is essential in the development of patient trust and satisfaction since the patients will feel more secure with the knowledge of details surrounding their upcoming procedures. The utilization of anatomical models thus represents a critical advancement in surgical preparation, one that is especially significant in the era of personalized medicine today. The deployment of simulation and training models also attests to the benefits of customization to surgical environments. Utilizing customized simulation tools, future as well as experienced surgeons can practice in a risk-free environment that mimics true-to-life experiences. These adaptive training models offer repetitive training, which allows the medical professionals to practice and sharpen their skills and build confidence before actual surgeries are performed. This advantage not only contributes to overall skill enhancement of healthcare providers, but also leads to enhanced patient care, as surgeons who are highly skilled are likely to achieve better results. With the rapidly changing landscape of surgical education, the advent of these customized training tools marks a pivotal moment in sustaining commitment to continuous improvement within the health care community. As a whole, these simulations play an important role in optimizing surgical planning, ultimately achieving better patient safety and care (Figure 8.10).

8.3.3. Examples of Custom Tools in Use

The runaway development of technology in the medical sector has led to the groundbreaking innovation of personalized surgical tools that highly enhance surgical accuracy and patient outcomes. A few of the advances are patient-specific instrumentation and custom surgical guides for particular anatomies. These devices allow surgeons to take precise paths through complex anatomical structures, thus eliminating the risk associated with traditional surgery. By employing advanced imaging techniques, surgeons can create guides that are specially designed to meet the specific anatomy of a patient, enabling procedures previously considered too complicated. Such personalized devices eventually transform the surgical world through increased success rates and maximized patient recovery times, representing an important transition towards ever more custom-oriented methodologies in medical procedures. Other than custom surgical guides, pre-surgical planning is increasingly based on the application of anatomical models that resemble patients' specific anatomical characteristics. Surgeons can practice and visualize complex procedures using the models prior to actual surgery. By creating three-dimensional images of the patient's anatomy through advanced imaging technology such as MRI and CT scans, surgeons can plan their approach better and more accurately. Not only does this enhanced planning method allow them to conduct the surgery with greater confidence, but it also decreases the chances of unforeseen complications. Finally, the use of patient-specific anatomical models in surgery planning showcases the importance of individualized care in the healthcare sector and serves to lift the levels of surgery, as well as improving patient safety. The virtual reality environment forms the foundation of training models employed by medical practitioners to improve their skills before use in operating rooms. Use of virtual reality (VR) and augmented reality (AR) technologies in medical training is also increasing, providing an interactive environment which can accurately mimic real-world surgical operations. The simulation enables trainees to practice intricate techniques in a zero-risk environment, building enhanced understanding of uncomplicated and complex surgical processes. As highlighted in recent literature, the intersection of VR/AR technology in surgical training is the ultimate level of modernization of educational practices in medicine, particularly in specialized fields where learning by doing is critical (Dellavalle et al., 2020). Of greater significance, such advancements not only enhance the training process but also prepare surgeons adequately to benefit from the ergonomic design of new tools and instruments, therefore leading to improved surgical outcomes (Das et al., 2017).

8.4. PRE-OPERATIVE PLANNING USING ANATOMICAL MODELS

The inclusion of anatomical models in pre-operative planning is a big leap forward for surgical precision and patient care. Surgeons can use 3D models from imaging tests to see complex anatomical structures before the procedure, and it would be easier to understand the unique character of each patient's anatomy. This planning process allows for individually customized surgical guides and instruments unique to the patient, thereby enhancing the accuracy of cuts and reducing operating time. Use of physical models, particularly those that mimic soft tissue behavior, is now an essential adjunct to numerous areas of surgery. New developments pinpoint the importance of handling soft tissue manipulations in urology and minimally invasive surgery, where conventional techniques may be insufficient (Bart et al., 2006). Therefore, pre-operative planning with anatomical models significantly enhances surgical procedure and optimizes the overall effectiveness of medical treatment. Moreover, the use of simulation and training models in surgery allows for a more diversified learning experience among medical professionals. These models are not just vital tools in pre-operative planning but also provide useful training to enhance surgical skills. By having access to realistic, patient-specific anatomy models, surgeons can practice complicated procedures without taking any risk. Not only does this improve performance during operations, but it also makes novice as well as veteran surgeons more confident. Furthermore, application of such models allows complications to be estimated, and other methods investigated, ultimately encouraging a culture of ongoing improvement of surgical techniques and approaches (Kalová et al., 2019). Anatomical models are therefore integral to the development of surgical competence as well as informing intra-operative planning. Patient-specific instrumentation created from intra-operative planning with anatomical models has significantly altered surgical outcomes. By creating specially tailored instruments based on the specific anatomical specifications of the patient, medical professionals are able to enhance the accuracy and precision of surgical operations. The customized approach not only diminishes the risk of surgical complications but also provides improved recovery times following the operation and patient satisfaction. With increasing and ever-more surgery systems adopting high-level technology, utilization of pre-operative planning equipment, such as anatomical models, is set to increase, resulting in increasing medical device and surgical planning innovations. This step towards ever more individualized surgical methods thus emphasizes the necessity for ongoing study and innovation within this field, resulting in safer and more effective surgery in a variety of patient groups (Bart et al., 2006; Kalová et al., 2019) (Figure 8.11).

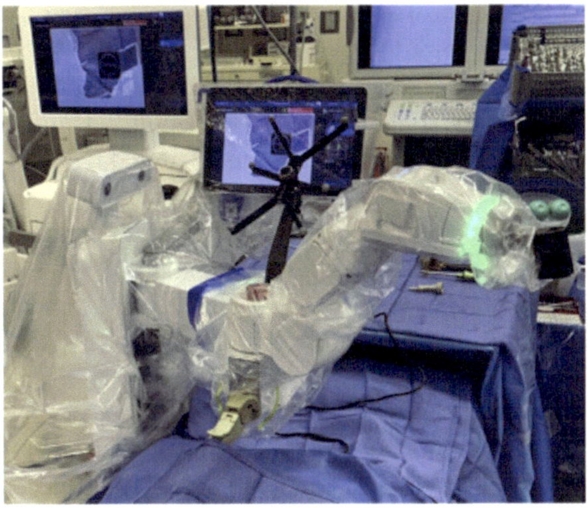

Figure 8.11. Recent innovations emphasize the importance of addressing soft tissue manipulations in domains such as urology and minimally invasive surgery, where conventional approaches may fall short.

Source: https://ars.els-cdn.com/content/image/1-s2.0-S2667099223000385-gr2.jpg.

8.4.1. Importance of Anatomical Accuracy

In the very complex field of surgical intervention, the significance of anatomical accuracy cannot be overlooked. While surgeons work to provide maximum outcomes, the use of instruments such as individualized surgical guides and instruments has become a necessity. These devices are created so that they can be tailored to the unique patient's particular anatomical structures, thereby improving the accuracy of surgery. These tailored approaches significantly reduce complications and support quicker rates of recovery. Furthermore, the application of computer-assisted orthopedic surgery (CAOS) systems is modern innovation within this field, where technologies can easily align surgical instruments with the patient's own anatomy, enabling higher precision (Kalová et al., 2019). Therefore, the adoption of these customized solutions is pivotal to limiting intraoperative errors and increasing general surgical efficacy. Pre-operative planning through comprehensive anatomy models plays an important role in maximizing surgical procedures. Using three-dimensional (3D) imaging and printing technologies, surgeons are able to create accurate replicas of a patient's anatomy to guide surgical planning. These accurate models do more than allow one to envision complex anatomical relationships; they also offer a medium by which to rehearse the operation before actual surgery. Surgical models have the ability to reduce unforeseen complications by allowing the surgical team to anticipate complications and adjust their strategy accordingly. Literature has found many applications of 3D printing in surgical use, such as surgical guides and implants, which have demonstrated reduced operative time and improved patient outcomes (Annemans et al., 2016). It is concerned with the necessity of anatomical accuracy in pre-operative planning as a premise for successful complex surgical procedures. In addition to enhancing surgical accuracy, the development of simulation and training models is crucial in preparing medical professionals with experience for real-world applications. The models provide a hands-on experience that closely simulates the nature of operating rooms, on which students can practice on anatomically accurate models. Surgical trainees are, by the use of the models, able to refine their skills in a safe environment, leading to enhanced knowledge of human anatomy and surgery. As these technologies evolve, they also provide an environment in which anatomical accuracy is always encouraged so that future surgeons are equipped to work with complex cases. This blend of education and technology is ultimately central to the creation of a surgical team that continually prioritizes patient safety and produces successful treatment results throughout their practices.

8.4.2. Types of Anatomical Models

The role of anatomical models in modern surgical interventions is two-fold, with implications both in planning and during the execution of medical interventions. One of the most significant applications is the use of patient-specific surgical guides and instruments tailored to the patient's specific anatomy. They offer improved navigation through complex structures, yielding optimal results. Pre-operative planning itself is revolutionized by anatomy models since they enable surgeons to visualize the anatomical landscape in three dimensions. For example, volumetric imaging techniques like CT and MRI generate three-dimensional models that enhance spatial awareness of a surgeon regarding relationships within the body (Kalová et al., 2019). This intense preparation not only improves surgical accuracy but also reduces the risk of complications, thus benefiting both practitioners and patients. In surgical education, simulation and training models are excellent means of exercising surgical skills in a safe environment. These models, typically made to simulate human anatomy, facilitate the learning process by allowing trainees to repeat various procedures several times. Through these advanced training modalities, surgeons can sharpen their proficiency and manage challenging scenarios before entering the operating room.

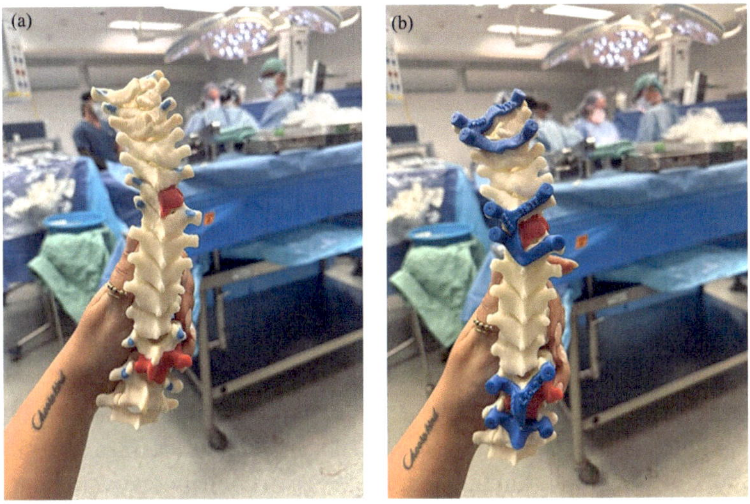

Figure 8.12. The role of anatomical models in modern surgical practices is multi-faceted, impacting both planning and execution of medical procedures.

Source: https://journals.sagepub.com/cms/10.1177/18632521251318552/asset/c9918475-9933-47f4-8c4f-0ed630b41e85/assets/images/large/10.1177_18632521251318552-fig3.jpg.

The fidelity of these models has significantly enhanced, with the addition of soft tissue dynamics and dissimilar anatomical presentations. As the literature has suggested, modeling for computer-assisted surgical devices has revolved around models that are integrated with soft tissue management, critical for use in urology and minimal invasive surgical procedures (Bart et al., 2006). Such integration of anatomical modeling into teaching programs eventually culminates in improved quality of care in practice. In addition, patient-specific instrumentation is a significant advance for the application of anatomical models in planning operations. With precise models created using a patient's own information, surgeons can create instruments and implants designed specifically to a patient's unique anatomy. Not only does this customized method streamline surgery, but it also aims to augment postoperative success and restrict the duration of recovery. The integration of such technology is compatible with current trends in personalized medicine, emphasizing tailored interventions that react to an individual patient's physiology. Complexity issued by soft tissues can also be addressed by using sophisticated surgical navigation systems, which monitor movement skillfully during procedures (Bart et al., 2006). Therefore, the integration of individualized anatomical models in surgical planning not only enriches conventional methods but also expands what is possible with medical device design (Figure 8.12).

8.4.3. Case Studies Demonstrating Effectiveness

Innovation in surgical planning has been impacting patients' outcomes more and more, particularly by utilizing personalized surgical instruments and guides. These personalized devices enable surgeons to perform sophisticated surgeries with better precision and less invasion. Case study testimonials, e.g., orthopedic procedures, have shown that the use of these personalized instruments could lead to shorter operation times and better implant positioning, thereby resulting in better patient recovery. Moreover, the use of such personalized devices lowers the risk of complications as they are adjusted to match the unique anatomical structures of every patient. These developments not only optimize surgical efficiency but also enhance patient-centered principles, which are an example of how personalized practices in medical devices can contribute towards improved surgical quality and satisfaction. Pre-operative planning utilizing anatomical models is another great innovation that has proven to be beneficial in the majority of surgical specialties. Surgeons, through the utilization of 3D-printed replicas of a patient's anatomy, can plan extensively prior to the procedure. Planning helps analyze surgical techniques as well as potential complications that could arise during the procedure. Case studies illustrate that the application of these models of anatomy leads to fewer surgical errors and shorter patient recovery times. Surgeons have reported higher levels of confidence with surgeries involving these models, which also works well towards training new professionals in the field. These new practices reflect a shift towards a more aware and more knowledgeable process of surgical planning, ultimately making overall surgical procedures more efficient and safer. The incorporation of training and simulation models into surgical education and preparation also recognizes the effectiveness of advanced technologies in medical equipment. The models provide a safety-free environment for surgical trainees to practice and experienced surgeons to refine techniques without compromising patient safety. Case studies proving the effectiveness of such training models demonstrate that students undergoing simulation-based training have better technical skills and decision-making skills during actual surgeries. The benefits of such training extend to technical proficiency, as the models have a tendency to promote teamwork and communication between surgical teams. Therefore, the integration of advanced simulation tools arbitrates an improved-informed surgery practice, ultimately allowing for an excellence-based culture in surgical outcomes and patient safety within healthcare settings.

8.5. SIMULATION AND TRAINING MODELS

Surgical planning has increasingly depended on the utility of training and simulation models, which represent new ways of translating complex clinical data into effective surgical plans. Through the integration of these models, surgeons can visualize pathologies through detailed anatomical representations, which can be done with three-dimensional printing technology. These advances have a direct impact on patient care, particularly in congenital heart disease, where individualized models make possible precise preoperative assessment and enhancement in surgical skills. Importantly, use of anatomical models in training medical professionals improves experience-based learning, hence bridging the gap between theoretical knowledge and practical application. As can be observed through case studies, innovative technologies regularly reshape the way in which trainees engage with advanced procedures, eventually driving innovation in surgical practice and in patient care, underlining the significance of effective training models in modern medicine (Anwar et al., 2018). For further enhancement of surgical precision, multimodal simulation environments are being increasingly utilized for preoperative planning. Such environments integrate multiple sensory modalities, for instance, haptic feedback and immersive visualizations, in order to provide an integrative interaction with the surgical process. For instance, in the case of hip arthroplasty, utilization of haptic feedback provides surgeons with the ability to feel tactile feedback regarding the anatomy, thereby providing a better sense of comprehending intricate relationships between bone structures. Such paradigms of training not only improve technical skills but also facilitate the development of critical decision-making abilities in real operating room settings. With improvement in training, shifting towards multimodal interfaces is a paradigm shift from traditional training methodologies, emphasizing a more integrated model of surgical training that keeps pace with the evolving technological advancements in medical devices (Caldwell et al., 2006). In the end, the significant shifts in surgical training models are part of a larger movement toward customized and streamlined patient care. Individualized surgical guides and patient-specific instrumentation are among the leaders of this change, allowing for tailored surgical solutions founded on individual anatomical differences. Simulation and training model use extends beyond mere technical readiness; it also promotes a sense of teamwork among multidisciplinary teams with greater communication. As medical systems advance with these technologies, the effects on pedagogic approaches and clinical practices are vast. Thus, further evolution of simulation modes not only promises to revolutionize surgical planning but also emphasizes the urgency of ongoing research and development in medical technologies to meet the evolving demands of diverse patient groups and realize the best results in operating rooms (Anwar et al., 2018).

8.5.1. Purpose of Simulation in Surgery

The introduction of high-level simulation into surgical practice is a significant shift in the planning and execution of surgical procedures. Breakthroughs in tailor-made surgical guides and instruments facilitate enhanced accuracy of interventions, ultimately resulting in improved patient outcomes. Through the employment of anatomical models during pre-operative planning, surgeons gain enhanced visual representation of complex anatomical features in three dimensions, thereby reducing intraoperative complications. This advanced understanding is crucial when working with precise anatomical variations in individual patients. For instance, application of multimodal environments has been promising in the development of interactive, immersive simulations that facilitate enhanced surgical preparation, as noted in current research on haptic technology (Caldwell et al., 2006). These developments underscore the significance of simulation in surgery, not just as a training platform but as a revolutionary learning tool for surgical residents. Simulation and training models have emerged as crucial components of surgical training, providing a valuable skill-acquisition and assessment platform. They offer the chance for repeated repetition in a risk-free environment where surgeons can master their craft without the pressures one labors with in the operating room. Features like haptic feedback and interactive scenarios offer realistic training experiences, which enable learners to enhance their procedural proficiency. In congenital heart disease, three-dimensional printing as a learning and training tool has also gained popularity, with the potential to enable learners to navigate complex anatomical models (Anwar et al., 2018). This not only promotes technical proficiency but also promotes collaboration among multidisciplinary teams. Accordingly, the continuous improvement in simulation technology upgrades the training of healthcare professionals by inculcating a culture of competency and assurance among newbie surgeons. Patient-specific instrumentation is at the forefront of individualized surgical therapy, highlighting the eerie capabilities of simulation technologies. By designing personalized instruments and guides that exactly fit each patient's anatomy, surgeons can significantly upgrade the speed and accuracy of surgical methods. This optimization directly improves surgical results while reducing patients' recovery periods. In addition, the use of virtual simulation during pre-operative planning gives surgical teams a clear plan of action, allowing them to foresee problems and produce effective strategies beforehand. Such innovative strategies reflect a larger movement in orthogonally tackling the orthogonality of current surgeries, demonstrating how simulation influences not only immediate clinical practice but also the future direction of surgical development. As orthogonally underscored by the emergence of personalized medicine, the integration of technology and planning eventually serves the common purpose of enhancing patient care and safety (Figure 8.13).

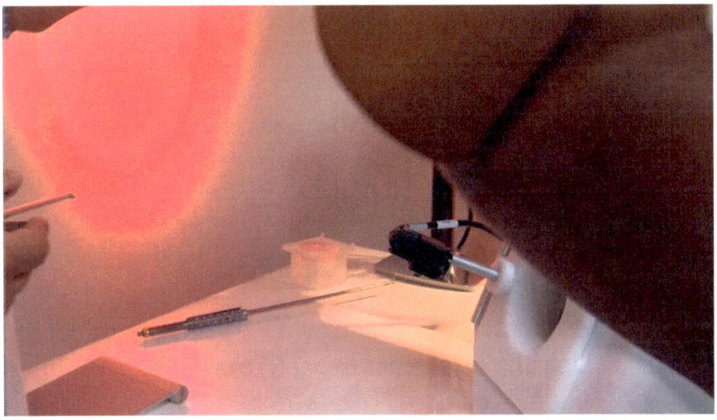

Figure 8.13. Simulation and training models have emerged as essential components of surgical education, providing an effective platform for skill acquisition and assessment.

*Source:*https://cf-images.us-east-1.prod.boltdns.net/v1/jit/4988507115001/809f8f03-19be-4da1-a6d6-e50a72563979/main/1280x720/41s429ms/match/image.jpg.

8.5.2. Types of Simulation Models

In the industry of medical devices and surgical planning, there are many types of simulation models that have a vital function to fulfill in ensuring both procedure efficacy and education of the healthcare professionals. One particularly significant model is the utilization of custom made surgical guides and instruments, which are produced according to the individual anatomy of certain patients. This procedure not only streamlines the surgical process but also improves outcomes by allowing surgeons to visualize and plan their course of action beforehand. Through creating such tailored guides, experts are capable of anticipating potential complications and modify their techniques, accordingly, thus saving time in the operating room and reducing the potential for errors. Also, technological advancements in 3D printing have enhanced the accuracy of such customized instruments, rendering them even more viable for routine surgical procedures, enhancing the general quality of care delivered to patients in different settings.

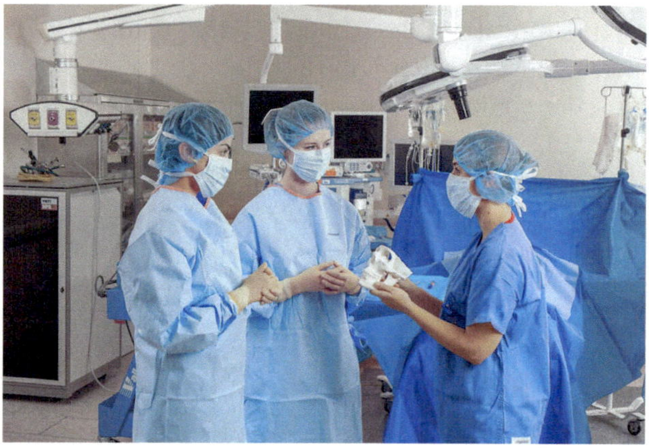

Figure 8.14. Pre-operative planning significantly benefits from the integration of anatomical models, which allow surgeons to explore complex anatomical structures before entering the operating room.

Source: https://blogs.gwu.edu/himmelfarb/files/2023/02/3d-printing-surgery-form-labs.jpg.

Pre-operative planning has a lot to benefit from the utilization of anatomical models that allow surgeons to explore complex anatomical structures before the operating theater. By utilization of high-fidelity 3D models from patient-specific imaging, such as CT or MRI scans, surgeons are able to perform in-depth examination of the surgical site. Such a level of preparation is done to enable more understanding of the surgical environment and contribute to making informed decisions regarding incisions, instrument selection, and potential ways of accessing the surgery. The interactive dynamic between the models replicates live surgical situations, providing valuable feedback that reinforces the surgeon's skill and confidence. Pre-operative planning using anatomical models therefore highlights the potential of simulation models to enhance surgical results such that experts become better equipped to manage the nuances of individual cases. Simulation and training models also highlight the paradigmatic potential of advanced technologies in surgical training. Such models allow medical practitioners to rehearse surgery in a mimic environment, sharpening skills without endangering patient safety. Virtual reality simulations, for instance, provide experiential training that mimics real surgery conditions, permitting practitioners to repeat practice endlessly until proficiency is achieved. Patient-specific instrumentation also raises the realism of such models through the use of actual anatomical information, making training more useful and effective. This personalized training not only equips surgeons with the technical expertise required but also prepares them for handling unexpected complications in real operations. The incorporation of simulation training in surgical education reflects an innovative vision aimed at surgical greatness and patient protection, ultimately converting into improved health outcomes for various medical specialties (Figure 8.14).

8.5.3. Impact on Surgical Outcomes

The use of advanced medical devices in surgical planning is transforming the method and performance of operations in the operation theater. Among the advances is the use of customized surgical guides and instruments that give accurate alignment and orientation to surgeons during complex procedures. These personalized instruments are derived from the specific anatomy of the patient, leading to a more controlled and efficient surgery. Studies have determined that patient-specific plans can result in reduced operation times and improved outcomes since surgeons have fewer variables to deal with in the operating room. Furthermore, the use of patient-specific guides enhances the patient's overall experience by possibly reducing postoperative complications and recovery time. Consequently, the role of these devices in enhancing the precision of surgery is central to an understanding of their broader impact on surgical outcomes in the field of medicine today. In the field of pre-operative planning, high-end imaging technology has shown anatomical models to greatly improve surgeons' comprehension of intricate cases. With three-dimensional (3D) printed models, experts are in a position to visualize the fine details of a patient's anatomy, a benefit that comes in useful for complex procedures, i.e., those carried out in maxillofacial or orthopedic surgery. These models provide a tangible representation of the patient's unique features, allowing sophisticated surgical plans to counteract threats introduced by space uncertainty. Review of surgical publications puts into focus that these visual aids not only enhance surgical planning but are also an element in intraoperative choice-making. Thus, the use of anatomical models is linked to improved surgical efficacy and enhanced surgical team confidence, substantiating the belief that proper pre-operative preparation has a direct relationship with successful outcomes in surgery (Annemans et al., 2016). Training and simulation models play key roles in preparing surgical teams for deployment within actual contexts. Through providing platforms where experienced surgeons and trainees can hone their skills, such models facilitate proficiency in surgical techniques without the immediate risks associated with live surgery. The capacity for practice using simulators allows for improved understanding of workflow within a surgical technique, which increases proficiency and reduces errors when conducting actual surgeries. Current evidence indicates that the use of simulation in surgical education not only enhances technical skill but also promotes intercommunication between surgical teams, resulting in additional patient safety and outcome gains. Furthermore, training models are supported by the use of patient-specific instrumentation, permitting smoother translation of skill within the operating room. Consequently, all these technologies combined underscore the importance of complete training as a major determinant of surgical success (Bini et al., 2019).

8.6. PATIENT-SPECIFIC INSTRUMENTATION

Surgical developments have witnessed the utilization of patient-specific instrumentation as a critical driver in the increase of the scope of operations, with precise solutions utilized to fit individual anatomy and maximize surgical outcome. This theoretical framework enables the surgeon to use customized surgical guides and instruments that have been uniquely created for individual patients' anatomy. Personalization not only maximizes surgical precision but can also potentially reduce operative time and complications. With the introduction of patient-specific designs, the surgical team is better equipped to manage complex anatomical differences among different patients. The innovation is an indication of going towards patient-centered care in surgery practice, pointing to the importance of personalized care in enhancing procedural effectiveness and efficiency. The existing focus on patient-specific instrumentation is very much in compliance with the overall direction of value-based healthcare, where outcomes are increasingly tied to individualized care and improved patient experience. Pre-operative planning has evolved a lot, particularly aided by anatomical models obtained using sophisticated imaging techniques and 3D printing technologies. The ability to create precise anatomical copies allows one to perform extensive simulation prior to the actual surgery, leading to more informed decision-making. Surgeons can assess anatomy differences they may encounter during surgery, which can result in optimally maximized surgical planning and reduction of intraoperative surprise. Existing literature indicates that such preparation will result in a considerable reduction in surgical time and procedural overall success rates increase, paralleling clinical and cost improvement in outcomes pertaining to the use of patient-specific models. With

3D printing becoming the buzz in operating rooms, it is a prime example of how sophisticated technology bridges the space between preoperative planning and operative execution to achieve improved patient outcomes and institutional effectiveness (Annemans et al., 2016). Patient-specific instrumentation use in surgical procedures is the critical advancement in the medical devices and surgical planning space. Sophisticated simulation and targeted training models are necessary to ensure that surgical teams will be able to effectively employ the customized instruments created uniquely for each patient. These types of learning techniques not only assist in the development and refinement of surgical competence but also emphasize the importance of introducing surgical personnel to the specifics of each individual case. Further, the utilization of customized operating instruments has been linked to reductions in operating room preparation time according to recent clinical research of orthopedic cases (Bini et al., 2019). The outcomes show that there is a meaningful decrease in processing time, which has a significant impact on operational efficiency and resource utilization. By further improving training modalities alongside the implementation of patient-specific devices, the medical community can create safer and more effective surgical procedures for patients and clinicians.

8.6.1. Definition and Significance

In contemporary medical practice, the combination of newer technologies has revolutionized the planning of surgery, particularly through the use of customized surgical guides and instruments. Not only do these technologies enhance the precision of surgery but also reduce the risk associated with standard approaches. Through the employment of patient-specific instrumentation, surgeons are able to tailor their approach to adapt to distinct anatomical variations, leading to better overall surgical outcomes. The customizing process is generally founded upon wide-ranging pre-operative imaging, making it possible to fabricate guides that fit perfectly the patient's unique anatomy. Thus, such surgical devices constitute a pivotal nexus between advanced technology and practical execution in the operating room, demonstrating their indispensable role in modern surgical planning. Pre-operative planning cannot be overemphasized, as it has a direct relationship with the success of surgery and recovery rate. Through the utilization of anatomy models developed from advanced imaging techniques, such as DICOM images, operating teams can preview complex structures before they arrive in the operating room. Preoperative visualization allows surgeons to rehearse complex procedures, identify potential problems, and optimize best practices particular to the patient's specific needs. Furthermore, virtual environments with haptic feedback are emerging as important training platforms, in which real-time manipulation and assessment of surgical conditions may be conducted. These simulations not only enhance the skill set of the surgeon but also enhance the understanding of the operating field, ultimately leading to improved patient care and outcomes (Arnez et al., 2012). Incorporating simulation and model training into surgical training bridges the gap between theoretical and applied knowledge. Medical staff can perform realistic simulations of various surgical scenarios, perfecting their skill in a manner that does not carry the ethical cost of real procedures. These training models enable testing of new surgical approaches and error and correction, in order to reach competency. With the growth of the medical device market, the use of such methods grows, especially in the resolution of the diverse challenges presented by complex cases. By investing in high-cost training programs and advanced surgical planning software, medical centers and hospitals can ensure that clinicians are provided with the competency to manage the intricacies of today's surgical procedures (Bowers et al., 2009) (Figure 8.15).

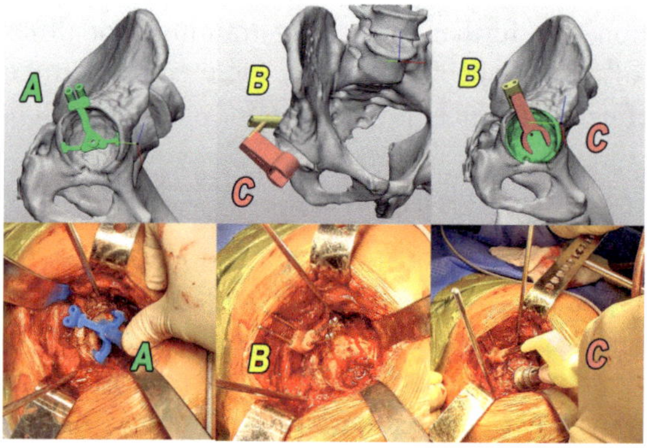

Figure 8.15. By employing patient-specific instrumentation, surgeons can tailor their approaches to individual anatomical variations, improving overall surgical outcomes.

Source: https://media.springernature.com/lw1200/springer-static/image/art%3A10.1186%2Fs12893-023-02281-3/MediaObjects/12893_2023_2281_Fig3_HTML.png.

8.6.2. Development Process of Patient-Specific Tools

The development of patient-specific devices for the surgical field has revolutionized preoperative planning and execution. With the fabrication of patient-specific surgical guides and instruments, clinicians can now tailor procedures based on individual patient anatomy. Personalization enhances accuracy in surgery, reduces operative time, and reduces postoperative morbidity. The process begins with advanced imaging techniques, where volumetric images obtained through MRI or CT scans are used to create tailored surgical blueprints. With these technologies, surgeons can view the patient's individualized anatomical landmarks, thereby facilitating designs that adapt to personal specifications intraoperatively. These technologies are the foundations of the world of medical devices, leading the way to more complex surgical techniques with an emphasis on outcomes and safety for the patient. To further improve surgical methods, preoperative planning has grown more advanced through the use of anatomical models, which are tangible representations of patient-specific data. With these models, multidisciplinary teams can rehearse complex procedures, bringing about greater familiarity and less time in the operating room.

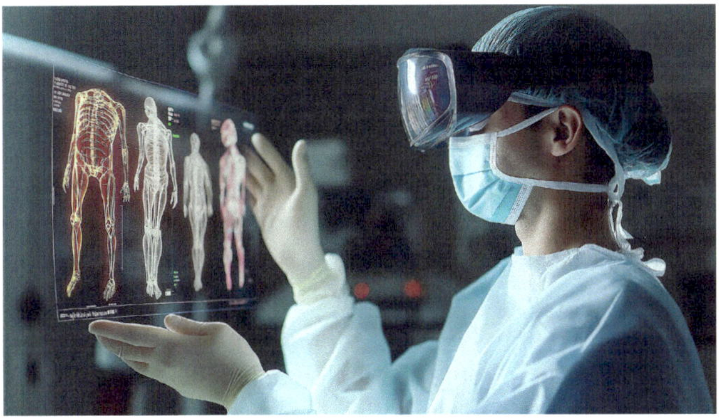

Figure 8.16. Patient-specific instrumentation embodies the pinnacle of innovation in surgical planning, bridging the gap between advanced technology and personalized medicine.

Source: https://s3.amazonaws.com/production.scholastica/article/127691/large/adobestock_956861332.jpeg?1740947687.

The development of these anatomical models is accomplished with sophisticated software that translates imaging data into 3D models so practitioners can actually see and interact with the anatomy. In addition, simulation and training models give surgeons the power to practice operations and iron out potential issues in a risk-free environment. This training not only enhances surgical proficiency but also promotes a working relationship between surgical teams, promoting harmonious planning and execution of patient-specific devices in surgery. Patient-specific instrumentation is the pinnacle of innovation in surgical planning, bridging the gap between high technology and personalized medicine. Creating such instrumentation involves advanced collaboration among different stakeholders, such as surgeons, biomedical engineers, and material scientists. The intricate design process is performed by iteratively testing and optimizing to ensure congruence with both the surgery technique and the patient's individual anatomy. Incorporating systems like Computer-Assisted Orthopedic Surgery (CAOS), which integrate imaging modalities and real-time data evaluation, has greatly increased the success of surgical intervention (Kalová et al., 2019). Moreover, the rise of autonomous surgical systems, as embryonic as it is, promises to redefine the very definition of surgical practice with increased precision and convenience, transgressing boundaries inherent in manual practice (Das et al., 2017). Ultimately, ongoing evolution of patient-specific instruments contributes to not only maximizing the results of surgery but also revolutionizing the art of medicine (Figure 8.16).

8.6.3. Clinical Applications and Success Stories

Medical device clinical use during surgical planning has altered procedure behavior, resulting in significantly improved patient outcomes. Customized surgical instruments and guides, for example, have been instrumental in enhancing precision during surgery, reducing time as well as the complications associated with employing traditional processes. Utilizing patient-specific anatomical data, guides provide surgeons with the ability to navigate complex surgical spaces more accurately. This tailored approach has been supported in effective case studies wherein the meticulous planning and execution enabled by such tools have minimized complications, made recovery periods easier, and enhanced patient satisfaction levels overall. These advanced applications of technology by way of pre-operative planning with anatomical models are a reflection of the commitment of healthcare systems towards evolving surgical techniques, a key aspect in achieving patient care effectively. Pre-operative planning using anatomical models has emerged as a core aspect in surgical success as well. These models are a three-dimensional representation of an individual patient's specific physiology, allowing surgical teams to visualize and plan in advance. Hospitals have sworn to higher quality in surgical performance when they use these models since they facilitate better communication among multidisciplinary teams. Furthermore, advances in training and simulation models subject prospective surgeons to realistic conditions, thus facilitating higher levels of comprehension in complex cases. This combined approach not only makes the surgical techniques more robust but also is an area where learning from the experience in actual clinical practice gets the highest importance, thereby reducing intraoperative errors to lesser extent and ultimately impacting patient safety adversely. Patient-specific instrumentation has been another innovation in the practice of surgical planning, demonstrating how personalized medicine is revolutionizing conventional practice. This innovative approach streamlines surgical tools implemented based on the individual details of patients' anatomy, enhancing the overall effectiveness of surgical procedures. Evidence from the healthcare systems utilizing these approaches shows a major decrease in procedure time and revision surgery needs, underscoring actual value addition within surgical practice through tailoring. Furthermore, financial gains through increased efficiency and optimization of resources are also considerable; healthcare organizations increasingly recognize that current best practices with the application of technology provide long-term benefits in the delivery of care (Johnson et al., 2011). This complete realization of patient-specific practice reinforces a drive towards advancing surgical planning that is efficient and responsive to individual patients' needs.

8.7. CONCLUSION

The evolution of medical devices has significantly transformed surgical planning, ultimately leading to patient-oriented practices. Precision medicine has led us into an era in which the incorporation of customized surgical guides and instruments is paramount, as they optimize the precision of surgical procedures. Patient-specific instrumentation enables surgeons to tackle complex surgical topographies, ultimately reducing operative time and improving postoperative recovery. The intersection of advanced imaging modalities has facilitated the easy development of personalized surgical plans taking into account the patients' specific anatomy, thus making therapy as effective as possible without inflicting unnecessary trauma on surrounding tissues. Pre-operative assessment has evolved towards emphasizing patient-specific factors that, in return, contribute to maximizing therapeutic efficacy and patient satisfaction, based on numerous guidelines (Lori et al., 2021). Surgical training has also been totally revolutionized with the emergence of simulation and training models. These devices are essential to the training of medical practitioners to equip them for real-life surgical operations by providing a risk-free environment to practice and improve their skills. Using realistic anatomical models, professionals can familiarize themselves with intricate procedures, enhancing their technical expertise and confidence in the operating room. It not only increases surgical competency but also adds to greater insight into patient-specific variables that influence outcomes. Additionally, focus on simulation-based training mirrors the personalized results that modern medical technology is engineered to offer in surgical planning, which plays a critical role in framing a new generation of proficient surgeons skilled in the operation of cutting-edge technologies (Matthew et al., 2021). Ahead, surgical planning has a future of continuing to push boundaries, utilizing the latest technology to better address patient needs and enhance clinical outcomes. Continued medical device research and development will naturally lead to even more sophisticated surgical planning methods taking full advantage of data visualization and artificial intelligence, paving the way for predictive analytics in support of personalized care. By combining multi-disciplinary perspectives, there can be constant optimization of surgical procedures such that interventions are ever evidence-based and responsive to the individual situations of every patient. Collectively, the integration of personalized tools, simulation, and precise pre-operative planning constitutes a solid foundation for surgical dominance, emphasizing the integration of innovation and patient care (Lori et al., 2021).

8.7.1. Summary of Key Points

The use of advanced medical technologies in planning for surgery has transformed the management of complicated procedures. The key to this transformation is the development of patient-specific surgical guides and instruments that support delivering more precision in the course of surgery. These technologies, which are founded on patient anatomy-data-based information, facilitate customized interventions aimed at the unique shape of a human's anatomy. By utilizing 3D printing technology in creating these guides, surgeons can offer even greater accuracy in cutting the bone and implant placement. The importance of having a precise and detailed pre-operative plan cannot be overstated, as it can minimize the risk for complications and improve patient care, and thus custom surgical guides are highly valuable tools in today's operating rooms. Pre-surgical planning has been greatly enhanced by the development of anatomical models replicating the surgical site. They enable surgeons to visualize complex anatomy relationships and practice correct techniques before actually being in the operating room. Technologies used to generate these models are usually DICOM images of digital tomographic scans, yielding very high-resolution representations of anatomy of the patient. This meticulous planning process allows surgeons to rehearse operations virtually, honing their technique and anticipating potential complications. Training using simulation and models also raises not only the surgeons' confidence but also their skill level, which indirectly translates to improved surgical performance and patient safety. The use of these models in surgical planning is a major leap in the practice, emphasizing accuracy and preparedness. In addition, patient-specific instrumentation has been a significant surgical planning innovation that provides added personalization and efficiency in procedures. This technique individualizes instruments to a patient's anatomy, allowing for more natural and direct interaction with the characteristics of the surgical site. Such precision reduces the risk of mistake and invasiveness, thereby enhancing patient recovery processes. The partnership of industry with academia, particularly in those states that have a solid underpinning of high-end industries, encourages such technological revolution in surgical procedures. The partnership supports ongoing research and development to fine-tune these technologies in order to make them integral parts of surgical planning and execution to further advance the standards of healthcare in medical practices (N/A, 2016).

8.7.2. Future Trends in Medical Devices and Surgical Planning

The use of new technologies and the manufacturing of medical devices is leading towards the revolution in surgical planning. Integration of the three-dimensional printing is one of the important future trends that allows patient-specific anatomical models to be produced. This technology is revolutionizing the dynamics of surgical preparation due to the possibility of customized surgical guides and instruments. By exactly replicating complex anatomical structures, surgeons can see and rehearse operations in a manner that optimizes accuracy and reduces complications. Three-dimensional printing is not only advantageous to patients but is a superb teaching device for inexperienced surgeons, allowing more awareness of anatomical variation and surgical technique. As noted in current studies, such innovative approach has already begun to improve patient treatment and surgical methods significantly, ushering in a new era of personalized health care solutions (Anwar et al., 2018). Among the trends in surgical planning is the growth in application of computer-aided orthopedic surgery (CAOS) systems, which significantly boost the precision of surgical procedures. These systems make use of advanced imaging techniques, including volumetric images from MRI and CT scans, to construct precise models of patients' anatomy. With such a large amount of knowledge, pre-operative planning is improved, and it becomes possible for surgeons to carry out intricate procedures with more confidence (Kalová et al., 2019). Further, CAOS systems are transforming to incorporate dynamic kinetic information about joints and their corresponding movements, offering surgeons a holistic view of the musculoskeletal system. These technologies allow patients to expect increasingly optimized surgical success, reducing intraoperative errors, as well as post-operative recovery periods. This alignment of technology and surgery anticipates a future where precision medicine is the standard. Furthermore, no part of planning future surgery can be overemphasized when it comes to thinking about the role simulation and training models have. These models serve as a bridge between theory and practice, providing useful platform opportunities for practitioners to ready their skills in the absence of risk. Through the utilization of high-fidelity simulations, surgeons are able to engage in real-life simulations that mimic real surgical practices. This allows for great repetition and mastery of complex techniques before opening the operating room door. These innovations do not just enhance surgeon preparedness but also give patient safety, as the possibility of errors decreases with improved skills. With the ongoing changes in the healthcare landscape, the incorporation of simulation technologies into surgical education will be important in ensuring that healthcare professionals are capable of utilizing innovative tools and techniques to their advantage (Anwar et al., 2018).

8.7.3. Final Thoughts on the Importance of Innovation in Surgery

Surgical innovation assumes an increasingly critical role in enhancing patient results and advancing medical practice. As techniques improve, the use of tailored surgical guides and instruments particular to the individual patient anatomy provides a cornerstone of modern surgical planning. Custom surgical instrumentation allows surgeons to conduct procedures with higher precision, reducing the possibility of complications and achieving greater recovery durations. Furthermore, preoperative planning using anatomical models makes it possible to efficiently visualize each patient's own unique anatomical landscape. This not only aids the surgical team in their planning but also in discussions about the potential risks and benefits to the patient, ultimately leading to joint decision-making. These cooperative endeavors showcase the revolutionary shift in the surgical profession that focuses on customized medicine according to the specific requirements of patients and enhancing overall patient care experiences. Beyond customized instruments and anatomical models, simulation and training procedures also play a significant function in strengthening the surgical community. These technologies allow surgeons to develop their skills in a safe environment, which facilitates them to gain the technical skills needed for complex procedures. Through immersion in simulations of real operating-room scenarios, active practitioners can experiment with various techniques, becoming more adaptive and confident. Enhanced training by simulation accelerates learning as well as offers a platform for continuing professional growth. As medicine strives to adopt increasingly advanced technologies, a culture of ongoing education and skill development among surgical teams is essential in maintaining high standards of patient safety and satisfaction. These training programs are, in the ultimate analysis, an expression of the bigger imperative of surgical innovation. The relevance of surgical innovation is underscored by the convergence of technology and humanity, seen in the application of patient-specific instrumentation. The continually evolving character of the medical devices industry implies a complex interplay between regulatory frameworks, innovation, and site-specific practice traditions, as is evident with respect to EU regulation of medical devices (Altenstetter et al., 1995). Surgeons leverage evidence-based information and advanced technologies to create patient-specific solutions, which lead to improved surgical results and quality of life. This marriage of science with personalized attention incites a radical shift in the world of surgery, inviting breakthroughs that resonate on an emotional level across societies. As it is evident from New Hampshires push for innovation-led development through interdisciplinary convergence between industry and academia (N/A, 2016), the pursuit of excellence in surgery is an expression of the importance of innovation in ensuring that patient care remains at the forefront of medical innovation.

REFERENCES

1. Altenstetter, C. (1995). Regulating healthcare technologies and medical supplies: A comparative overview. https://core.ac.uk/download/5079662.pdf (accessed on 14th October 2025).
2. Annemans, L., Gemmel, P., Tack, P., Victor, M., et al. (2016). 3D-printing techniques in a medical setting: A systematic literature review. https://core.ac.uk/download/84043719.pdf (accessed on 14th October 2025).
3. Anwar, A., Barach, B., Bhatla, A., Biglino, G., Biglino, I., et al. (2018). 3D printing is a transformative technology in congenital heart disease. https://core.ac.uk/download/212858839.pdf (accessed on 14th October 2025).
4. Arnez, V., Corney, J., Govea-Valladares, E., Hernandez, C., et al. (2012). A novel haptic model and environment for maxillofacial surgical operation planning and manipulation. https://core.ac.uk/download/9559140.pdf (accessed on 14th October 2025).
5. Bart, S., Baumann, M., Berkelman, P., Bolla, M., et al. (2006). Medical image computing and computer-aided medical interventions applied to soft tissues. Work in progress in urology. http://arxiv.org/abs/0712.2100 (accessed on 14th October 2025).
6. Bini, S. A., Bowden, D. E., Callahan, M., Capra, M., et al. (2019). Implementing a perioperative efficiency initiative for orthopedic surgery instrumentation at an academic center: A comparative before-and-after study. https://core.ac.uk/download/323062983.pdf (accessed on 14th October 2025).
7. Bowers, R., & Ross, K. (2009). A review of the effectiveness of lower limb orthoses used in cerebral palsy. https://core.ac.uk/download/9024488.pdf (accessed on 14th October 2025).
8. Burity, J., da Fonte, I. B., & de Melo, P. B. (2014). Radiological Society of North America (RSNA) 3D printing Special Interest Group (SIG): Guidelines for medical 3D printing and appropriateness for clinical scenarios. https://core.ac.uk/download/212867900.pdf (accessed on 14th October 2025).
9. Burton, M. J., Ramke, J., Marques, A. P., Bourne, R., Congdon, N., Jones, I., Ah Tong, B. A. M., et al. (2021). The Lancet Global Health Commission on global eye health: Vision beyond 2020. *The Lancet Global Health, 9*, e489–e551. https://doi.org/10.1016/s2214-109x(20)30488-5 (accessed on 14th October 2025).
10. Caldwell, D. G., Gray, J. O., Petrone, M., Testi, D., et al. (2006). A haptic-enabled multimodal interface for the planning of hip arthroplasty. https://core.ac.uk/download/104526.pdf (accessed on 14th October 2025).

11. Culclasure, D. F., & Eckhardt, L. (2025). Southwest Research Institute assistance to NASA in biomedical areas of the technology. https://core.ac.uk/download/pdf/85233530.pdf (accessed on 14th October 2025).
12. Culclasure, D. F., & Eckhardt, L. (2025). Southwest Research Institute assistance to NASA in biomedical areas of the technology utilization program final report, 1 Feb. 1969–24 Aug. 1970. https://core.ac.uk/download/pdf/85236539.pdf (accessed on 14th October 2025).
13. Das, N., & Yip, M. (2017). Robot autonomy for surgery. http://arxiv.org/abs/1707.03080 (accessed on 14th October 2025).
14. Dellavalle, R. P., Obagi, Z. A., & Rundle, C. W. (2020). Widening the scope of virtual reality and augmented reality in dermatology. https://core.ac.uk/download/287622747.pdf (accessed on 14th October 2025).
15. Feinstein, J. A., LaDisa, J. F., & Taylor, C. A. (2010). Aortic coarctation: Recent developments in experimental and computational methods to assess treatments for this simple condition. https://core.ac.uk/download/213079154.pdf (accessed on 14th October 2025).
16. Fortina, P., Kricka, L. J., Park, J. Y., & Polsky, T. G. (2015). The future of laboratory medicine–A 2014 perspective. https://core.ac.uk/download/54509579.pdf (accessed on 14th October 2025).
17. Gallego, G., Hall, J., Haas, M., & Viney, R. (2025). *Reducing the Use of Ineffective Health Care Interventions. CHERE Working Paper 2010/5.* https://core.ac.uk/download/pdf/6376811.pdf (accessed on 14th October 2025).
18. Johnson, C. W. (2011). Identifying common problems in the acquisition and deployment of large-scale software projects in the US and UK healthcare systems. https://core.ac.uk/download/110438.pdf (accessed on 14th October 2025).
19. Kalaskar, D., Leong, J., & Provaggi, E. (2017). Applications of 3D printing in the management of severe spinal conditions. https://core.ac.uk/download/79531622.pdf (accessed on 14th October 2025).
20. Kalová, M., Kubíček, J., Oczka, D., Tomanec, M., et al. (2019). Recent trends, technical concepts and components of computer-assisted orthopedic surgery systems: A comprehensive review. https://core.ac.uk/download/287649034.pdf (accessed on 14th October 2025).
21. Khumawala, B. M., Li, S., Visich, J. K., Zhang, C., et al. (2006). Radio frequency identification technology: Applications, technical challenges and strategies. https://core.ac.uk/download/56735577.pdf (accessed on 14th October 2025).

22. Kupelian, P. A., Meeks, S. L., Shah, A. P., Willoughby, T. R., et al. (2011). Expanding the use of real-time electromagnetic tracking in radiation oncology. https://core.ac.uk/download/323076551.pdf (accessed on 14th October 2025).
23. Lerner, L. B., McVary, K. T., Barry, M. J., Bixler, B. R., Dahm, P., Das, A. K., Gandhi, M. C., et al. (2021). Management of lower urinary tract symptoms attributed to benign prostatic hyperplasia: AUA guideline part II—Surgical evaluation and treatment. *The Journal of Urology, 206*, 818–826. https://doi.org/10.1097/ju.0000000000002184 (accessed on 14th October 2025).
24. N/A. (2016). *New Hampshire University Research and Industry Plan: A Roadmap for Collaboration and Innovation.* https://core.ac.uk/download/215517669.pdf (accessed on 14th October 2025).
25. Page, M. J., Moher, D., Bossuyt, P. M., Boutron, I., Hoffmann, T., Mulrow, C. D., Shamseer, L., et al. (2021). PRISMA 2020 explanation and elaboration: Updated guidance and exemplars for reporting systematic reviews. https://doi.org/10.1136/bmj.n160 (accessed on 14th October 2025).

CHAPTER 9

MICROFLUIDICS AND LAB-ON-A-CHIP DEVICES

Contents

INTRODUCTION

Microfluidics is a revolutionary technology that has greatly contributed to numerous scientific and medical disciplines by enabling manipulation of minute quantities of fluids at the microscopic level. It is marked by its ability to manipulate fluid flows within microchannels with dimensions typically less than a millimeter. Its evolution has enabled advancements in molecular biology, diagnostics, and chemical synthesis, among others. These capabilities are of paramount importance in enhancing sensitivity and efficiency in processes previously constrained by traditional methods. Miniaturization and integration of devices onto chip surfaces enable scientists to conduct sophisticated analyses on small samples, thereby reducing costs and time involved in experimental procedures. Microfluidics has therefore enabled pioneering uses from elementary research to real-world applications in medicine, environmental monitoring, and many more (Abate et al., 2017). Through being part of the growing movement towards point-of-care diagnostics, microfluidics has introduced lab-on-a-chip devices with the whole laboratory process in portable configuration. These technologies employ microfluidic technology for performing multiparametric analysis with speed and accuracy, typically generating outputs that otherwise would take significant time and investment using conventional laboratory equipment. Applications of these include nucleic acid amplification, protein detection, and cell sorting, now facilitated by miniaturized microfluidic platforms. This portability offers real-time diagnostic capability within different environments, from clinical settings to remote locations. The transition towards lab-on-a-chip technology not only enhances diagnostic efficiency but also completes gaps in access to high-level diagnostics that are essential in infectious disease management and biochemical studies (Abate et al., 2017). Moreover, microfluidics is not only applied in diagnostics but finds applications in future fields such as personalized medicine and targeted drug delivery. The ability to control biological constituents at the microscale enables scientists to tailor therapies based on patient-specific profiles, maximizing efficacy and minimizing side effects. Additionally, combining microfluidic systems with advanced imaging and sensing technology holds the promise to provide effective diagnostic tools that provide real-time proof of biological processes. Challenges continue to exist, particularly when it comes to the impact of external conditions on data quality, such as in iris recognition where external conditions can have the potential to degrade results. Nevertheless, the continued development of microfluidic technology promises to overcome challenges, paving the way for breakthroughs that transform the landscape of biomedical study and healthcare provision.

Definition and Overview

Microfluidics is a significant interface of life sciences and engineering that makes it possible to handle fluids at the microscale. As the science and technology of fluid-handling systems for small amounts of fluid—on the order of nanoliters to picoliters—microfluidics enables biochemical environments to be controlled with high precision. Microfluidics has enabled the development of lab-on-a-chip devices through which various laboratory functions are integrated on one platform. Through miniaturizing the processes, lab-on-a-chip devices minimize time and cost considerations that typically accompany conventional laboratory processes as well as enable real-time analysis and high-throughput screening. Microfluidic systems' inherent flexibility and efficiency make them of invaluable use in a variety of applications ranging from medical diagnostics to drug delivery, which highlights their status as a game-changer in scientific research today.

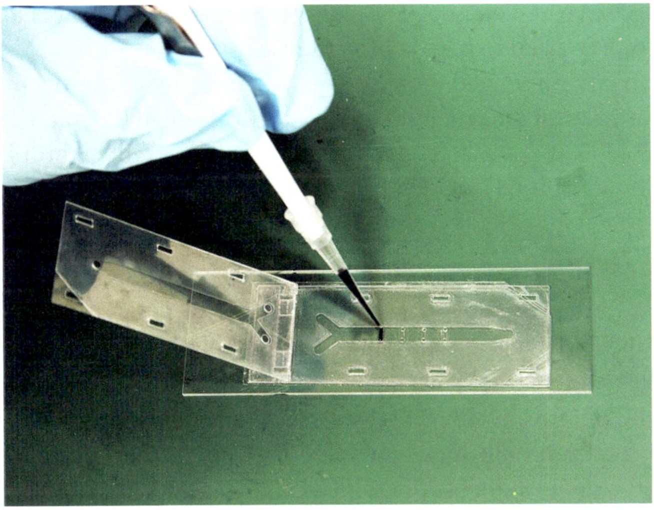

Figure 9.1. Microfluidics represents a critical intersection of engineering and life sciences, facilitating the manipulation of fluids at the microscale.

Source: https://upload.wikimedia.org/wikipedia/commons/thumb/a/ac/Microfluidic_Device_%286842746147%29.jpg/1200px-Microfluidic_Device_%286842746147%29.jpg.

The development of programmable biochemistry, as exemplified in systems like BioScript, is a significant advancement in the area of microfluidics. BioScript is a domain-specific language designed to make biochemical processes carried out on microfluidic devices easier and more user-friendly. Its innovative syntax allows for human understandability while offering a robust type of system for preventing prevalent errors encountered in biochemical interactions and ensuring efficient and safe experiments. In addition, the compiler optimizes concurrent execution of biochemical processes to ensure greater efficiency on complex microfluidic arrays. Scientists are able to achieve high-fidelity results that picture the actual applications of these technologies through simulation and real platforms. This not only broadens the use of microfluidics among practitioners in the life sciences but also accelerates the establishment of sophisticated applications in the field of biochemistry (Brisk et al., 2018). Ongoing research in microfluidic technologies has revealed promising trends, notably tailoring application-specific integrated microfluidic systems. Researchers are increasingly interested in designing multifunctional microfluidic platforms, such as those based on rotating disk technology (Lab-CD) and nanoliter dispensing technology. These platforms accommodate a high level of experimental design, such that researchers can tailor their approaches to fit specific research and diagnostic needs. Their versatility ensures that they can be applied to the varied demands of various applications of life sciences, from diagnostics to environmental monitoring. With continued improvement of such platforms, they reveal the potential of wider utilization in laboratories and show how microfluidics is ready to become a tool of considerable worth in scientific research and innovation (Ducrée et al., 2004) (Figure 9.1).

Historical Development

The history of microfluidics and lab-on-a-chip technology in the past can be followed to the early success in miniaturizing and microfabricating equipment in the late 20th century. Early research was focused on creating simple systems that would be able to handle volumes of liquids at the micro-scale because of the need for faster and more efficient analysis from biology to chemistry disciplines. Techniques such as photolithography, used widely in semiconductor manufacturing, formed the basis for the fabrication of sophisticated channel architectures that define microfluidic devices. As scientists began to think about applications for these devices, the integration of passive and active devices expanded the potential for what could be achieved in diagnostics and analysis and highlighted the potential for microfluidics to play a central role in future health technologies and environmental monitoring. In subsequent years, tremendous progress was made towards understanding the micro-scale fluid dynamics that resulted in the development of more sophisticated devices for special purposes. Acoustofluidic devices, for instance, have evolved to enhance sample manipulation and separation capabilities in microfluidic systems. Improvements in automated platforms with the ability to manage complex processes provided researchers with the capability of dynamically controlling and optimizing sample handling. A good illustration is the application of closed-loop systems to achieve effective sample collection and processing, which ultimately saves waste and precious biological material. As illustrated, this paradigm shift brought with it a new era of research possibility in diagnostics, particularly with the establishment of integrated platforms that simplify processes involving sample preparation and analysis, as presented in pioneering work in the field (Benett et al., 2015). Microfluidics applied to the diagnosis of cancer is but one illustration of the profound impact that has been brought about by developments in the past on current medical technology. Deformation-based circulating tumor cell (CTC) microchips are one critical innovation for early cancer detection, with fluid control at the micro-scale allowing for effective sample separation and analysis. Historical investigations on the flow regimes in CTCs have served to explain the mechanism behind their response in microgeometries, culminating in the optimization of device structure for better performance (Chen et al., 2015). Understanding parameters such as critical pressure and channel geometry has been instrumental in refining these filtration devices. With developments in the microfluidics technology, future research and development will be guided by lessons learnt from past progress, paving the way towards more functional and long-lasting diagnostic devices within a clinical environment (Figure 9.2).

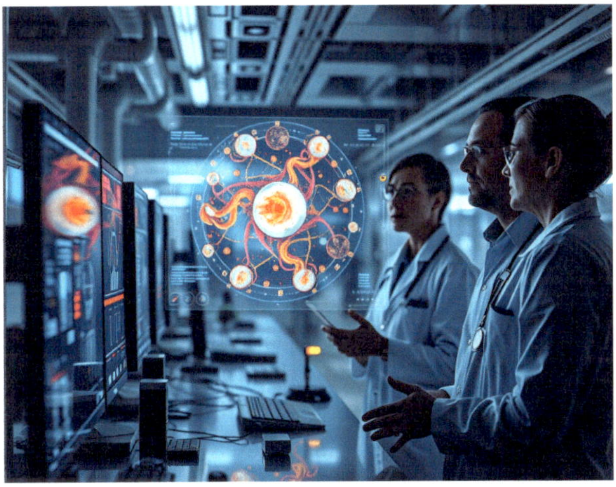

Figure 9.2. The evolution of automated platforms capable of complex processes empowered researchers with the ability to control and optimize sample handling dynamically.

Source: https://i0.wp.com/ajithp.com/wp-content/uploads/2025/02/image-18.png?fit=1024%2C768&ssl=1.

Importance in Modern Science

The function of lab-on-a-chip systems and microfluidics cannot be overstated in the context of current science, as they are the ideal fusion of advanced technology and innovative biomedical uses. The systems enable scientists to manipulate and analyze minute quantities of fluids, an important requirement in numerous fields of research, including personalized medicine and diagnosis.

The technologies enable rapid and cost-effective analysis, making them relevant tools in the biomedical research field. For instance, microfluidic devices can be utilized for the high-throughput screening of drugs in order to accelerate the process of therapeutic drug development. Through the enablement of point-of-care diagnostics, microfluidics represents the trend towards decentralized healthcare in order to achieve enhanced access to early medical intervention in developed and resource-constrained communities. Besides healthcare, the application of microfluidics also influences environmental monitoring and chemical analysis. The ability to perform complex fluid manipulation in miniature systems is very serious in applications while evaluating contaminants and in environmental toxin detection. This flexibility has gained much interest from industries where sustainability and public health are key factors, and thus the need for instant diagnostic devices independent of the traditional laboratory settings. The flexibility of lab-on-a-chip technology makes it possible to tailor applications to suit precise market needs and supports cross-disciplinary interactions between chemists, biologists, and engineers. The evidence of ongoing progress in photonics and material science toward the design of more effective lab-on-a-chip devices is testimony to the extent to which the scientific community has accepted the application of microfluidics in research and development activities. The educational significance of microfluidics and lab-on-a-chip technologies also contributes to their relevance in contemporary science. Organizations like the Boston University Photonics Center have placed a priority on collaborative research activities that combine education and practical application, as indicated by their yearly reports focusing on grants and innovation. The ability to engage students in research endeavors involving microfluidics promotes a new generation of scientists capable of meeting critical issues facing the world. Moreover, via initiatives such as National Science Foundation-supported sites for Research Experiences for Undergraduates and for Teachers, the budding scientists directly engage with the latest technologies, making them ready to pursue careers in inter-disciplinary research. Ongoing transmission of knowledge between the academic sector and business houses is imperative in sustaining the pace of microfluidics technology development and, in turn, ensuring its consistent utility in science and innovation (N/A, 2013, 2015).

9.1. PRINCIPLES OF MICROFLUIDICS

The principles of microfluidics are based on the precise handling of fluids on the micro level, typically in channels with diameters ranging from tens to hundreds of micrometers. This is in accordance with the laws of fluid mechanics, i.e., laminar flow, which is realized under low Reynolds numbers characteristic of micro-scale environments. In microfluidic systems, the absence of turbulence allows regular flow regimes, thereby promoting interactions among discrete fluid volumes without chaotic mixing in bulk systems. Hence, microfluidics can facilitate creating highly controlled environments needed for complex biological reactions, analytical processes, and chemical syntheses important in diagnostics and drug delivery applications. One of the prime applications of microfluidics is combining it with lab-on-a-chip devices, which consolidate different laboratory procedures onto a single microchip. Microfluidics renders experimental procedures much more effective by allowing quick analysis with an extremely small sample volume. For instance, in research biomedicine, microfluidic devices can be utilized to study cell activity under controlled environments, such as in experiments studying leukocyte extravasation. The ability to create structured flow paths enables researchers to simulate physiological conditions, allowing for detailed simulation of biological processes (Navarrete et al., 2018). These advancements illustrate how microfluidics enables new experimental setups that yield consistent and reproducible results. The building of microfluidic systems also often includes diverse materials such as polydimethylsiloxane (PDMS) and glass, which, depending on the desired application, possess distinct advantages. PDMS, for instance, is also used because it is biocompatible and easy to produce, hence suitable for creating channels and chambers in lab-on-a-chip devices. Fluid-solid interaction can also be effectively controlled through the modification of the surface by employing different surface modification techniques, hence enhancing such device performance by avoiding nonspecific adsorption and improving fluidic behavior. As such, the progressive development of microfluidic technologies continues to transform areas from clinical diagnostics to monitoring the environment, with an indication of the immense influence of the mastery of microfluidics principles in modern science (Ahmad et al., 2018).

9.1.1. Fluid Dynamics at the Microscale

Microscale fluid dynamics is a key area for the development of microfluidics and lab-on-a-chip technologies. At the microscale, the behavior of fluids is quite different from what is seen at the macroscopic scale, mainly due to the dominance of surface tension effects and the diminishment of Reynolds numbers. These conditions lead to unique flow characteristics such as laminar flow, where the fluid travels in parallel layers with minimal disturbance among them. The laminar flow plays a crucial role in the accurate control of fluid motion and mixing processes in microfluidic channels to facilitate applications from biochemical assays to drug delivery systems. Additionally, the understanding of microscale fluid dynamics enables one to develop novel devices that can perform advanced fluid manipulations with great efficiency and reliability, a requirement for the success of lab-on-a-chip technology. Additionally, continuous phase and droplet interactions in microfluidic devices highlight the intricacy of microscale fluid dynamics. Techniques such as droplet-based microfluidics exploit these interactions for applications including high-throughput screening and single-cell analysis. Recent advances have introduced means to elevate mixing and reaction rates by specific injection of immiscible droplets into microfluidic channels.

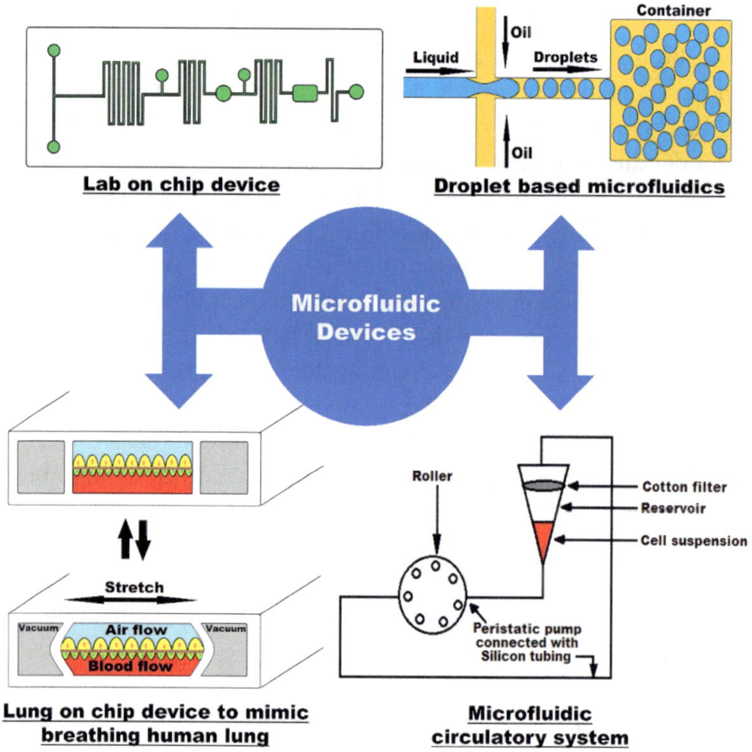

Figure 9.3. The study of fluid dynamics at the microscale plays a pivotal role in advancing microfluidics and lab-on-a-chip technologies.

Source: https://www.mdpi.com/biosensors/biosensors-12-00459/article_deploy/html/images/biosensors-12-00459-g001.png.

Through research, it has been found that the degree of mixing can be accurately controlled by varying the frequency of injection of droplets and the geometric channel parameters. The ability to control mixing at the microscale highly improves not only the precision of reaction conditions but also the efficiency of sample processing, demonstrating the crucial relationship between fluid dynamics and device functionality in lab-on-a-chip applications (Motosuke et al., 2018). In addition to mixing, droplet generation and manipulation in microfluidic devices are critical aspects of microscale fluid dynamics. Recent research has focused on computational methods, such as the color gradient lattice Boltzmann model, which provide clues on mechanisms of droplet formation for real-world applications in microfluidics. This enables one to make better sense of droplet formation in various flow conditions and allow them to simulate conditions that allow them to construct devices such as flow-focusers and microfluidic step emulsifiers. The translation of complex fluid behaviors into manageable computational frameworks permits experimental confirmation and optimizes device configurations for specific applications. Harnessing droplet dynamics, thus, not only opens up new frontiers in microfluidics but also inspires the development of versatile lab-on-a-chip devices to address a range of scientific and medical challenges (Rocca et al., 2017) (Figure 9.3).

9.1.2. Surface Tension and Capillary Action

In microfluidics and lab-on-a-chip technology, the principles of capillary action and surface tension have to be understood. Surface tension is a consequence of the attractive intermolecular forces among liquid molecules at the interface and manifests itself as a higher tension at the surface as opposed to the liquid body itself. This physical property is very dominant in explaining fluid behavior in microchannels, as it decides how liquids interact with surfaces and amongst themselves. In microfluidic systems, fluid flow control is often most sensitively dependent on surface tension. Through manipulation of the surface tension by various chemical treatment or surface modification, optimal flow performance can be obtained, optimizing the reactions and separations in the confined spaces. A sophisticated comprehension of these factors has the potential to create new possibilities in lab-on-a-chip devices, introducing more efficient and responsive devices for numerous applications. Capillary action, the capacity for a liquid to rise or fall in a constrained space due to surface tension, further contributes to the worth of microfluidic systems. This is utilized in microfluidic devices to provide fluid transportation without any type of external pumps, leading to advances within the creation of passive fluidic systems that perform successfully at microscopic scales. This feature is particularly valuable in applications where precision is most critical, such as in biochemical assays or drug delivery. Fluids move through a series of channel geometries, where capillary forces dictate their velocity and direction, facilitating coordinating mixing, splitting, or retention of samples in the device. Moreover, progress in material science enables the fabrication of surfaces with predesigned wettability, enhancing capillary action and the way for sophisticated microfluidic applications. Surface tension and capillary action control also enhance electrowetting device functionality, which are now ubiquitous in microfluidic applications. Electrowetting flips the surface tension of fluids when subjected to an electric field, allowing dynamic control over the motion of droplets on a substrate. This capability is particularly powerful in designing lab-on-a-chip devices, allowing rapid switching between different operational states—such as droplet generation, fusion, or division—ahead of multiple applications in the field of biotechnology. As testified to in the literature, control mechanisms are to be found in interactions of fluid dynamics and electrostatics, understanding the limitations and modifications of the electrowetting equation being required for optimization (Baret et al., 2005). As scientists continue to investigate the interaction among surface tension, capillary action, and electrowetting, the future of microfluidics promises even greater control over fluids for a range of forthcoming applications (Akhil et al., 2013) (Figure 9.4).

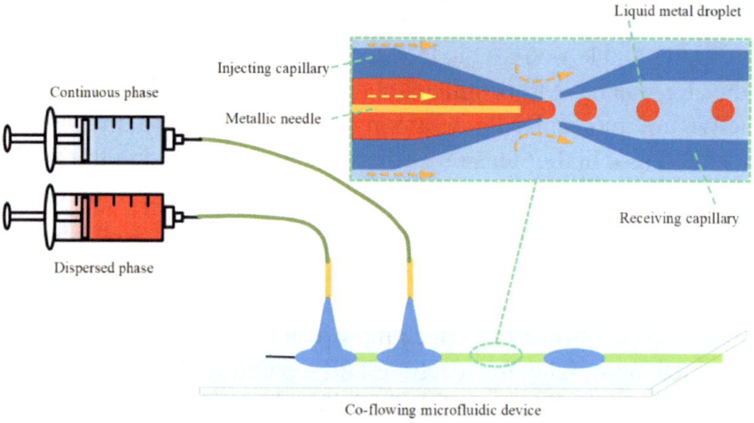

Figure 9.4. In microfluidic applications, precise control over fluid movement is often critically dependent on surface tension.

Source: https://www.mdpi.com/micromachines/micromachines-11-00169/article_deploy/html/images/micromachines-11-00169-g001.png.

9.1.3. Flow Control Mechanisms

Flow control components are the fundamental building block of microfluidics and lab-on-chip systems since they govern the fluid behavior at microscopic levels. The flow control components exploit various principles such as pressure-driven flow, electrokinetic flow, and surface tension to control the liquids with high precision. Pressure-driven flow can be blended with pumps to attain a constant flow rate in order to realize precise mixing and reaction time for biological diagnostics. Electrokinetic transport is greatly useful in the case of low volume since it has the capability to achieve high transport speeds by utilizing electric fields, which are necessary for cell sorting or analyte detection-based applications. With the addition of these forces, microfluidic devices are capable of emulating very complex biological milieus at very high throughput with decreased sample sizes, thus paving the way towards cutting-edge diagnostics and therapeutic applications (Abate et al., 2017).

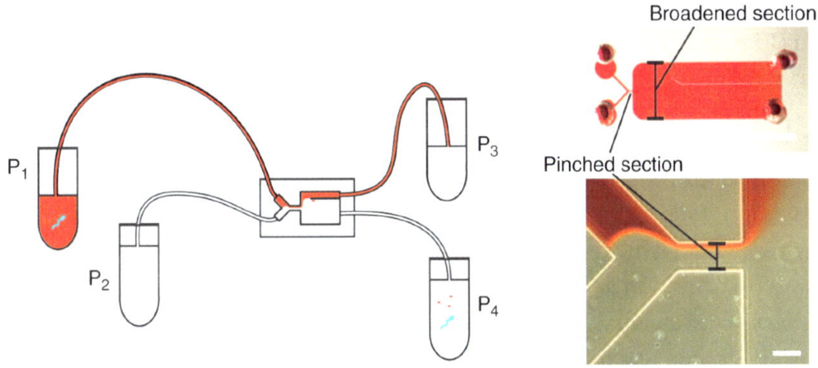

Figure 9.5. Flow control mechanisms are a fundamental aspect of microfluidics and lab-on-a-chip devices, as they dictate the behavior of fluids at microscopic scales.

Source: https://www.mdpi.com/micromachines/micromachines-12-00391/article_deploy/html/images/micromachines-12-00391-g001.png.

Flow control system design and implementation also play crucial roles to optimize performance in lab-on-a-chip devices. Some of the geometries employed to tailor fluid motion and interaction include microchannels and valves. Passive flow control, through capillary forces and hydrophobic/hydrophilic patterns, ensures robust and convenient system designs that do not require an external power source. Conversely, active flow control devices like pneumatic or electroactive valves provide programmable and command-driven control over fluid pathways. Their flexibility can improve the operation of lab-on-a-chip devices in applications ranging from drug delivery to biological analysis. Given that control overflow is key to developing stable and efficient microfluidic systems, research goes on to explore new approaches that further foster flow stability and response times (Abate et al., 2017). Furthermore, the performance of flow control devices will directly contribute to data quality in information gathered from microfluidic devices, particularly in delicate analyses like molecular diagnostics. Variabilities in the flow can lead to additional noise and artifacts, which will complicate the interpretation of results. For instance, image processes such as iris recognition systems can be adversely affected by compromised image data due to variable fluid flow and environmental conditions. Accordingly, the evolution of flow control technologies is vital for maximizing analytical performance as well as bringing devices into strict compliance for laboratory and clinical use. Better flow control eventually translates to the accuracy and dependability of diagnostic procedures, with microfluidic and lab-on-a-chip devices capable of operating under various conditions while still maintaining their performance and integrity (Abate et al., 2017) (Figure 9.5).

9.2. LAB-ON-A-CHIP TECHNOLOGY

The evolution of lab-on-a-chip technology has transformed the application of analytical and diagnostic use in biomedicine, environmental studies, and food safety. The underlying technology, microfluidics, provides fine control of minute amounts of fluids in integrated devices. The technology, besides performing fast assays and analysis, reduces the requirement of reagents to a minimum, ultimately reducing costs with effectiveness. With ongoing studies into new approaches in this area, technologies such as nucleic acid amplification and single-cell analysis become increasingly feasible with real-time measurement being achievable and more applied in point-of-care settings. The advancements call to mind the potential of lab-on-a-chip technologies to overcome the limitation associated with traditional laboratory approaches, paving the way for widespread use in various fields of research and diagnosis, as highlighted in recent studies (Abate et al., 2017). Further, the impact of lab-on-a-chip technology permeates into fundamental fields of biodefense and public health, where it is critical to identify pathogens rapidly. For instance, electrowetting on dielectric (EWOD) has been used to develop digital microfluidics platforms, which have been promising for the detection of airborne pathogens at rapid rates, an important application in military and security. Such platforms are effective in collecting and concentrating biological matter, delivering very sensitive assays that can be performed in under 10 minutes. This capacity for rapid analysis is particularly important in those instances where swift response to biological hazard is urgent. The integration of magnetic separation technologies with lab-on-a-chip platforms further enhances sensitivity and specificity, rendering these devices inevitable in epidemiological monitoring and crisis management schemes aimed at mitigating the transmission of infectious diseases (Coudron et al., 2019). In addition to biomedical applications, lab-on-a-chip technology has novel environmental monitoring and food safety applications. Execution of multiple assays in parallel in a compact package allows for comprehensive assessments of many environmental contaminants, including waterborne pathogens and crop produce. As there is growing public concern with foodborne illnesses, fast and reliable test systems become a vital need. Lab-on-a-chip technologies, not only enable identification of pathogenic microorganisms but also integrate the process of food safety evaluation. With greater access to advanced diagnostic technologies, the technology encourages proactive measures for the guarantee of public health and food security. The modularity of lab-on-a-chip platforms and their increasing sophistication put them in the forefront of next-generation analytical devices, beginning a new chapter on precision and reliability across many areas (Abate et al., 2017) (Figure 9.6).

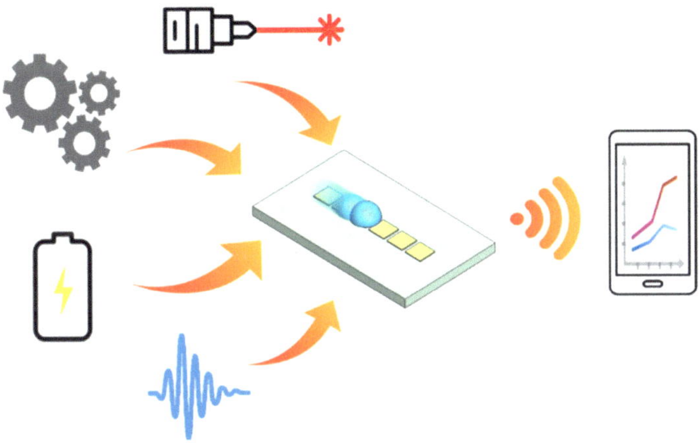

Figure 9.6. The development of digital microfluidics platforms that employ electrowetting on dielectric (EWOD) has shown promising results in the rapid detection of airborne pathogens, crucial for military and security applications.

Source: https://media.springernature.com/lw685/springer-static/image/art%3A10.1007%2Fs10404-019-2294-y/MediaObjects/10404_2019_2294_Fig9_HTML.png.

9.2.1. Definition and Functionality

The microfluidics and lab-on-a-chip (LOC) devices are a revolutionary branch of scientific research and diagnostics. Microfluidics entails the manipulation of fluids at the micrometric scale, allowing accurate control over chemical reactions and biological assays. LOC devices, however, incorporate a number of laboratory processes into one chip, integrating processes such as sample preparation, analysis, and recording of data. By reducing the assay time and sample volume drastically, these devices enhance experiment efficiency and allow for high-throughput screening. Thus, the name microfluidics is not used in the context of fluid manipulation alone; it encompasses an entire system for many applications in medicine, environmental monitoring, and food safety. Microfluidic devices become meaningful due to the capability of performing complex tasks in confined spaces.

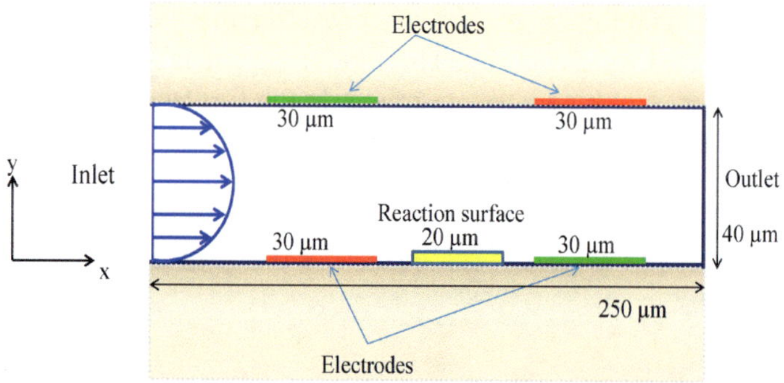

Figure 9.7. Innovations like AC electro-osmosis (ACEO) exemplify the evolving methodologies within microfluidics.

Source: https://www.mdpi.com/micromachines/micromachines-11-00342/article_deploy/html/images/micromachines-11-00342-g001.png.

They make use of principles like passive and active flow control to aid in the flow and blending of fluids, enabling interactive dynamics commonly needed in biological research. Technologies like AC electro-osmosis (ACEO) are a prime example of the advancements made in microfluidics methodologies. ACEO enables the control of microflows by causing fluid motion through electric fields, which can be used to improve mixing and pumping functions. These advancements also attest to a growing need for multifunctionality in microfluidic devices since researchers continue to engineer novel applications demanding intricate fluid dynamics and transport characteristics, thereby striving towards more integrated systems behaving in a lab-within-a-channel manner. More importantly, the clinical applications of microfluidic devices cannot be overstated. For instance, microfluidic devices for isolating and studying circulating tumor cells (CTCs) from blood samples have been constructed for cancer diagnosis and therapeutic monitoring, a key application. A continuous flow optimized microfluidic device for capturing viable CTCs showcases the capability to recover over 85% of such cells from large volume blood samples within minutes with minimal destruction of cell integrity for further examination (Wu et al., 2012). This highlights one of the main characteristics of microfluidics: the ability to integrate precision engineering and the needs of biology so that such devices can become indispensable tools in personalized medicine. As this field continues to develop, the relationship between definition and function will be imperative in developing future biomedical applications (Figure 9.7).

9.2.2. Components of Lab-on-a-Chip Devices

Lab-on-a-chip (LoC) systems are complex systems that integrate multiple laboratory functions onto a single microchip, transforming the landscape of analytical chemistry and biology. A key component in the devices is the system of microfluidic channels that allows for the controlled manipulation of fluids at the microliter or nanoliter scale. Such channels are typically fabricated in materials such as polydimethylsiloxane (PDMS) or glass, leaving space to create sophisticated channel geometries allowing for transportation, mixing, and reaction of fluids in confined areas. Microfluidics miniaturization not only conserves reagent consumption and prevents waste but also enhances the speed and resolution of biochemistry analysis, pushing the limits of diagnostic capability in applications like molecular diagnostics and point-of-care testing, as reported by Abate et al. (2017). Sensor integration is another equally vital component of lab-on-chip devices required for real-time detection and monitoring of varied analytes. These sensors can entail a range of technologies, including optical, electrochemical, and calorimetric methods, which are each optimized to detect specific biochemical interactions. Microfluidic calorimeters, for instance, have been demonstrated to be suited for high-throughput biochemical determination with extremely minute sample volumes, allowing for dense metabolic investigation. Fabrication of microfluidic calorimeters, exemplified by the merging of hard- and soft-polymer microfluidics, demonstrates enhanced thermal resolution and robotic sample handling capabilities. This technology allows the precise measurement of reaction heat and enthalpic changes, showing the widespread applications of sensors in LoC technologies as cited by Axelrod et al. (2009). Finally, lab-on-a-chip devices' operation is facilitated by advanced actuator systems and electronics control. These factors play a critical role in fluid flow control, for instance, via micropumps and microvalves, which regulate the movement of samples along the channels precisely. The combination of acoustic, magnetic, and electrostatic principles is typically applied to develop such actuation systems so that researchers can carry out processes that used to be cumbersome via automation. Smart control system integration adds functional characteristics to LoC devices, making them universal for a broad range of applications from drug screening to field monitoring. Ultimately, the integration of microfluidic channels, sensors, and actuating systems provides a symbiotic arrangement that imparts meaning to the efficiency and utility of lab-on-a-chip technology for modern science (Figure 9.8).

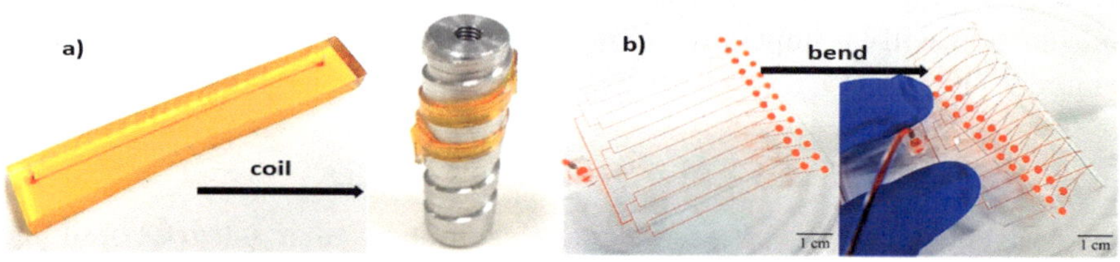

Figure 9.8. The development of microfluidic calorimeters, characterized by a combination of hard- and soft-polymer microfluidics, demonstrates enhanced thermal sensitivity and automated sample manipulation capabilities.

Source: https://www.mdpi.com/micromachines/micromachines-10-00830/article_deploy/html/images/micromachines-10-00830-g009.png.

9.2.3. Comparison with Traditional Laboratory Techniques

The introduction of microfluidics and lab-on-chip systems represents a dramatic deviation from traditional laboratory practices, primarily due to their potential for miniaturization and automation. Unlike traditional techniques involving extensive manipulation and greater sample quantities, microfluidics enables the manipulation of picoliter to nanoliter volumes of fluid. This reduction not only minimizes reagent loss but also accelerates reaction rates, a characteristic that makes it a preferred approach for quick-result applications. Moreover, traditional methods involve exclusive skilled personnel and additional room to fit equipment, making them restrictive in accessibility within some settings. The efficiency improvements exhibited by microfluidic devices have revolutionized diagnostics so that point-of-care can now be carried out in settings that were previously impractical (Abate et al., 2017). Microfluidic devices' relative sensitivity and specificity provide an additional advantage over traditional laboratory approaches. In molecular diagnostics, for example, conventional methods are apt to struggle with the requirements of high-resolution analysis of complex biological samples. Microfluidics facilitates sensitivity by embracing more effective assay designs that minimize background noise and maximize target detection levels. This is particularly important in applications such as nucleic acid amplification and protein detection, where microfluidic devices have been shown to yield quicker and more precise results than conventional laboratory procedures. The ability to accommodate multiple analytical operations within a single microfluidic device is an additional luxury that makes processes easier, which is notably different from the sequential nature characteristic of traditional approaches (Abate et al., 2017). The environmental quality issues facing conventional methods such as those associated with conventional imaging techniques emphasize the revolutionary nature of microfluidics. For instance, techniques that utilize accurate imaging can be critically affected by noise and stray reflections, undermining data quality, and precision in results. Microfluidic devices, on the other hand, can be designed to counteract such complications with internal controls considering fluctuating environmental conditions. By doing so, microfluidics not only enhances reliability of results but also fosters innovation in the field of various scientific disciplines. The more obvious benefits of microfluidics, including reduced analysis time, improved sensitivity, and operational flexibility, make it a desired alternative to traditional laboratory protocols.

9.3. APPLICATIONS IN BIOMEDICAL FIELDS

Applications of microfluidics and lab-on-a-chip devices in the biomedical sciences have revolutionized diagnostics and treatment regimens. These technologies are capable of dealing with minute volumes of liquids, thus enabling high-throughput analysis of biological samples. The convergence of various laboratory functions on a chip, microfluidics enables rapid, low-cost testing, which is imperative in clinic settings. For instance, the capability of conducting multiple assays simultaneously can greatly speed up patient diagnosis and subsequent treatment alternatives. Moreover, miniaturization of devices enables point-of-care analysis, where one gets the results in real-time at the site of patient care, thus addressing the need for time-critical interventions. Such advantages testify to the revolutionary potential of microfluidic devices in ensuring greater healthcare efficiency and patient outcomes. In addition to diagnostics, microfluidic technology has also emerged as central tools for drug discovery and drug-delivery systems. By providing the potential to precisely control dosing and release of drugs, researchers can tailor drug formulations for optimal therapeutic benefit. Microfluidic devices also allow the simulation of complex biological environments, which means researchers can study the interaction of drugs at a cellular level, critical for the consideration of pharmacokinetics and pharmacodynamics. Moreover, this technology can enhance the effectiveness of targeted drug delivery, hence minimize side effects, and maximize efficacy. For example, the union of inertial focusing technologies has ensured tremendous advances in waterborne pathogens like Cryptosporidium parvum concentration, with extremely high recovery rates while being scalable for other microbiological applications and infectious disease research (Bridle et al., 2016). This possibility illustrates the broad scope for microfluidic systems to address critical biological problems. Additionally, the application of microfluidics in biometric systems, as in iris recognition, indicates that it can be employed in security and authentication procedures. The quality of eye image data deteriorates under less-than-optimal conditions, particularly when images are captured with visible wavelength illumination, which introduces noise and complicates segmentation. Current studies have shown that application of advanced segmentation methods, such as the Circular Hough transform, significantly improves the performance of iris recognition systems under challenging conditions (Ahmad et al., 2018). Such cross-pollination between microfluidics and biometric technology showcases interdisciplinarity of innovation in the biomedical field, where mechanical engineering, optics, and biology are consolidated to enhance the reliability and effectiveness of personal verification systems. These cross-disciplinary advances underscore the wide-ranging significance of microfluidics to numerous alternative applications, much beyond traditional biomedical applications (Figure 9.9).

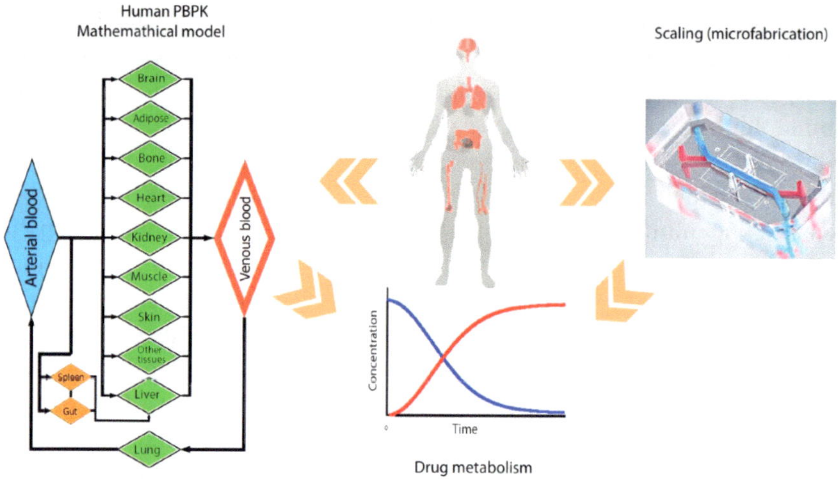

Figure 9.9. Microfluidic devices can simulate complex biological environments, allowing researchers to study drug interactions at a cellular level, which is vital for understanding pharmacokinetics and pharmacodynamics.

Source: https://pub.mdpi-res.com/micromachines/micromachines-07-00162/article_deploy/html/images/micromachines-07-00162-g001.png?1539571416.

9.3.1. Disease Diagnostics

In disease diagnostic science, microfluidics and laboratory-on-a-chip technology are a paradigm shift that enhances efficiency and accuracy of diagnostic testing. Traditionally, medical diagnostics were bulk laboratory tests that were costly and time-consuming, typically hindering prompt patient treatment. Microfluidic system development makes laboratory functions available in miniaturized form on one chip, allowing for quick molecular analysis to be applied in a variety of environments, from point-of-care. The technologies not only streamline the workflow but also allow different diagnostic tests to be incorporated into a single platform with the ability to increase the throughput of valuable information without loss of precision. This skill is particularly relevant in infectious disease management, where diagnosis at the right moment can significantly improve patient outcome and avoid the transmission of disease-causing pathogens (Abate et al., 2017). The use of microfluidics in molecular diagnostics offers increased sensitivity and specificity that aids the detection of diseases at an earlier stage.

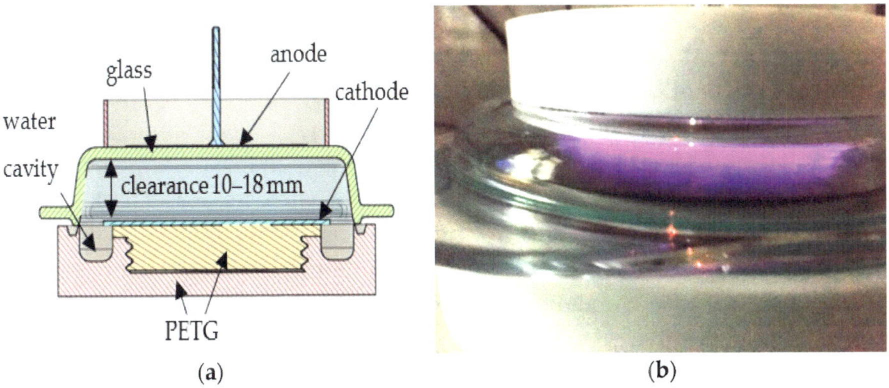

Figure 9.10. Utilizing all-glass substrates for microfluidic networks allows for enhanced sterility and functionality while maintaining low-cost, mass-production capabilities.

Source: https://pub.mdpi-res.com/applsci/applsci-13-06365/article_deploy/html/images/applsci-13-06365-g001.png?1684838887.

Advanced technologies such as next-generation sequencing and nucleic acid amplification depend heavily on such technologies that enable quick and precise analysis of genetics. Automated sample preparation processes reduce the chances of contamination and human error, hence increasing the precision of results. Therefore, healthcare workers are able to achieve actionable information earlier, which is particularly in situations with critical care. Furthermore, the capability of conducting high-resolution melting analysis and protein detection also showcases the multi-functionality of lab-on-a-chip devices, making them valuable assets in modern diagnostics (Abate et al., 2017). One of the most notable examples of the efficiency of lab-on-chip technology can be seen in the development of microfluidic systems incorporating on-chip optical detection, for instance, recent developments. Utilization of all-glass substrates in microfluidic networks allows for higher sterility and function at low-cost mass fabrication. Integration of chemiluminescent biochemical reaction within microenvironments has strong promise in real-time disease diagnosis. Immobilization of specific enzymes, such as horseradish peroxidase, on chemically modified channel surfaces allows these devices to detect major biomarkers with sensitivity. Testing has now successfully shown to be able to identify hydrogen peroxide as low as 18 μM, showing the potential of technology to identify disease markers with high specificity. With these advances, microfluidics is now altering disease diagnostics into a new field, paving the way towards more effective healthcare strategies (Figure 9.10).

9.3.2. Drug Development and Delivery

The advancement of medicines has been significantly enhanced by the advances in microfluidics and lab-on-a-chip (LOC) technologies. The technologies have precise control of microscale fluid dynamics, which enables the manipulation and analysis of ultra-small amounts of biochemical reactions. The accuracy is paramount in optimizing drug formulation, enhancing bioavailability, and predicting pharmacokinetic behaviors. Microfluidic systems are able to rapidly screen various drug compounds under a controlled setting, accelerating the process of drug discovery by allowing researchers to assess the effectiveness of various drug candidates simultaneously. Further, because they have the ability to automate and use less reagent, LOC devices offer a cost-effective alternative to classic laboratory procedures that are essential in an era where research funding is increasingly constrained, eventually providing the way forward from laboratory settings to patient treatment methods involving personalized medicine (Joshi et al., 2016). Drug delivery systems are also revolutionized by the use of microfluidics, which enables the creation of advanced delivery platforms that enhance therapeutic efficacy. Drug delivery systems may be designed to be responsive to specific physiological requirements, with controlled release of the drug to the site of action, which is particularly beneficial in treating chronic disease and cancer. With the utilization of microfluidic channels to establish controlled release profiles, these systems are able to minimize side effects and maximize therapeutic effect. Advances such as organ-on-a-chip technologies also allow for the production of more representative *in vitro* models of human tissue, which increases the capacity to predict drug response as well as to perform toxicology studies. Therefore, understanding interactions within biological systems has the capability to greatly improve drug delivery mechanisms and outcomes beyond traditional methods that were typically non-predictive (Joshi et al., 2016). Integrating microfluidic technologies with drug development and delivery not only drives research and clinical expertise but also provides a distinct chance to transform drug engineering and drug administration. For instance, the combination of microfluidics with wearable technology can lead to smart drug delivery systems that monitor patient parameters in real time and adjust dosing accordingly. Such systems are reminiscent of projects such as 'Scent Whisper,' where microfluidics is engaged in personal communication through smell. By facilitating the convergence of therapeutics and diagnostics onto a single platform, researchers are opening the way for more efficient, patient-focused therapies. This emerging convergence demonstrates the centrality of microfluidics to the future of pharmacology, paving the way for a future of more integrated drug development and delivery better aligned with present-day healthcare needs.

9.3.3. Personalized Medicine

Personalized medicine is a new paradigm of taking care of medical health, in which clinical interventions and medical therapy are tailored to the individual-specific genetic, environmental, and lifestyle factors. Microfluidics and lab-on-a-chip (LOC) devices play a very significant role in promoting such personalized approaches by maximizing diagnostic procedures. These technologies facilitate rapid and efficient molecular-level analysis, thereby enabling efficient interventions in a variety of medical disciplines, such as oncology and infectious diseases. With microfluidics, clinicians are able to achieve a more sensitive biomarker detection, which ultimately leads to more targeted patient stratification and treatment protocols. This level of individualization not only enhances therapeutic efficacy but also minimizes undesirable effects, emphasizing the work of technological advancement in realizing the objectives of personalized medicine (Abate et al., 2017). The capability of microfluidic systems to perform several analyses in reduced scale supports the broader ambitions of personalized medicine. For example, such devices are capable of conducting complicated assays in which nucleic acid amplification and protein detection are done from very small sample amounts, and hence they are perfectly suited for use in point-of-care. Through the development of improved sample preparation techniques and fast transition to diagnostic output, lab-on-a-chip devices enable medical practitioners to provide timely and precise medical evaluations. This real-time feedback loop is instrumental in personalized medicine as it enables clinicians to modify treatment protocols in real time in accordance with real-time patient feedback, hence optimizing care efficacy as well as patient outcomes (Abate et al., 2017). Furthermore, platforms such as droplet microfluidics have been able to bring single-cell analysis doors to discovering patient-specific disease pathophysiology. Such technologies allow for label-free and noninvasive profiling of cellular metabolism, most critically in oncology, where cell-type distinctions between proliferating and quiescent cells are relevant to therapeutic choice. By leveraging technologies that detect metabolic states without causing cell damage, researchers are able to more acutely delineate cellular heterogeneity of tumor microenvironments. This information can be correlated with genomic profiles to design more suitable targeted therapies to the biochemical topology of your disease, further supporting microfluidics as a means to advance personalized medicine (Figure 9.11).

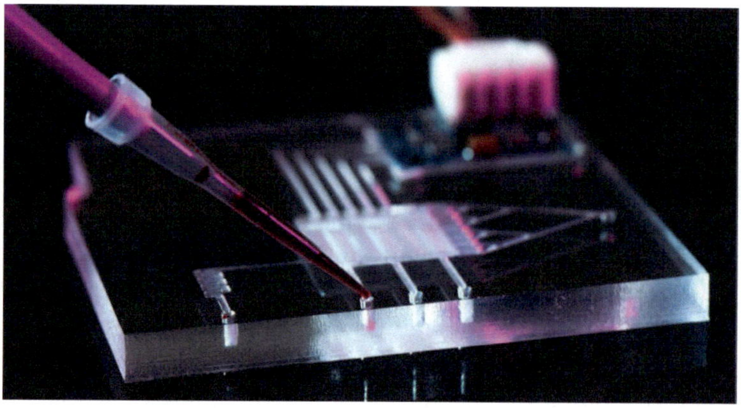

Figure 9.11. The integration of microfluidics and lab-on-a-chip (LOC) devices plays a pivotal role in enabling such personalized approaches by streamlining diagnostic processes.

Source: https://www.alineinc.com/wp-content/uploads/2024/07/Untitled-design-2024-07-05T164917.886-1024x536.jpg.

9.4. APPLICATIONS IN ENVIRONMENTAL MONITORING

The integration of microfluidics and lab-on-a-chip technology in environmental monitoring is a breakthrough in analytical science, enabling faster and more sensitive detection of pollutants and pathogens. The advanced systems can be designed to analyze samples from different environments like water bodies, soil, and air, saving time and labor compared to traditional techniques. For example, microfluidic networks etched into glass substrates have been utilized in new developments to facilitate robust chemical reactions in tiny channels to detect toxic materials, like heavy metals or dissolved gases, at trace concentrations. Such capability is critical in addressing environmental concerns, where real-time monitoring and quick decision-making can be made possible in pollution management and disaster prevention, showing the capability of microfluidic technology in enhancing environmental protection efforts (Caputo et al., 2017). The use of microfluidics in environmental monitoring also covers research on biodiversity and ecosystem health. Through equipping these tools with cutting-edge molecular diagnostics, scientists are now able to assess water quality and microbial diversity at never-before-seen speeds and with greater precision. This is most critical in ecosystems where changes in environmental conditions—caused by climate change or human processes—can have dramatic repercussions for vegetation and animals. Microfluidics has the capacity to enable direct analysis of nucleic acids from a wide range of organisms under field conditions, thus aiding in determining microbial community dynamics and resilience. Developments in this area include systems for delivering results on time, enhancing ecologists and environmental scientists, a great deal in studies and conservation, thus leading to well-informed strategies in biodiversity management and ecosystem recovery (Abate et al., 2017). In addition to tracking pollutants and quantifying biodiversity, microfluidic devices will also revolutionize food safety in environmental monitoring. Having the capability to screen food commodities against contaminants like pesticides and microbial pathogens in real-time is invaluable given the direct effect on public health. Lab-on-a-chip devices can be employed in various environments in food production and distribution to facilitate point-of-care analysis to provide food safety management. These devices become particularly useful in a more integrated food economy where transportation distances can create many contamination hazards. Moreover, the small size of these devices makes it possible to integrate them with other food safety devices at little cost. With rapid and uniform detection of foodstuffs, microfluidic technologies can potentially reduce significantly the risk of foodborne diseases and food security as a whole (Caputo et al., 2017).

9.4.1. Water Quality Testing

Water quality monitoring is vital for both environmental health and public safety. Traditional methods of testing water typically are slow processes, which may not have the necessary sensitivity required for the detection of trace-level contaminants. This is where microfluidics and lab-on-a-chip devices step in as game-changers, as they can significantly reduce the complexity of the test process. These technologies enable timely analysis by integrating several laboratory functions onto a single chip, thus enabling real-time water quality monitoring. Miniaturization through these technologies enables high-throughput testing, increasing efficiency and facilitating more universal water quality tests in various environments. Microfluidic technology has emerged as a key technology for improving accuracy and sensitivity in water quality testing in recent studies. For instance, some devices are able to conduct colorimetric assays to detect impurities such as glucose, with outstanding accuracy comparable to traditional plate readers that is critical in fulfilling regulatory needs and protecting public health. New advances, including 3D-printed microfluidic devices, not only reduced the cost of water testing but also improved optical clarity, thereby enabling better impurity detection such as heavy metals and pathogens. This versatility means that microfluidic devices can be employed over a spectrum of applications, from laboratory to field applications, to guarantee water samples are assessed rapidly and effectively. Moreover, the integration of advanced algorithms with microfluidic technologies allows for increased solid data evaluation and interpretation of water quality data. Intelligent systems can enable automatic processing and transfer of pertinent information, which ensures fast response to suspected contamination incidents. Incorporating machine learning models in these devices is also capable of predicting sources and trends of contamination over time, thus enhancing proactive measures in water management. There are challenges involved, especially standardizing these devices in different contexts and realizing effectiveness in negating environmental factors that tend to influence the results of tests. Yet, as microfluidics continues to evolve, the possibility of greater water quality assessment becomes an extremely real potentiality, fostering greater environmental stewardship and public health.

9.4.2. Air Pollution Analysis

Air pollution is a serious worldwide issue with serious human health and environmental impacts. Air quality management is so complicated that it requires the most up-to-date analytical technologies that are capable of monitoring and analyzing airborne pollutants in real-time. Microfluidics and lab-on-a-chip devices have proven to be revolutionary technologies in this respect. These devices enable the manipulation of minute volumes of liquids in channels as small as micrometers to quickly analyze various pollutants at trace levels. The merging of various analytical processes into a single platform enhances the efficiency of air quality analysis with less reliance on huge laboratory facilities. These innovations play a key role in answering the urgent call for transportable air quality monitoring systems that can facilitate response to pollution events in a pre-emptive way and empower citizens with rights to real-time information regarding their environmental health. The applications of microfluidic technology exceed those of routine air quality monitoring; they introduce new methods for the detection of biological agents of threat and airborne pathogens. As demonstrated by recent developments, such as the electrowetting on dielectric (EWOD) technique, lab-on-a-chip systems are capable of efficiently screening and identifying airborne biological agents of national security interest, including chemical and biological warfare (CBW) agents. This development is significant in light of airborne pathogen threats and the need for quick, effective detection systems that function in varying conditions. Through the integration of immunoassay capability on portable microfluidic systems, researchers have successfully achieved quick detection times with minimal requirements for samples. That efficiency not only enhances readiness for response but also displays enormous potential for the application of microfluidics in revolutionizing public health protection measures for air pollution and biological hazards (Coudron et al., 2019). Furthermore, the intersection of lab-on-a-chip and microfluidic technologies with wearable technology is a critical frontier area in air pollution measurement. As shown by pioneering efforts like Scent Whisper, which stem from microfluidic concepts, these wearable devices have the ability to empower personal air quality experiences by correlating smell stimuli with environmental data. This new communication method through scent unveils the therapeutic applications inherent in the monitoring of air quality and presents a new way of enhancing the wellbeing of people. The potential development of similar technologies towards the measurement of air quality at localized levels can allow individuals to make informed decisions regarding their surrounding environments. With the blending of art, science, and technology, the study of odor communications in air pollution defines new paradigms for user interaction and awareness, bridging environmental science and human experience (Tillotson et al., 2005).

9.4.3. Soil Contamination Detection

Determination of soil contamination is critical to environmental monitoring and responsible agricultural production. Traditional methods of soil analysis require large amounts of time, labor, and, in most instances, significant laboratory space that is not suitable for real-time assessments in the field. Due to these drawbacks, lab-on-a-chip technology and microfluidics have been developed as cutting-edge solutions that facilitate quick and efficient identification of soil contamination. These technologies miniaturize sample sizes and enable the integration of an array of analytical functions within a compact platform. By using micro-scale fluid manipulation, they provide the ability to enhance sensitivity and specificity of heavy metal and organic pollutant contaminant detection for environmental health and safety. Soils toxicity tests using microfluidics incorporate advanced analytical techniques such as capillary electrophoresis (CE). Portable CE systems provide a streamlined means for *in-situ* analysis, thus transcending the limitations of conventional laboratory settings. The systems employ electric fields to demagnetize soil sample components, making precise determination of contaminants possible in real time. Its portability and affordability have made it more available for field testing, which can create environmental awareness and remedial action. Additionally, the technical advancements in conjunction with sensor technologies offer potential improvements in automatic monitoring systems, thereby catalyzing an aggressive approach in soil quality and safety management. The importance of bridging these technology gaps cannot be overstated, as they have an immense influence on the efficacy of contamination detection across different environmental conditions (Cranny et al., 2013). Moreover, lab-on-a-chip devices are revolutionizing detection of soil pathogen through such techniques as single-cell sequencing. Using droplet microfluidics, researchers can encapsulate individual cells and analyze their genomic information, important in learning the impact of microbial contamination in soils. New technology advancements enable fast sequencing of mixed cell populations, enhancing the capacity to establish the presence of toxic pathogens that may compromise crop yields and soil health. These methods are enhancing the identification of specific pollutants to previously unprecedented levels, enabling the design of specific remedial strategies. This shift to high-throughput, low-bias soil analysis methods not only benefits agricultural production but also makes significant inroads into broader ecological studies of soil ecosystems and their roles in maintaining life (Abate et al., 2018).

9.5. CHALLENGES IN MICROFLUIDICS

Microfluidics has undoubtedly changed a lot of disciplines but is faced with extreme challenges that limit its broad applicability. Chief among these challenges is the complexity in device fabrication. The fabrication process for microfluidic devices requires sophisticated techniques such as soft lithography or injection molding, which are costly and time-consuming. Additionally, reproducibility and scaling up production are significant barriers. Variations in the microfabrication process can result in device performance variations, and thus reliability in clinical applications is an issue. This becomes particularly significant when using microfluidics for the purpose of molecular diagnostics, as the highest sensitivity and specificity are required to provide accurate results. If these fabrication challenges are not addressed, then the potential of microfluidic technology to the fullest in these applications, such as infectious disease management and biomedicine, can remain unfulfilled (Abate et al., 2017). But yet another major problem is the merging of microfluidic devices with detection systems. Microfluidics process samples more and reagents less, but they need sophisticated detection modalities to perform at the scale and speed required for sound analysis. Traditional analytical modes do not work in micro-scale settings, calling for detection modality innovations. For example, optical detection techniques could face challenges with decreased volumes of fluid, and electrochemical detection strategies could require microenvironment-specific recalibration. Moreover, their integration with microfluidic platforms introduces additional engineering complexities, which can deter new players in the market. Therefore, resolution of such integration problems is central in realizing the potential of lab-on-a-chip devices, especially in targeted molecular diagnostics and therapeutic monitoring applications (Bower et al., 2016). Also, biocompatibility of materials used in microfluidic devices is a great challenge, most importantly with biological samples. The biological fluid-device material interface can induce unwanted effects, i.e., protein adsorption or cell destruction, which can compromise the sample integrity and, consequently, the result. Identification of materials that are not only cell-compatible but also easy to manufacture is a challengingly difficult task for researchers. Long-term stability of the materials under various operating conditions is an additional issue. Though microfluidics is applied more extensively in personal medicine, where states of tissue *ex vivo* must be maintained, biocompatibility of the material assumes extreme significance. Hence, it is necessary to surmount these material challenges in order to advance the efficacy and reliability of microfluidic devices towards clinic applications, for example, in cancer research and drug testing (Abate et al., 2017).

9.5.1. Fabrication Techniques

The evolution of fabrication processes in microfluidics has significantly influenced the design and application of Lab-on-a-Chip devices. Soft lithography is one of the building block processes that utilizes polydimethylsiloxane (PDMS) for creating complex microchannel networks. The process allows high-resolution patterning and rapid prototyping, allowing scientists to fabricate and design devices with the capability of manipulating small volumes of liquids accurately. These developments have introduced into microfluidic systems possibilities that are unattainable by conventional means, such as enhanced sensitivity and reduced operational cost in molecular diagnosis. Illustrative of these developments in molecular biology, such on-site testing becomes feasible in areas like infectious disease control and food safety, thus illustrating the widespread application of microfluidic technologies in many industries (Abate et al., 2017). In addition to soft lithography, hybrid integration approaches have also taken the forefront of microfluidic device manufacturing. At the forefront of these advances is hybridizing PDMS microfluidics with fused silica capillaries, offering new geometries to enhance functionality at the expense of leakage. Hybrid designs allow for the reuse of capillaries, enhancing the economic efficiency of experiments using multiple fluidic configurations. The modular design of these devices supports ease of use; using a simple three-step fabrication procedure that can be conducted in minutes, scientists are able to effectively streamline their work procedures. This integration not only supports traditional capillary electrophoresis but also maximizes coupling with mass spectrometry, and the resulting hybrid systems become extremely versatile tools in analytical chemistry (Dimov et al., 2009). Moreover, the ongoing exploration of fabrication techniques further expands the limits of what can be achieved in microfluidic operations. Techniques such as 3D printing and laser ablation are increasingly being explored, enabling more intricate designs and reduced production times. All of these advancements are likely to continue enhancing the functional capability of Lab-on-a-Chip devices with potential for performing more advanced analyses and gathering data in real time. As these methods evolve, they become the ideal candidates for expanding the realm of microfluidics, building more collaborations with fields like genomics and personalized medicine. Therefore, advancing fabrication techniques offers solutions to the existing problems and creates a platform for future technological innovations that can cure priority healthcare and environmental issues (Abate et al., 2017) (Figure 9.12).

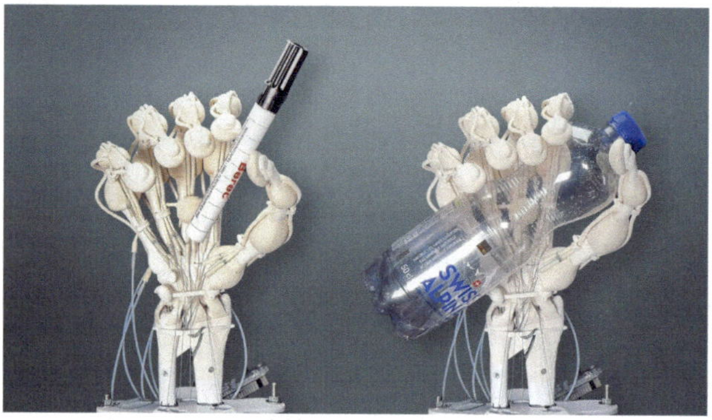

Figure 9.12. Techniques such as 3D printing and laser ablation are increasingly being explored, enabling more intricate designs and faster production times.

Source: https://www.plasticsengineering.org/wp-content/uploads/2023/11/1_Hand-robot_credit_Zurich-ETH_Thomas-Buchner-1200x675.jpg.

9.5.2. Integration with Other Technologies

The union of microfluidics and lab-on-a-chip devices with other emerging technologies has led to significant advances in virtually every field of research. The systems are particularly worth their while in molecular diagnostics, where they enhance the capability to conduct rapid and efficient analysis. Developments in molecular biology in the past couple of years have made it necessary to simplify processes such as protein detection and nucleic acid amplification. Therefore, microfluidic technology evolved as a crucial tool that not only reduces the time and cost needed for conventional methods but also enhances sensitivity and functionality. Such characteristics provide chief aid for effective interventions in applications ranging from infectious disease management to food safety, marking the revolutionary potential of integrating microfluidics with existing biomedical technologies (Abate et al., 2017). Moreover, the incorporation of advanced computational methods within microfluidic device design has revolutionized the way scientists approach channel networks and fluid flow.

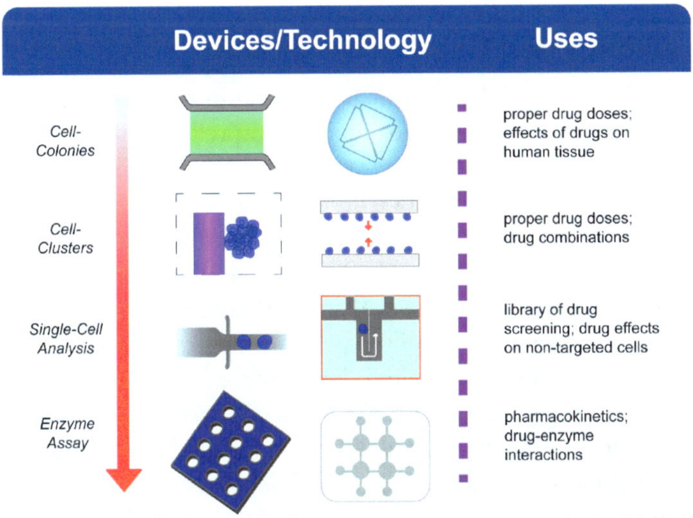

Figure 9.13. The introduction of algorithms like directed placement signifies a breakthrough in the mechanical layout of microfluidic systems.

Source: https://www.mdpi.com/ijms/ijms-19-02731/article_deploy/html/images/ijms-19-02731-g004.png.

The emergence of methodologies like Directed Placement is a paradigm shift in the mechanical design of microfluidic devices. The breakthrough enables component proximity and minimizes fluid channel lengths considerably and optimizes area usage. As such, scientists can utilize more minimalist and effective designs that are nonetheless functional. With the interaction of computational design tools with biological functions, integration allows scientists to overcome current limitations in microfluidic technology, with the performance of the devices being improved and easier to produce (Brisk et al.,

2019). Integration with other new technologies, such as artificial intelligence and biosensing, extends the scope of possible applications for lab-on-a-chip systems further. By leveraging AI, researchers can analyze vast quantities of data generated by microfluidic assays to help them make more informed decisions in diagnostics and medicine. In addition, biosensing technologies are evolving towards real-time monitoring of simultaneous biological events in microfluidic systems. This helpful association not only speeds up scientific discovery but also brings in greater accuracy in diagnostics and therapeutic action. With the further advancement of microfluidics, integration with these technologies will increase even more extensively, ushering in the era of more available, speedy, and customized medical treatment (Abate et al., 2017) (Figure 9.13).

9.5.3. Scalability and Commercialization

Scalability and commercialization of lab-on-a-chip devices and microfluidics are essential parameters that govern their widespread adoption in the clinical as well as consumer markets. With advancements in microfluidic technology, scientists are increasingly focused on creating devices that accurately replicate complex biological systems. Organ-on-a-chip technology has been a significant advancement and has allowed for more accurate drug screening and toxicology testing. Such innovations have caused microfluidic devices to be adopted in research centers, hospitals, and clinics as the need for integrated diagnostic devices grows. However, it is tough to break these laboratory achievements to achieve commercialization, for example, the need for comprehensive validation, compliance with regulations, and devising sustainable business models that achieve production costs and consumer interaction (Rainer et al., 2015). Commercialization of lab-on-a-chip products is also hindered by complexity and operational demands of the point-of-care testing. The in-box diagnostic opportunity provided by these products is enormous, but their complex design may place constraints on usability and ease of access. Market strategies must resolve the trade-off between innovativeness of features and design usability to enable market penetration and consumer confidence. Furthermore, the incorporation of disposable elements can limit scalability, increasing cost in an industry that is growing ever more cost-sensitive. A platform strategy, as has been debated in current scholarship, focuses on the evolvability of systems and modularity as solutions to such concerns, allowing users to gradually transition between device generations without diminishing user appeal (Atraktchi et al., 2016). To be able to overcome the path to commercialization, the coupling of smart technologies with microfluidic devices is paramount. The combination of mobile devices with lab-on-a-chip systems presents distinct possibilities for real-time diagnostics and targeted medicine. Still, commercial success demands breaking through technical hurdles relating to the coupling of software and hardware pieces of equipment in an effective manner. A robust interface system for these devices is necessary to facilitate user interaction and extend the range of lab-on-chip system functionality in various applications. Strategic interface design makes devices versatile and scalable and, ultimately, contributes to a market situation in which innovation can thrive without sacrificing practicability, thus promoting new opportunities in medical diagnostics and therapeutics (Atraktchi et al., 2016).

9.6. FUTURE TRENDS IN MICROFLUIDICS

The future of microfluidics holds the promise of transforming several fields, primarily through enhanced molecular diagnostics. With the development in molecular biology, the integration of microfluidic technologies will facilitate simplified analysis protocols to offer rapid and efficient intervention against infectious diseases and biodefense. The compact nature of lab-on-a-chip devices enables the possibility of point-of-care applications, minimizing the need for large-scale laboratory equipment. Besides, improved sensitivity and reduced operating costs are sure to enhance the access to these technologies. As stated by Abate et al. (2017), microfluidics makes new methods possible, including nucleic acid amplification and next-generation sequencing, which provide valuable tools for high-throughput analysis. This transformation not only creates deeper understanding of biological systems but also enhances public health interventions to new threats, driving a new era of individualized medicine and diagnostics. Beyond molecular diagnostics, interest is growing in the design of simple programming languages tailored to biochemistry. The development of such platforms as BioScript is a typical example of this phenomenon, attempting to unite biochemists and engineers through a plain and easy language. By introducing an easy syntax for biochemical operations of complex types, BioScript invites effortless adoption by practitioners in the life sciences. The bringing forth of a type-safe method discourages faults—particularly chemical interaction faults—from arising, providing strength to safety regulation within microfluidic experimentation. As development goes on, the versatility of BioScript will enable scientists to take advantage of future microfluidic technologies in a more optimized way, making experiment conduct more streamlined and spurring innovation in the field, as described by Brisk et al. (2018). Finally, the future also promises better miniaturization and integration of microfluidic devices with advanced technologies such as artificial intelligence and machine learning. By combining these technologies, researchers will tend to optimize predictive capability and automation of the experimental process. Integration will provide real-time capability for data analysis, such that better clinical decision-making will result from faster decision-making. Ongoing development of microfluidic sample preparation platforms supporting sample-in, answer-out workflows will be a key component. These advances will not only accelerate the pace of scientific inquiry but also extend the application of microfluidics to the entire mainstream research domain, including food safety and environmental monitoring. As microfluidics comes along, its marriage with computer technologies will indeed transform biological analysis to be conducted in a new era of efficiency and accuracy.

9.6.1. Advances in Materials Science

Recent advances in materials science have been central to the optimization of the functionality and performance of microfluidics and lab-on-a-chip systems. The incorporation of new materials, such as biocompatible polymers and nanomaterials, has enabled the fabrication of smaller, more precise components that permit intricate manipulations of fluids. These materials offer advantages such as increased chemical resistance and improved surface properties, which are essential in most biological applications. For instance, the development of polymeric substrates with tailored properties can significantly improve the operation of microfluidic devices by ensuring reproducible fluidics and avoiding destructive interactions with samples. Therefore, material science development directly influences the capacity of lab-on-a-chip technologies to perform complex analysis on a micro scale and facilitate the creation of personalized medicine, diagnosis, and therapeutic applications. Furthermore, innovation in new processing techniques, along with traditional manufacturing methods, has led to innovation in microfluidics. Techniques such as 3D printing and soft lithography are being applied more regularly to create complex channel geometries previously difficult to make. This allows for the design of passive components such as tapered microchannels, which utilize hydrodynamic effects to attain efficient particle separation in mixed samples. Research indicates that such arrangements can optimize sample throughput while minimizing use of resources, fulfilling the increasing demand for automating biomedical applications (Abidin et al., 2017). As these processing methods continue to improve, they significantly lower production costs and time, facilitating its increased application in numerous healthcare settings. The area of programmable biochemistry has also significantly expanded, driven mostly by advances in materials science. The creation of domain-specific languages, such as BioScript, serves to illustrate how materials and software can be combined to create user-friendly interfaces for life sciences applications. Beyond making laboratory procedures easier, the innovation also enhances the efficiency and safety of biochemical reactions using an effective type of system that minimizes biochemistry error possibilities (Brisk et al., 2018). With increasing ability of the microfluidic platforms to incorporate such intelligent programming functions, lab-on-a-chip devices as a whole become more resilient and versatile, facilitating use in diverse biological applications and towards an increasingly automated, high-accuracy approach to scientific research and diagnosis (Figure 9.14).

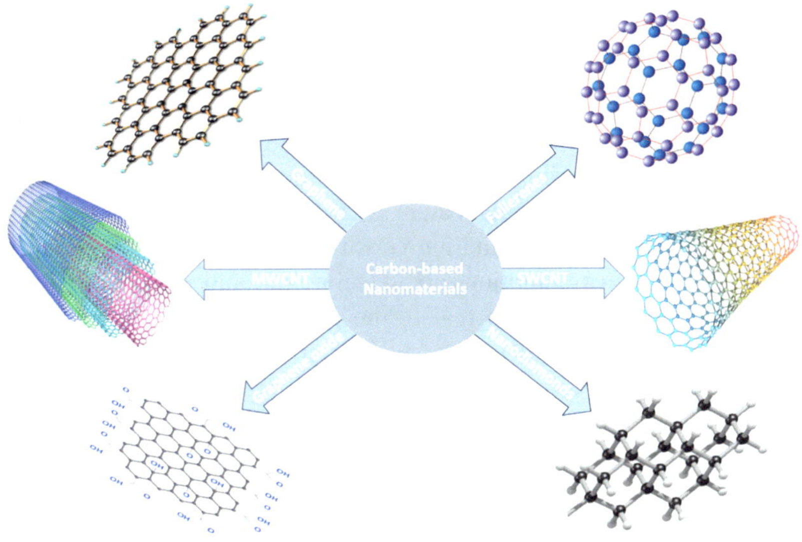

Figure 9.14. The integration of novel materials, such as biocompatible polymers and nanomaterials, has enabled the development of smaller, more precise components that facilitate intricate fluid manipulations.

Source: https://www.mdpi.com/polymers/polymers-17-00893/article_deploy/html/images/polymers-17-00893-g001.png.

9.6.2. Integration with Artificial Intelligence (AI)

Incorporation of artificial intelligence (AI) into microfluidics and lab-on-a-chip systems is a revolutionizing phase in lab medicine that enormously enhances the capabilities of such technologies. AI systems offer high-level data analysis and pattern recognition, which are crucial because experimental data volume continues to rise. Such innovations offer scientists the chance to automate processes that were originally labor extensive, thus improving effectiveness and precision in diagnosis and research applications. By leveraging AI's predictive capabilities, researchers can gain insights into biological processes and interactions at micro-scale levels. This development aligns with the historical trend of predicting future laboratory medicine advancements, as evidenced by reflections on past expectations regarding technological evolution in medical laboratories (Fortina et al., 2015). Consequently, the integration of AI with microfluidics not only enables efficient operations but also paves the way for revolutionary approaches towards patient diagnostics and customized medicine. However, full realization of AI potential within microfluidics is challenging, especially at the initial phase of technological development. At this stage, there is uncertainty regarding potential use and targeted markets, and therefore firms are unable to accurately determine the value of inventions. The lack of prototypes for new AI-powered devices hinders the ability to discern applications and users (Gérald et al., 2025). These challenges support the argument for interdisciplinary collaboration where technologists collaborate intimately with domain specialists to counteract cognitive biases that can restrict innovative thinking. By fostering an exploratory culture and facilitating constructive conversation, stakeholders can dislodge dominant assumptions about technology and explore broader uses. Such collaboration is crucial to realize the potential of AI in optimizing the functions of microfluidic devices. As AI and microfluidics gain more synergy, it is important that the ethical and regulatory problems raised by such technologies are tackled. The implementation of AI-driven decisions in automated laboratory settings raises issues on accountability, bias, and reliability, which should be critically examined. The laws must not lag behind technological advancements in order not to hinder it while upholding standards of ethics. The integration of AI into lab-on-a-chip technology also necessitates ongoing professional education and training to ensure they can utilize these advanced systems effectively. Thus, while the possibilities for AI to revolutionize microfluidics are huge, it is important to embrace its integration from a comprehensive perspective that balances not only technical feasibility but also the sociocultural implications of the type of change such integration would bring.

9.6.3. Potential for Point-of-Care Testing

The development of microfluidics and lab-on-a-chip technology is a revolutionary promise for point-of-care testing (POCT) with the offer of rapid diagnostics that will be able to make a significant contribution towards patient care. Previously, the employment of central laboratory testing has resulted in delays that can have a detrimental effect on clinical decision-making. Microfluidic technology facilitates sample processing and analysis to be carried out in the site of care, thus decreasing the amount of time tests need to take before providing results. This immediacy not only promotes early medical interventions but also bypasses logistical challenges in shipping samples to remote laboratories. The possibility of quick diagnostics is even more pertinent in emergency medical states, where time is crucial, hinting at the central role microfluidics can have in contemporary healthcare settings. Furthermore, the flexibility of microfluidic systems increases their application in POCT across various medical specialties, including the care of infectious diseases and chronic condition monitoring. By enabling the concomitant testing of numerous tests on a single chip, these devices streamline the diagnostic process, enhancing efficiency and reducing costs from standard testing methods. Emerging technologies powered by advancements in molecular biology spur new methodologies for rapid testing, such as nucleic acid amplification and protein detection. This versatility is especially important in resource-constrained settings or rural locations where full-scale healthcare services are not readily available. The incorporation of microfluidics into POCT not only keeps advanced diagnostics democratized but also aligns with the principles of personalized medicine and patient-focused care.

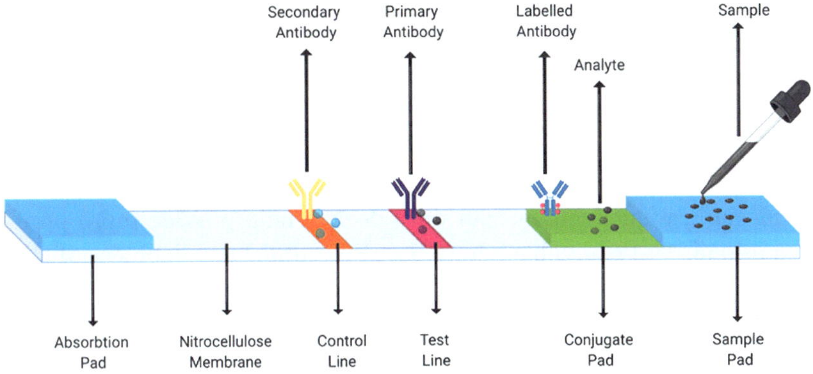

Figure 9.15. The advancement of microfluidics and lab-on-a-chip devices signifies a transformative potential for point-of-care testing (POCT), offering rapid diagnostics that can significantly enhance patient care.

Source: https://www.frontiersin.org/files/Articles/602659/fbioe-08-602659-HTML/image_m/fbioe-08-602659-g004.jpg.

The merge of lab-on-a-chip technology with POCT also provides opportunities for bringing health monitoring and preventive care far more advanced. These technologies can be integrated with wearable technologies to conduct continuous or periodic health monitoring, enabling proactive healthcare approaches. Real-time biomarker monitoring can lead to earlier diagnosis of diseases, which can lead to significantly improved outcomes for the patient. The capability of the systems to monitor diseases like diabetes or cardiovascular diseases on a continuous basis is particularly useful as they can monitor critical health parameters continuously. Whereas the health environment is becoming progressively embracing of technological innovations, microfluidics is to shape the future of POCT by provoking precision, accessibility, and management of general well-being (Abate et al., 2017; Navarrete et al., 2018) (Figure 9.15).

9.7. CONCLUSION

Briefly, the emerging technology of lab-on-a-chip and microfluidics devices is leading the forefront of technologies poised to revolutionize numerous sectors, most notably healthcare and diagnostics. By miniaturizing advanced laboratory processes, these technologies provide greater precision and enhanced sensitivity, ultimately saving time and cost over traditional approaches. As populations grow more expectant of more efficient and targeted healthcare measures, microfluidics present themselves as key players towards fulfilling these needs. The capability to carry out rapid diagnostic tests, in addition to the potential for performing high-throughput analyses, makes these devices critical components of modern medical procedures. In addition, the scope of applications for microfluidics transcends the realm of routine diagnostics to novel drug design and targeted medicine, especially in the field of oncology. The ability to store tissue samples in an *in vivo*-like state allows scientists to probe normal and pathological tissue biology in ways previously unimaginable, as recent studies have shown. Not only does it help provide more profound insights into disease pathophysiology but also into the development of tailored treatments for patients with cancer, rendering microfluidics a tantalizing alternative to traditional animal models (Bower et al., 2016). In this context, the integration of microfluidic technologies with clinical practice can lead to improved patient outcomes through targeted therapy. Further, with molecular biology breakthroughs aligning with the capabilities of microfluidics, the potential for radical applications becomes increasingly apparent. From the amplification of nucleic acids to targeted protein measurement, these technologies are a manifestation of biology-technology convergence driving innovation across industries from infectious disease management and food safety (Abate et al., 2017). Point-of-care diagnostics driven by microfluidics have not only increased accessibility but have also enabled timely interventions that are essential in emergency and resource-scarce settings. As research and development continue to push the field further, the future of microfluidics promises a great deal of innovation that will revolutionize the game in molecular diagnostics and therapeutic delivery.

9.7.1. Summary of Key Points

In talking about the landscape of microfluidics and lab-on-a-chip chips, one of the most powerful currents is their design and functionality. The breakthrough of continuous-flow microfluidic devices has transformed applications in biological sciences significantly. Among the principal concerns is the manual design nature of such devices, which is both technically arduous and demands understanding of biological mechanisms. The arrival of Directed Placement, a revolutionary algorithm, counters this weakness. By optimizing the physical arrangement of fluidic components, it enhances the connectivity of channels and reduces the overall channel length by up to 91% while simultaneously increasing area utilization by 8% on average. Not only does this innovation ease the design process but it also transcends obstacles that have thus far hindered increased application of microfluidic technology in the laboratory setting, a big leap toward enhanced efficiency and performance in lab-on-a-chip technology (Brisk et al., 2019). Enhanced progress in microfluidic technology is achieved through automated and modular integration of platforms, which ensure precise sample handling. The ability to process small quantities effectively is an important feature, especially in situations where sample materials are limited or expensive. A novel microfluidic architecture allows the processing of samples of 0.15 ml to 1.5 ml and facilitates the automation of operations such as collection of samples, priming of systems, and cleaning. The closed-loop system coupled with fluid handling automation renders sample processing effective without the production of excess wastage.

Interestingly, the design can be used with a variety of microfluidic devices, such as acoustofluidic setups, which expand the range of applications, particularly in size-separation operations with biological samples. With the implementation of real-time feedback in experiments, researchers enjoy improved sample collection, significantly contributing to the device's performance and reliability (Benett et al., 2015). With future breakthroughs in microfluidics, the intersection of design, automation, and application presents a focus area for continued research and development. The ability to integrate several functions into one platform enhances the functional use of lab-on-a-chip devices, thereby expanding their potential area of applications in various disciplines, from diagnostics to environmental monitoring. Emphasizing stable device-to-device connections and stable performance reiterates the need for a general framework for ensuring smooth transition between the laboratory and chip environments. These developments in design approaches and optimization of operational processes provide the gateway to radical innovations in microfluidics, enabling increased research and development towards broad breakthroughs that can affect healthcare and the biological sciences. These developments, thus, reflect one of the ongoing efforts to enhance the technology in microfluidics and apply its applications to daily life (Benett et al., 2015; Brisk et al., 2019).

9.7.2. Implications for Future Research

The field of microfluidics and lab-on-a-chip (LoC) devices holds tremendous promise in shaping biomedical research and diagnostics, particularly in the fields of personalized medicine and point-of-care testing. Upcoming research must address more sophisticated biological constituents that can interact dynamically within microfluidic systems. For instance, the situation of creating microfluidic devices that are able to mimic biological conditions holds potential to make us understand complex biological processes such as leukocyte extravasation. By advancing methods in centering as well as guiding cells in microchannels, researchers are able to mimic artificially physiological conditions required for accurate experimental outcomes. This new approach not only further enhances our capacity for analyzing cellular interactions but also paves the way for better diagnostic approaches, demonstrating the merit of microfluidics in healthcare solutions in the 21st century (Navarrete et al., 2018). Moreover, the integration of microfluidic technology with other fields, such as wearables and environmental sensors, offers a fertile ground for interdisciplinarity and innovation. From the study of microfluidics in wearables, where sensitive material can transmit information based on physiological parameters, subsequent research should revolve around synergistic applications of such technologies. This is through producing platforms with capacity to transmit real-time information for the monitoring of health status or environmental dynamics. Through this, researchers can be capable of developing more integrated solutions towards health and environmental management.

The versatility and promise of microfluidic devices to address global health issues, thus, may prove to be the deciding factor, which highlights the imperative for continued research into integrating them with emerging technologies (Tillotson et al., 2005). Lastly, the implications for ongoing research extend into the arena of sustainability and the ethics of developing microfluidic technologies. With increasing demand for rapid, low-cost diagnostics, the manufacturing and end-of-life disposal environmental impact is still a significant concern. Future research should explore green materials for designing microfluidic devices, along with technologies that minimize waste generation during the product life cycle. Ethical concerns regarding data privacy and potential misuse of health-related information generated by lab-on-a-chip systems should not be neglected either. Resolution of these issues will guarantee that microfluidics development is beneficial to society and in accordance with ethical guidelines. This multifaceted emphasis on sustainability and ethics is an essential part of emerging research agendas for microfluidics and lab-on-a-chip technology (Navarrete et al., 2018).

9.7.3. Final Thoughts on the Impact of Microfluidics

Microfluidics and lab-on-a-chip technologies' revolutionary power have become the essence of modern scientific advancements, particularly in the fields of health and environmental observation. Miniaturizing common laboratory operations, the chips enable one to carry out intricate analysis using much smaller amounts of samples and reagents. Application of microfluidics in the concentration of waterborne pathogens such as Cryptosporidium parvum and Giardia lamblia shows its effectiveness in achieving high levels of recovery that even surpass traditional processes like centrifugation (Bridle et al., 2016). Second, the accessibility of the devices facilitates decentralized testing, which is needed for emergency health response and regular diagnostics. Such promise emphasizes how profoundly microfluidics affects, not only to enhance scientific processes but also to extend diagnostic capabilities to populations globally. As wonderful as pathogen detection is, however, microfluidics has transformed molecular diagnosis, becoming firmly integral to the nature of current biomedical science and medical devices. Technological developments in this field have enabled high-speed analyses which are crucial for effective intervention measures in various fields including infectious disease control, food safety, and biodefense (Abate et al., 2017). With enhanced sensitivity and efficiency, the arduous process of protein analysis and nucleic acid amplification can now be done without disruption on one chip. This advancement not only saves time and cost but also represents a paradigm shift towards point-of-care diagnostics, thereby allowing timely clinical judgments to be made. The streamlined sample-in, answer-out diagnostic model further facilitates the use of such technologies in resource-limited settings where traditional laboratory setup may be lacking. Finally, the microfluidics growth curve is poised to influence a variety of non-medical industries, highlighting opportunities in environmental science and biotechnology. Its application in cell analysis and sorting is the opening door to research that leaves the door open for advancements in personalized medicine and the development of therapies. The convergence of microfluidic technologies also makes real-time measurements of environmental parameters possible, facilitating the search for sustainability and public health. As long as scientists keep working on and refining these devices, the contribution of interdisciplinary collaboration will be crucial to realizing their full potential. The development that is ongoing in microfluidics will usher in an era where procedures in the lab are not only more efficient and accurate but also inherently more accessible, thereby transforming our way of scientific inquiry and healthcare delivery.

REFERENCES

1. Abate, A. R., Demaree, B., Lan, F., Weisgerber, A., et al. (2018). An ultrahigh-throughput microfluidic platform for single-cell genome sequencing. https://core.ac.uk/download/323062457.pdf (accessed on 14th October 2025).
2. Abidin, Z. Z., Anuar, M. R., Dahlan, S. H., Lim, Y. C., et al. (2017). Tapered microchannel for multi-particles passive separation based on hydrodynamic resistance. https://core.ac.uk/download/154349688.pdf (accessed on 14th October 2025).
3. Aghaamoo, M., Digman, M. A., Kamalakshakurup, G., Lee, S., et al. (2019). Label-free metabolic classification of single cells in droplets using the phasor approach to fluorescence lifetime imaging microscopy. https://core.ac.uk/download/286362561.pdf (accessed on 14th October 2025).
4. Ahmad, A. S., Ahmar, A. S., Asmuni, H., Hishamudin, M., et al. (2018). Iris segmentation. https://core.ac.uk/download/19162806.pdf (accessed on 14th October 2025).
5. Akhil, V., Harneet, K., Parveen, L., Saleem, M., et al. (2013). Microfluidic mechanics and applications: A review. https://core.ac.uk/download/20492585.pdf (accessed on 14th October 2025).
6. Al Atraktchi, F. A. Z., Dimaki, M., Kjærgaard, C., Madsen, M., et al. (2016). Evolvable smartphone-based platforms for point-of-care *in-vitro* diagnostics applications. https://core.ac.uk/download/83999630.pdf (accessed on 14th October 2025).
7. Axelrod, B. W., Johannessen, M. L., Roukes, M., Murphy, R., Recht, D., Thorsen, T., Fon, W., et al. (2009). High-sensitivity microfluidic calorimeters for biological and chemical applications. https://core.ac.uk/download/4882823.pdf (accessed on 14th October 2025).
8. Baret, J. C., & Mugele, F. (2005). Electrowetting: From basics to applications. https://core.ac.uk/download/pdf/11459959.pdf (accessed on 14th October 2025).
9. Benett, W. J., Bora, M., Burklund, A., Fong, E., et al. (2015). A microfluidic platform for precision small-volume sample processing and its use to size separate biological particles with an acoustic microdevice. https://core.ac.uk/download/323063130.pdf (accessed on 14th October 2025).
10. Bower, R., Dawson, A., Green, V., Greenman, J., et al. (2016). Microfluidics: The fur-free way towards personalized medicine in cancer therapy. https://core.ac.uk/download/151160881.pdf (accessed on 14th October 2025).

11. Bridle, H., & Jimenez, M. (2016). Microfluidics for effective concentration and sorting of waterborne protozoan pathogens. https://core.ac.uk/download/96883805.pdf (accessed on 14th October 2025).

12. Brisk, P., Crites, B., & Kong, K. (2019). Directed placement for mVLSI devices. https://core.ac.uk/download/323311285.pdf (accessed on 14th October 2025).

13. Brisk, P., Curtis, C., Lesani, M., Loveless, T., et al. (2018). BioScript: Programming safe chemistry on laboratories-on-a-chip. https://core.ac.uk/download/323311195.pdf (accessed on 14th October 2025).

14. Caputo, D., Costantini, F., de Cesare, G., Gardeniers, H., et al. (2017). An all-glass microfluidic network with integrated amorphous silicon photosensors for on-chip monitoring of enzymatic biochemical assay. https://core.ac.uk/download/144472954.pdf (accessed on 14th October 2025).

15. Chen, X., Xu, J., & Zhang, Z. (2015). Entry effects of droplet in a micro confinement: Implications for deformation-based CTC microfiltration. http://arxiv.org/abs/1601.01932 (accessed on 14th October 2025).

16. Coudron, L., Johnston, I., McCluskey, D., McDonnell, B., et al. (2019). Fully integrated digital microfluidics platform for automated immunoassay; a versatile tool for rapid, specific detection of a wide range of pathogens. https://core.ac.uk/download/287581383.pdf (accessed on 14th October 2025).

17. Cranny, A., Green, N. G., Harris, N., Lewis, D., et al. (2013). Review on the development of truly portable and *in-situ* capillary electrophoresis systems.

18. Dimov, I. K., Ducrée, J., Lee, L. P., Riaz, A., et al. (2009). Hybrid integrated platform of PDMS microfluidics and silica capillary for effective CE and ESI-MS coupling. https://core.ac.uk/download/11309615.pdf (accessed on 14th October 2025).

19. Ducrée, J., Koltay, P., & Zengerle, R. (2004). Microfluidics: An enabling technology for the life sciences. https://core.ac.uk/download/11309631.pdf (accessed on 14th October 2025).

20. Fortina, P., Kricka, L. J., Park, J. Y., & Polsky, T. G. (2015). The future of laboratory medicine–A 2014 perspective. https://core.ac.uk/download/54509579.pdf (accessed on 14th October 2025).

21. James, S. W., Partridge, M., Tatam, R. P., Tothill, A., et al. (2017). Fabrication and optimization of a fused filament 3D-printed microfluidic platform. https://core.ac.uk/download/77602512.pdf (accessed on 14th October 2025).

22. Joshi, P. N. (2016). Cells and organs on chip—A revolutionary platform for biomedicine. https://core.ac.uk/download/322426977.pdf (accessed on 14th October 2025).

23. La Rocca, M., Lauricella, M., Montessori, A., Stolovicki, D., et al. (2017). Regularized lattice Boltzmann multicomponent models for low capillary and Reynolds microfluidics flows. http://arxiv.org/abs/1711.02003 (accessed on 14th October 2025).

24. Morales Navarrete, P. (2018). Development of flow focusing device for the visualization of leukocyte rolling adhesion. https://core.ac.uk/download/214845386.pdf (accessed on 14th October 2025).

25. Motosuke, M., Sakurai, R., & Yamamoto, K. (2018). Concentration-adjustable micromixer using droplet injection into a microchannel. http://arxiv.org/abs/1808.04509 (accessed on 14th October 2025).

26. N/A. (2013). *The Boston University Photonics Center Annual Report 2013–2014.* https://open.bu.edu/bitstream/2144/29752/1/Photonics-Center-Final-Annual-Report-2013-2014-v2.pdf (accessed on 14th October 2025).

27. Piat, G., & Gillier, T. (2025). Exploring over the presumed identity of emerging technology. https://core.ac.uk/download/pdf/6618787.pdf (accessed on 14th October 2025).

28. Rainer, A., Perestrelo, A., Águas, A., Barbulovic-Nad, A., Chang, Y., Chen, H., Das, R., et al. (2015). Microfluidic organ/body-on-a-chip devices at the convergence of biology and microengineering. https://core.ac.uk/download/210536597.pdf (accessed on 14th October 2025).

29. Tillotson, J. (2005). Scent by a wireless web. http://ualresearchonline.arts.ac.uk/4908/29/J.Tillotson_paper_WALES.pdf (accessed on 14th October 2025).

30. Wu, A., Sturm, J., D'Souza, J., Loutherback, K., Liu, L., & Austin, R. (2012). Deterministic separation of cancer cells from blood at 10 mL/min. https://core.ac.uk/download/pdf/290604.pdf (accessed on 14th October 2025).

CHAPTER 10

CURRENT TRENDS AND EMERGING TECHNOLOGIES

Contents

INTRODUCTION

The convergence of advanced technologies has triggered revolutionary advancements in the field of biomedical engineering, an age of emerging evolution. In this realm, traditional practices are being supplemented by techniques that integrate materials science, computing, and medicine. New-age techniques such as 4D printing and intelligent materials are transforming the method of designing and producing medical devices. These technologies enable the creation of dynamic structures that are capable of modifying themselves in real time according to changes in the body, enhancing therapeutic efficacy and patient outcomes. Besides, research on biopolymers has gained strength since their ability to act as biodegradable alternatives to synthetic polymers for medical devices has been promoted. This shift to such eco-friendly materials is also part of a larger paradigm of responding to environmental concerns without trading off the quality of healthcare solutions, which is a critical domain of concern in present biomedical science (Baranwal et al., 2022). Meanwhile, artificial intelligence (AI) is also assuming a vital role in enhancing design automation processes in biomedical engineering. By leveraging machine learning algorithmic processes and predictive modeling, AI streamlines device development and manufacturing processes. This combination facilitates rapid iteration and prototyping, which facilitate the rapid modification of designs to suit patient-specific requirements. In addition, hybrid manufacturing systems that combine traditional fabrication with novel technologies such as additive manufacturing enable unprecedented design freedom. These systems permit the production of complex geometries that were not feasible previously, thus expanding the scope of biomedical applications from implants to diagnostic devices. As these technologies converge, they have the ability to propel the world of biomedical engineering into an era of personalized medicine and on-demand capability. Another necessity trend reshaping the future of biomedical engineering is the convergence of wearable and Internet of Things (IoT) medical devices into the healthcare fabric. These allow for continuous monitoring and real-time data capture and provide healthcare providers invaluable information about the health of patients. Therefore, there is a clearly visible shift towards preventive care, with interventions being actively given and not in a reactive state. This is made possible with the advancements in piezoelectric energy harvesting, making these devices sustainable to use without requiring constant replacement with new batteries (Sezer et al., 2020). The potential for enhanced patient engagement through feedback from real-time data is a step closer to more patient-centered care in healthcare. All these innovations in technology direct the need for endless innovation in biomedical engineering towards opening the door to innovations that address both effectiveness and sustainability in medicine.

Definition of Biomedical Engineering

The integration of engineering principles with biological sciences gives rise to a productive multidisciplinary field known as biomedical engineering. It is naturally defined by its function of promoting healthcare through the generation of new technologies and methodologies. As it emerges, the definition encompasses several elements such as tissue engineering, medical imaging, and bioinformatics, which are indicative of the broad area of application in improving patient care and understanding of complex biological systems. Emerging trends, such as the use of AI in design automation, show the efforts in biomedical engineering towards optimum efficiency and precision in medical device development and ultimately transforming the industry. Moreover, upcoming technology like 4D printing and smart materials reflect the implementation of engineering solutions in meeting dynamic healthcare needs and enabling tailored therapeutic interventions and thus emphasizing the utility of biomedical engineering in contemporary medicine. Expanding the definition of biomedical engineering also includes its core position to data-driven medicine.

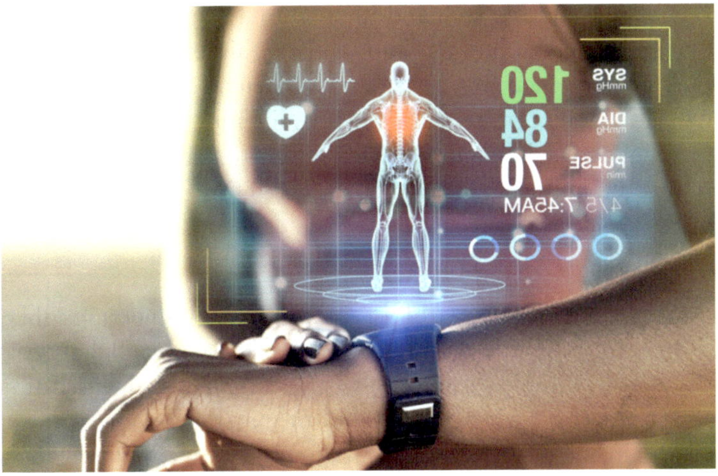

Figure 10.1. The introduction of wearable technology and internet of things (IoT) devices further integrates engineering solutions with daily healthcare practices, creating a seamless user experience that promotes patient engagement and proactive health monitoring.

Source: https://media.licdn.com/dms/image/v2/D5612AQHXUUifUqkAHA/article-cover_image-shrink_720_1280/article-cover_image-shrink_720_1280/0/1713831871929?e=2147483647&v=beta&t=7h-HVtmt-8F9PqIh1yGlnZa6zYzQozG-8BE62VJLCFyk.

The addition of computational science and engineering (CSE) to it is a breakthrough since it provides the tools for simulation of biological systems and understanding of their complicated processes, which traditional experimental methods tend to struggle with achieving. With biomedical engineering riding the wave of opportunity, that powerful computing makes possible, especially in the face of challenge imposed by extreme-scale computing and the data revolution, capabilities in predictive modeling are extended and personalized medicine approaches encouraged (Biros et al., 2016). Through this convergence, therefore, is made possible the development of sophisticated diagnostic tools and treatment protocols all with a direct effect on patient outcomes and a push beyond previous possibilities within health care. Besides, the landscape of biomedical engineering is being reshaped by the integration of traditional manufacturing methods with cutting-edge technologies. Hybrid manufacturing systems are a case in point, coupling additive and subtractive methods to produce complex medical devices with enhanced efficiency and versatility. These advancements resonate deeply in the soul of biomedical engineering, delivering unprecedented heights in device customization and functionality. The emergence of wearable tech and Internet of Things (IoT) products further integrates engineering solutions into daily healthcare practice, giving an unbroken user experience that fosters patient engagement and early disease monitoring. The trends persist to thrive, consolidating the dynamic position of biomedical engineering in continually expanding its definition and application to address the pressing concerns of modern healthcare (Figure 10.1).

Importance of Current Trends

With the rapidly changing world of biomedical engineering, there is no underestimating the importance of emerging trends. Among all the breakthrough advancements, 4D printing is unique, which adds the element of time to the traditional 3D printing with the capability of materials to transform shape or function when subjected to environmental stimuli. This technology is particularly groundbreaking when it comes to designing adaptive medical devices with the ability to respond dynamically to shifts in body physiology. These technologies have the capability of enhancing patient outcomes by providing uniquely individualized treatment approaches that are more effective and reduce the burden of invasive procedures. Additionally, smart materials obtained by 4D printing provide for the development of tissue engineering scaffolds to mimic the natural sequence of cellular growth and differentiation, significantly enhancing regenerative medicine. The coming together of such technologies makes it vital to be current with such trends in order to advise on the future of medical solutions accordingly (Nagle et al., 1996). Artificial intelligence (AI) has remained a revolutionary force in design automation, revolutionizing how biomedical engineers innovate. The use of machine learning algorithms allows for rapid processing of massive data sets to improve the design and functioning of medical implants and devices. This integration with AI not only improves the automation of design but also enables the production of more intelligent, responsive systems that are capable of real-time monitoring and data analysis. AI's ability to recognize patterns and predict outcomes leads to a new generation of customized medicine, where therapies are tailored based on patient-specific profiles. Secondly, as design automation becomes increasingly sophisticated, it also makes hybrid manufacturing systems possible that utilize traditional fabrication techniques and sophisticated technologies. These technologies enable a more integrated and responsive process of production of medical devices, with preparedness to be in a position to deal with the evolving needs of healthcare (Geyter et al., 2009). Current trends also reveal the strategic role of wearables and the Internet of Things (IoT) in shaping the future of medical treatment and diagnostics. The development of wearable health monitors makes it possible to collect data in real-time, allowing for well-informed decisions by the patients and medical professionals. With advancing smart technologies and biometrics, convenient integration of devices into patient care is a pointer to the shift towards decentralized healthcare models, with heightened accessibility and convenience. Predictive analytics are made feasible by the streaming nature of data from these monitors, which, in turn, lead to preventative healthcare measures. Also, the collective capability of wearables and emerging technologies in AI and machine learning means superior algorithms can learn health tactics based on the patient's behavior. Tapping into and responding to these emerging trends is crucial for researchers and practitioners seeking to actualize the promise of enhanced health outcomes in a more digitalized world (Nagle et al., 1996) (Figure 10.2).

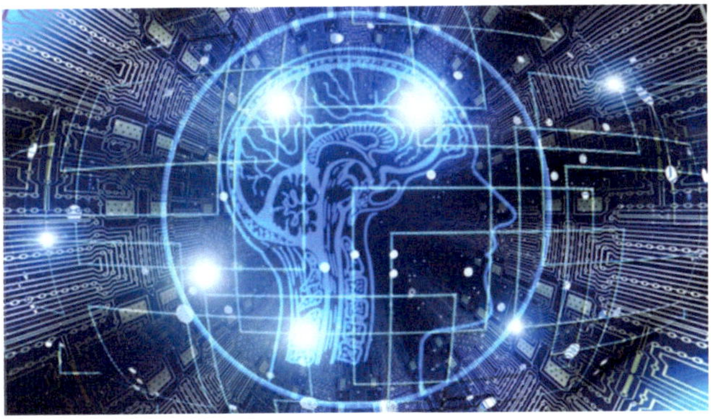

Figure 10.2. Artificial intelligence (AI) has emerged as a pivotal force in the automation of design processes, transforming how biomedical engineers approach innovation.

*Source:*https://res.cloudinary.com/engineering-com/image/upload/w_640,h_640,c_limit,q_ auto,f_auto/ai_design_digitrans_img01_phm0dc.jpg.

Overview of Emerging Technologies

The constant evolution in technology has driven the practice of biomedical engineering to new horizons, especially through innovation like 4D printing and the development of smart materials. The essence of 4D printing is the capability to produce structures that are able to change shape or function with time when exposed to external stimuli. This remarkable talent is particularly worth its weight in gold during scaffold production for tissue engineering, when dynamic behaviors can allow for improved compatibility with biological systems.

Combined with smart materials responsive to mechanical, thermal, or chemical forces, the potential for creating devices responsive to patient needs is enormous. Hence, not only do such technologies hold the promise of enhanced treatment effectiveness in their use, but they also bring with them new therapeutic techniques that have the potential to transform the patient experience within healthcare provision, exemplifying the dynamic nature of biomedical engineering innovations. Apart from the physical creation of medical devices, artificial intelligence (AI) is revolutionizing the design process of automation in biomedical engineering.

This groundbreaking technology enhances the development process through efficient work processes in designing, rapid prototyping, and ideal material selection based on desired parameters. AI processing considers vast amounts of data, providing insights used to drive optimized designs tailored to specific medical needs, reducing time to market for new devices. Furthermore, AIs predictive ability can facilitate the identification of issues beforehand through the process of design so that the engineers can potentially address issues prior to their occurrence. As the biomedical designs become more sophisticated, employment of AI not only improves efficiency but also facilitates the manufacture of personalized and precise healthcare solutions such that patient care is enhanced and the quality of treatment improved. The evolution of hybrid manufacturing systems is an essential trend in biomedical engineering since they blend traditional manufacturing techniques with innovative additive processes. This blending provides the capability to produce complex, personalized medical devices impossible using traditional means. By incorporating various manufacturing techniques, such as the synergy between subtractive machining and additive manufacturing, engineers have the ability to design high-performance parts with intricate geometries tailored to meet specific patient needs. Also, the introduction of wearable technology and IoT-based healthcare devices into this setting further indicates a broader shift toward individualized medicine. These interconnected systems have real-time monitoring and data collection from the patient, thus opening doors for a more preventative aspect of healthcare. In essence, the convergence of manufacturing innovations and smart technologies further broadens the field's capability to meet multiple medical requirements, driving the future of biomedical engineering.

10.1.4D PRINTING IN BIOMEDICAL APPLICATIONS

The integration of state-of-the-art manufacturing technologies is bringing about innovative solutions in biomedical engineering. Among these, 4D printing is an exciting technology that allows the creation of adaptive structures that respond to external stimuli and evolve over time. The technology involves the use of smart materials—those that can alter their shape or characteristics when subjected to certain conditions—and has profound implications in personalized therapy and medicine. For instance, researchers are looking into the way highly sophisticated self-assembling tissue engineering scaffolds can be engineered to detect physiological changes, stimulate cell growth, and assist in healing. Also, the union of 4D printing with concepts from the Fourth Industrial Revolution emphasizes the potential for developing extremely complex medical devices that are not just effective but also adaptive to the unique needs of specific patients, therefore revolutionizing traditional surgical methods and post-surgical care practice (Dehghanghadikolaei et al., 2019). Coupled with advancements in artificial intelligence, design automation in biomedical engineering is becoming increasingly sophisticated. AI can optimize personalization in 4D printing by predicting and optimizing the behavior of material under an immense number of parameters, thereby shortening the amount of time required to achieve functional medical products. Machine learning algorithms can browse large collections of information drawn from previous experiments and know the most effective designs and material combinations for specific medical applications. This 4D printing-AI association extends beyond typical manufacturing processes; it encourages hybrid production systems combining subtractive and additive production, synthesizing intricate biomedical devices to perform more than a single function in a single device. This development enhances the efficiency of diagnostics and treatments overall (Chou et al., 2019). Additionally, the integration of 4D printing with wearable and Internet of Things (IoT) devices is a revolutionary shift towards patient tracking and therapy. 4D printing materials can be embedded within wearable devices, which are now no longer confined to tracking just health parameters but also change their characteristics in real-time from user information. For example, a 4D printed wearable designed to change compression in response to swelling or other changes in the body would deliver optimal therapeutic benefit without the need for human adjustment. This dynamic interaction builds a more responsive health system that enables continuous feedback between practitioners and patients. The synergetic potential of 4D printing, smart material technology, and Internet of Things (IoT) technology enables a revolutionary trajectory for biomedical applications which will usher in next-generation health care focused on personalization and responsiveness (Chou et al., 2019; Dehghanghadikolaei et al., 2019).

10.1.1. Explanation of 4D Printing Technology

Taking 3D printing to the next level, 4D printing technology is one step ahead of traditional 3D printing in that it introduces time as an element, producing objects that are able to change shape or functionality when exposed to environmental triggers. It uses smart materials, which are capable of responding to change in heat, moisture, or light, thereby offering transformative technologies in numerous fields, particularly biomedical engineering. For instance, drugs may be released or properties of mechanics altered in medical implants on demand, significantly improving patient outcomes. Besides, the materials can be engineered to cause tissue regeneration and, therefore, underlining the potential of 4D printing technology to revolutionize personalized medicine by providing tailored solutions that evolve over time according to precise patient needs, an orientation matching trends pointing towards the transition of medical interventions towards more adaptive strategies (Dehghanghadikolaei et al., 2019). Additionally, the use of artificial intelligence (AI) in 4D printing design processes also works towards enhancing the speed and reliability of creating these interactive materials. AI programs make it easy to automate design through predicting how different configurations would respond to certain stimulations, which in turn maximizes the usability of printed materials. This process not only reduces prototyping time but also facilitates the creation of intricate geometries that were previously impossible through conventional manufacturing practices. This synergy between AI and 4D printing tracks the trend of intelligent manufacturing systems, where intuitive interaction between technology and human wisdom produces innovative designs and production. All these advances will also promote the development of the next generation of medical devices that will actually adapt in real-time to the patient's physiological status, hence boosting the texture of biomedical engineering (Rosa et al., 2019). The effect of the 4D printing technology extends beyond the single-use device since the addition of wearable technology and Internet of Things (IoT) provides new opportunities for remote patient monitoring and personalized medicine. Wearable tech with embedded 4D printed components can adapt to biometric signals to adjust their functions, and in this way, a more dynamic approach to health management is achieved. Smart bandages made of 4D printed materials that change their shapes to improve healing based on moisture levels as well as infection levels are an example. This adaptable capability not only enhances the efficacy of treatment but also changes patient engagement by offering personalized solutions to health. With ongoing progress in synergy among 4D printing, AI, and IoT, the potential of its widespread use in biomedical engineering becomes more evident, which will give rise to a shift towards more active and personalized medical interventions that are in line with the individualized health profiles of patients (Dehghanghadikolaei et al., 2019) (Figure 10.3).

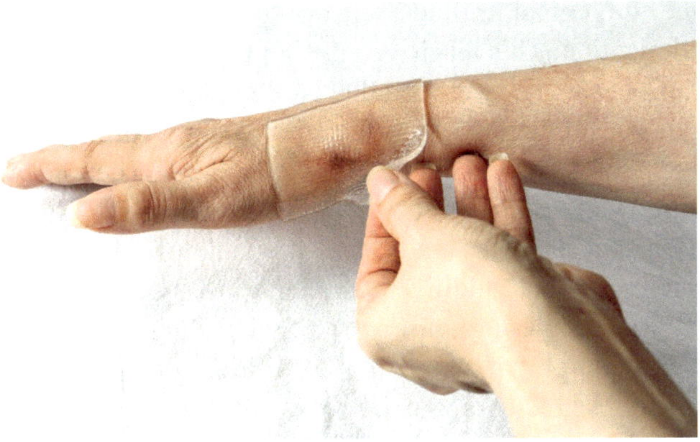

Figure 10.3. Medical implants can be designed to change their mechanical properties or release drugs on demand, significantly improving patient outcomes.

*Source:*https://www.azom.com/images/Article_Images/ImageForArticle_24126_17322730938169245.jpg.

10.1.2. Applications in Tissue Engineering

The intersection of sophisticated manufacturing techniques and tissue engineering is going through a revolution, particularly with the support of 4D printing. The emerging approach allows the fabrication of dynamic scaffolds that are able to respond to varied environmental stimuli, thus making tissue regeneration more efficiently than the traditional approaches. By incorporating shape-memory polymers and bioactive materials, these smart scaffolds can be engineered to respond to physiological conditions such as temperature or pH and thereby stimulate improved cell adhesion and tissue formation. These scaffolds can be engineered to change their shape or behavior over time, providing new opportunities in personalized medicine, where scaffolds may be tailored to the specific patient requirements after surgery. Not only do these technologies accelerate the healing process, but also enhance the effectiveness of regenerative therapies, making 4D printing a main technology in the greater field of tissue engineering (Geyter et al., 2009). Artificial intelligence (AI) is increasingly becoming a key element in tissue engineering application design automation. AI algorithms can efficiently analyze vast datasets, optimizing scaffold designs before their physical creation, thereby reducing material waste and production time. Through machine learning techniques, the properties of various materials can be precisely predicted, guiding engineers toward the best combinations for specific biomedical applications. In addition, AI-augmented virtual simulations enable scientists to foresee how tissues will respond to mechanical stressors and biological milieus, ensuring an evidence-based approach to scaffold optimization. This AI-driven design paradigm not only accelerates the fabrication of new tissue-engineered constructs but also ensures that they will meet the numerous functional, stability, and biocompatibility requirements that biomedical applications demand (Oliver et al., 2009). The integration of hybrid manufacturing systems within tissue engineering is a three-dimensional route for innovation that balances traditional methods of fabrication with cutting-edge technologies such as additive manufacturing. The complementary strategy allows for material layering with accuracy, tailoring the scaffold architecture to replicate the complex structure found in biological tissues. By synergistic fabrication, it is feasible to create scaffolds with excellent mechanical integrity and optimal biological properties. Further, the convergence of IoT and wearable biomedical devices enables real-time monitoring of healing, which can enhance the patient outcome via continuous data capture and analysis. As these technologies converge, a new era of smart, responsive medical devices surfaces that fulfills the requirements of personalized medicine, ultimately finding expression in improved therapeutic interventions and rehabilitation protocols in the tissue engineering field (Geyter et al., 2009).

10.1.3. Potential for Personalized Medicine

In the rapidly evolving climate of biomedical engineering, research in personalized medicine holds unprecedented promise to enhance patient outcomes. With the application of multi-dimensional information about an individual's biological profile—his or her genome, epigenome, transcriptome, and habits—healthcare providers are able to develop individually tailored treatment regimens compatible with each patient's unique profile. New data integration tools have become obligatory as scientists try to construct integrative models capturing the underlying disease intricacies. According to emerging trends, the integrated methods, which integrate diverse data sources, have the potential to contribute to essential insights, forecasting treatment effectiveness as well as selecting appropriate biomarkers with greater accuracy. The ability to combine such data marks a paradigm shifts in medicine, leading medical practice away from the same approach and towards increasingly individualized therapeutic regimens (Goldenberg et al., 2018). Furthermore, the integration of wearable technology and Internet of Things (IoT) devices has triggered the quantified self-movement, where health can be experienced in a richer sense. Through sensors tracking various aspects of health, one is able to quantify their body state in real time, leading to preemptive health management strategies. While these wearables are providing valuable information, they provide just a limited view, that being primarily physiological parameters.

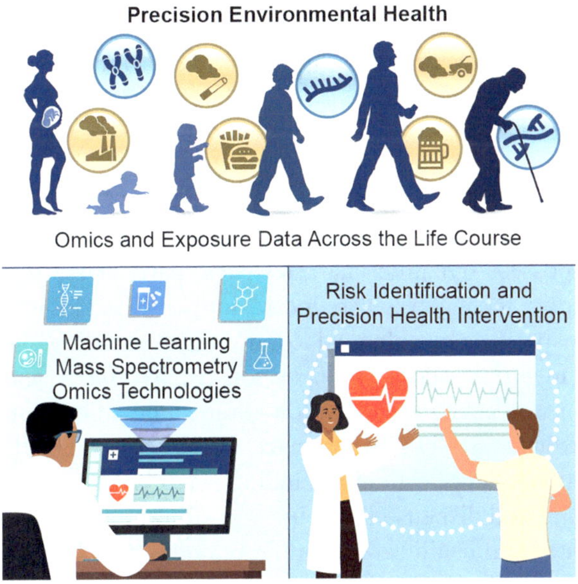

Figure 10.4. By leveraging multidimensional data about an individual's biological makeup—including their genome, epigenome, transcriptome, and lifestyle—healthcare providers can develop tailored treatment strategies that align with each patient's unique profile.

Source: https://www.cell.com/cms/10.1016/j.xgen.2024.100591/asset/279f3fa1-4280-47e4-aa8c-8a82466cd274/main.assets/fx1_lrg.jpg.

To augment the power of personalized medicine, social and environmental data must be included that can provide further context to the biometric data collected. For instance, collecting health-related data from social media usage can provide a more comprehensive view, not only of biomedical data but also of lifestyle determinants and social determinants, incorporating a holistic view of patient health (Haddadi et al., 2015). With continuing advances in personalized medicine, 4D printing and smart material-based hybrid manufacturing systems will revolutionize therapeutic interventions. Being able to fabricate biomimetic structures that respond dynamically to environmental stimuli, there is a promise of creating individualized medical devices and implants that adapt to patients' evolving needs. This bi-directional interdependence of patient data and customized manufacturing processes creates potential for real-time response to unique responses to treatment. In this manner, the interfacing between next-generation technologies in design automation and bioprinting renders personalized medicine not only possible but practical, with interventions that continuously evolve in concert with each patient's pathway toward health. With the incorporation of these advanced techniques, the future of personalized medicine is a transformative revolution in the manner in which medical healthcare can be delivered (Goldenberg et al., 2018) (Figure 10.4).

10.2. SMART MATERIALS IN HEALTHCARE

Material science breakthroughs have propelled the development of smart materials that possess dynamic characteristics, particularly in healthcare. As industries progress, the materials are increasingly utilized to innovate solutions that are responsive to physiological conditions, enhancing patient care and results. Smart materials such as bio-responsive hydrogels and electroactive polymers in biomedical engineering allow for the innovation of medical devices that respond instantaneously to user needs. These technological advancements usher in revolutionary applications, including smart bandages that can sense the status of a wound and dispense medicine accordingly. The interdependence of material attributes and healthcare technology points to a fundamental synergy between biology and engineering, providing a platform where preventive medicine becomes a reality. By unleashing the power of smart materials, emerging trends herald a shift toward adaptive, personalized health solutions that are in line with patient-centric design philosophy. The integration of 4D printing technology in the manufacturing of smart materials is one such turning point in healthcare solution customization. This new production process allows for the creation of materials that change shape or function over time in response to environmental cues, thus prolonging their utility in real-world applications. Having the capability to fabricate complex adaptive structures opens up new avenues for wearable sensors that monitor essential signs and adjust treatment regimes autonomously. For instance, scientists can create stents that sense the arterial conditions of individual patients through 4D printing, thereby improving clinical outcomes. Moreover, integrating these new fabrication techniques with artificial intelligence (AI) during design automation increases manufacturing effectiveness for intricate health devices. This convergence of technology significantly emphasizes ongoing development within the biomedical industry, leading to a more adaptive environment for healthcare in the long run.

Wearable and Internet of Things (IoT) devices have increasingly made use of smart materials to monitor and control personal health more effectively. The incorporation of interactive, responsive materials in the devices allows for the monitoring of health parameters with greater accuracy and provides real-time feedback to the individual and medical professionals alike. Sensor-integrated intelligent clothing can monitor biometrics such as heart rate, temperature, and activity level, enabling continuous health monitoring without disrupting the daily life of the users. In this context, studies on integrated systems comprising organic thin film electronic devices (OFEDs) are typical of the emphasis being laid on innovation when it comes to wearable technology. It not only improves the user experience but also facilitates improved communication between healthcare practitioners and patients, facilitating informed decision-making. With the integration of advanced materials and digital health technology, healthcare stands to revolutionize significantly, offering strong, flexible solutions customized to specific needs and improving overall health management.

10.2.1. Definition and Types of Smart Materials

The combination of innovative materials and engineering results in a variety of applications significant for advances in biotechnology and other fields. Intelligent materials, which exhibit dynamic sensitivity to environmental stimulus, are of particular interest in biomedical engineering. Intelligent materials are capable of changing their properties as a function of temperature, pressure, humidity, or electric field and thus have the potential to play a revolutionary function in medical devices and treatments. For instance, piezoelectric materials convert mechanical stress into electrical energy, showing considerable potential in energy-harvesting devices for wearable technology. Given the growing demand for more responsive and adaptive medical products, there is a need to comprehend and implement smart materials, especially drug delivery systems and tissue engineering, representing a leading trend in biomedical engineering (Dehghanghadikolaei et al., 2019). 4D printing is a great example of the shifting paradigm of smart materials, where structures can be fabricated to shift function or form over time. By incorporating material capable of responding to some stimulus, such as heat or moisture, 4D printing has the ability to create complex biomimetic structures that can transform in accordance with varying conditions of the human body. This versatility can potentially enhance the performance of biomedical devices to make them better at their therapy delivery or diagnostic functions. Furthermore, as 4D printing technology advances, it may open new avenues for personalized medicine, where the structures can be tailored to meet the unique physiological requirements of individual patients, hence being in close harmony with the ongoing trends in biomedical engineering (Debackere et al., 2025). In the future, the inclusion of smart materials in wearable and Internet of Things (IoT) medical devices is a gigantic area of healthcare innovation. With the inclusion of smart materials in wearable technology, engineers can design devices with live monitoring and data collection capacities, which can lead to early interventions for various health problems. For example, smart bandages that adapt to the environment of a healing wound or body chemistry-sensitive biosensors illustrate the promise of delivering improved patient results. In addition, as artificial intelligence becomes a more crucial part in design automation, the combination of AI and intelligent materials can lead to the creation of next-generation biomedical devices that are effective as well as extremely personalized, with a possible revolutionary transformation in medical treatment provision (Dehghanghadikolaei et al., 2019) (Figure 10.5).

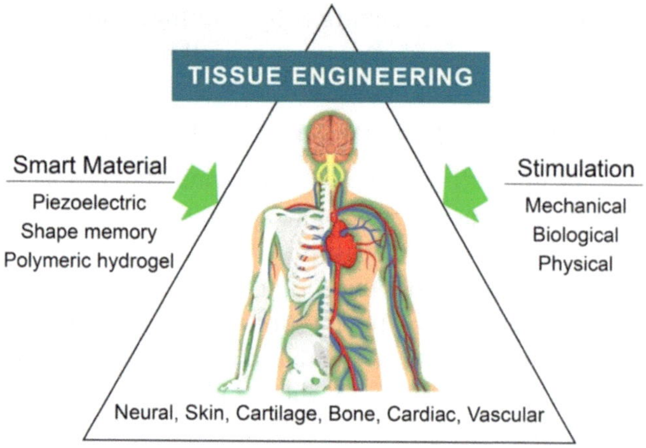

Figure 10.5. Smart materials, defined by their ability to respond dynamically to environmental stimuli, are particularly relevant in biomedical engineering.

Source: https://pub.mdpi-res.com/pharmaceutics/pharmaceutics-15-02356/article_deploy/html/images/pharmaceutics-15-02356-ag.png?1695268558.

10.2.2. Role in Drug Delivery Systems

The application of cutting-edge technologies in drug delivery systems best defines the evolving face of biomedical engineering. Modern methods such as 4D printing enable one to fabricate dynamic drug delivery systems that change their form in response to physiological conditions. With this method, not only can one release drugs in a controlled manner but also respond to the body's reaction to some stimuli, thereby achieving the highest therapeutic effectiveness. Utilizing smart materials, the systems have the potential to dynamically adjust dosages from real-time physiological inputs, thus mimicking biological processes to enhance patient outcomes. Such research into innovative applications marks a milestone shift in direction towards personalized medicine, whose treatment modalities are individually tailored to the patient's needs, ultimately transforming how therapies are designed and delivered. In addition, the integration of drug delivery systems with artificial intelligence (AI) is radically transforming design automation. AI accelerates drug development faster through enhanced identification of drug composition and delivery mechanisms with large datasets.

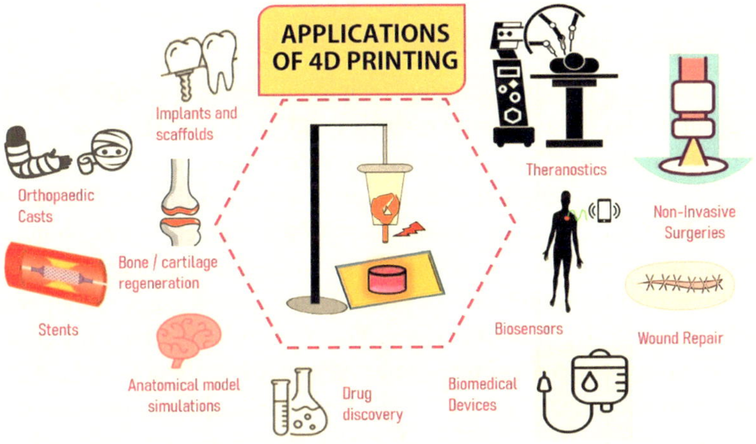

Figure 10.6. Modern methodologies such as 4D printing facilitate the development of dynamic drug delivery systems that can adapt to physiological changes.

Source: https://media.springernature.com/lw1200/springer-static/image/art%3A10.1007%2Fs13346-022-01200-y/MediaObjects/13346_2022_1200_Fig5_HTML.png.

Beyond this capability to speed up the process, it enhances targeting specificity in aimed tissues or cells. By employing predictive analytics from AI, scientists can predict pharmacokinetics and pharmacodynamics of novel drug formulations so that they achieve maximum therapeutic effect with side effects at an absolute minimum. The arrival of such smart design platforms advances the next generation of drug delivery where precision medicine expresses its best form and patient compliance is maximized by data-driven personalized interventions. The marriage with wearable devices and Internet of Things (IoT) only adds to the rising prominence of drug delivery systems in contemporary biomedical engineering. This integration enables real-time monitoring of medication adherence and physiological state, enabling timely intervention. Through the deployment of active sensing technologies on drug packaging, as proposed in some recent studies, the potential for developing an integrated drug delivery environment exists. Not only do the medicines become reusable through this technology, but also the quality and integrity of recovered medicines are ensured by continuous monitoring. By incorporating medicines into the IoT environment, the health care system can be transformed into an active system that enhances patient safety and maximizes clinical outcomes. This marriage of technologies is a crucial step in reinventing drug delivery paradigms of the modern era (Figure 10.6).

10.2.3. Impact on Prosthetics and Implants

Material science and manufacturing technology breakthroughs are having a dramatic impact on the field of prosthetics and implants. 4D printing, the next revolution after 3D printing, allows us to create responsive materials that adapt dynamically to environmental stimulation. This capability makes prosthetics sensitive to the movement and environment of the user, enhancing functionality and user comfort. For instance, intelligent materials can change rigidity or shape with respect to temperature or pressure and provide support depending on the requirements at the time of activity. This flexibility not only maximizes the user experience but also maximizes integration with daily activities. As a result of advances in manufacturing processes, these technologies are a historic shift towards more personalized, efficient, and responsive prosthetic technologies that embody the values of sustainable healthcare systems outlined in continuing research into pervasive health monitoring (Perez et al., 2015). The integration of artificial intelligence (AI) into design automation processes is another technology area that powerfully affects the manufacturing of prosthetics and implants. Artificial intelligence technologies enable the simulation and testing of prosthetic design, allowing developers to compare thousands of different variations in a matter of minutes that would have otherwise taken them months. Such an accelerated design process generates more imaginative and precise prosthetic solutions that fit individual anatomical and functional requirements. Also, AI can make it possible for the integration of information from patients past medical histories and current health statuses such that prosthetic devices are not only structurally stable but also ergonomically beneficial. The complexity of AI algorithms can be able to optimize automated manufacturing systems at lesser costs and greater accessibility, as required for larger-scale acceptance and implementation in healthcare settings (Abels et al., 2014). The integration of prosthetics with wearable and Internet of Things (IoT) technology has provided a new paradigm in patient rehabilitation and care. Incorporating sensors and connectivity features into prosthetic devices, medical practitioners can administer continuous monitoring and feedback to patients. Prosthetic devices can transmit usage information in real time, enabling practitioners to tailor back-up programs and monitor patient progress effectively. Furthermore, such data linking facilitates the merging of health records and clinical databases to facilitate more informed and personalized treatment plans. As paradigms for preventive and participatory medicine evolve, the merging of prosthetics, wearable technology, and IoT technologies underscores the importance of data to achieve the best outcomes for patient rehabilitation and health care management (Perez et al., 2015) (Figure 10.7).

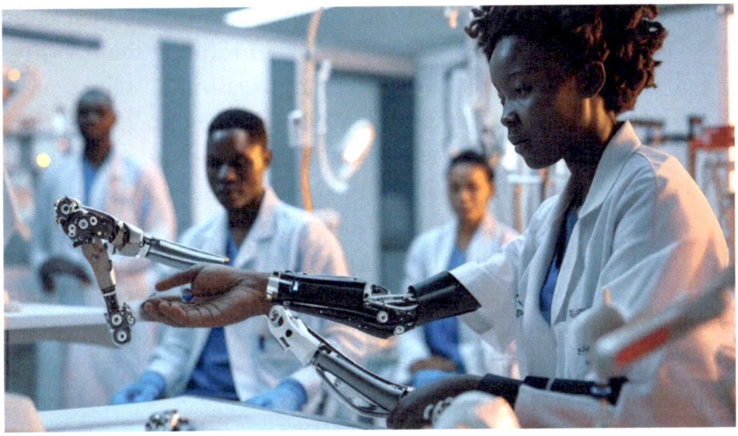

Figure 10.7. The integration of prosthetics with wearable and internet of things (IoT) technologies signifies a transformative shift in patient care and rehabilitation.

Source: https://media.licdn.com/dms/image/v2/D4D12AQG_sYKuxSeyng/article-cover_image-shrink_720_1280/B4DZfMFn5QGsAQ-/0/1751475761310?e=2147483647&v=beta&t=OsSLEeB2kV0HlK60R3chDycfhPkM2rklcefKS3c0ocI.

10.3. ARTIFICIAL INTELLIGENCE IN DESIGN AUTOMATION

With the era of quick-paced biomedical engineering, latest approaches like Artificial Intelligence (AI) for design automation are currently in the limelight when it comes to industrial innovation. The use of AI-based technologies in design automation allows the speed and accuracy of product engineering to reach levels hitherto unprecedented. This aspect becomes even more relevant in the context of the complexity of biomedical devices, which need to adhere to rigorous regulatory and performance specifications. For instance, computer codes are able to examine design solutions that can be overlooked by human designers and facilitate end-to-end examination of materials and manufacturing processes. With the optimization of the design process through performance modeling and predictive analytics, AI does not only guarantee faster time-to-market but promotes the creation of very personalized biomedical solutions appropriate for unique patient needs, thus enhancing overall healthcare delivery in the modern medical setting. With the domain still being increasingly automated, hybrid manufacturing systems stand to benefit enormously from a combination of the traditional approaches and advanced technologies like 4D printing and smart materials. The hybrids allow for simultaneous processing of several design needs, enhancing the capability of biomedical engineering techniques. AI is critical in this setting in terms of refining the hybrid systems, material behavior predictions, and enabling real-time adjustment during fabrication. For example, Ewart et al. (2019) describes how a hybrid strategy that involves additive and subtractive manufacturing processes can lead to improved outcomes over employing one approach alone. These technologies not only maximize efficiency but also solve complex geometrical problems in device design, ultimately leading to improved performance and functionality in biomedical devices. The opportunities for localized manufacturing and patient-specific devices are also gigantic, resulting in the age of personalized medicine. AI-based design automation is also ushering in the doors for integrated devices in the Internet of Things (IoT) platform in a smarter way. AI-enabled wearable medical devices are capable of capturing patient health data in real time and adjusting a device's functionality based on real-time biosignals autonomously. As Das et al. (2017) have pointed out, such precision inherent in robot-guided systems allows for improved surgical results through the facilitation of interventions that are tailored to the patient's individual physiological needs. These kinds of integration not only foster surgical precision but also challenge the cooperative nature of human surgeons with independent robotic systems. Combined, these advances detail how AI-based design automation is fueling revolutionary trends in medicine and steering the development of increasingly sophisticated and powerful biomedical engineering processes.

10.3.1. Overview of AI Technologies in Engineering

The present engineering field is better integrated with the latest technology that drives the development of various sectors, including biomedical engineering. Among these, artificial intelligence (AI) is the most visible as a revolutionary force. Most significantly, AI in design automation allows the creation of highly efficient systems that automate processes by minimizing human intervention. With learnable algorithms that can process extremely large data sets, AI enables the identification of the optimal designs and solutions for certain biomedical applications. This has important implications for fields such as prosthetics and implantable devices, where precision and customizability are paramount. Hence, AI not only increases efficiency but also significantly improves the quality of healthcare products, and thus why integration of such advanced systems into engineering applications focused on the medical sector is essential (Fluitman et al., 1996). Additionally, the technology of 4D printing and smart materials is a groundbreaking movement towards the development of adaptive and responsive biomedical devices. By using materials whose characteristics can be changed by environmental stimuli, engineers can design devices that better mimic biological functions. This new feasibility also extends to drug release systems that modify release behaviors in response to physiological conditions or external factors. Combined with AI, these materials can be engineered to anticipate patients' needs and significantly enhance therapeutic outcomes. The fusion of 4D printing technology and smart materials underscores the necessity for ongoing research and development in developing personalized treatment plans that cater to the complex needs of patients and thereby improve overall healthcare management (Bizopoulos et al., 2021). As engineering and AI continue to merge, hybrid manufacturing systems are a significant trend in biomedical applications. By combining conventional manufacturing techniques with sophisticated digital processes, these systems allow for the production of sophisticated medical devices that are scalable and customizable. By leveraging AI algorithms to balance and optimize production operations, engineers can achieve unprecedented efficiency while accommodating unique patient requirements. Even more so, wearable and IoT medical devices represent another example of convergence, allowing for real-time monitoring and data collection to drive individualized healthcare decisions. This convergence of technologies not only enhances the power of biomedical engineering but also facilitates data-based patient care, which provides impetus towards continuous improvement and innovation in this field (Fluitman et al., 1996).

10.3.2. Benefits of AI in Biomedical Design

The intersection of artificial intelligence (AI) and biomedical design is creating groundbreaking innovations in the field, particularly with the development of new materials and manufacturing methods. The most important breakthrough is the development of 4D printing, wherein materials change continuously in accordance with environmental stimuli, thereby enhancing their functionality in medical application. These smart materials may react to temperature or pH, allowing implants that are more integrated with biological systems or drug delivery systems that release medicine upon stimulation by specific stimuli. These developments suggest a highly promising future when the marriage of

AI and new material sciences gives rise to products not only meeting medical needs but also improving patients' outcomes through customized interaction. With advancing research, incorporating AI algorithms into these procedures will make sure that designs are not only efficient but also highly specific to individual patient profiles, thus solving unique medical problems effectively. In design automation, AI serves a key role in simplifying biomedical device development through sophisticated modeling and simulation methods. These technologies allow for rapid prototyping and testing before the development of physical prototypes, significantly shortening development cycles and employing large data sets to predict outcomes.

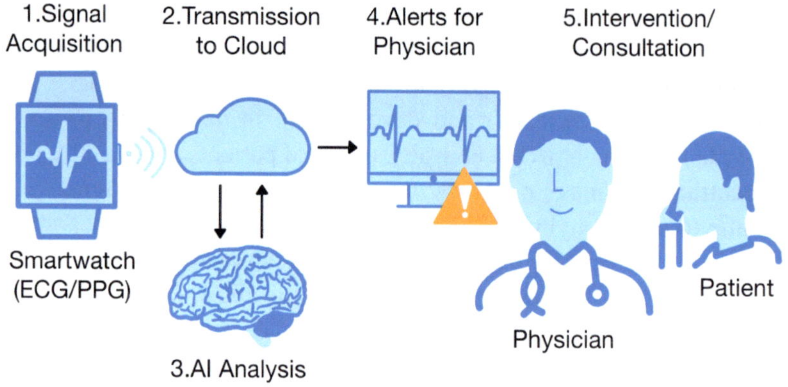

Figure 10.8. By automating the analysis of critical signals such as the RR interval and electrocardiogram (ECG), AI applications enhance diagnostic accuracy and facilitate timely interventions, ultimately reducing morbidity and mortality associated with cardiovascular diseases.

Source: https://pub.mdpi-res.com/biomedicines/biomedicines-13-01685/article_deploy/html/images/biomedicines-13-01685-g002.png?1752063021.

This predictive capacity is particularly relevant in cardiovascular well-being, where AI-driven monitoring devices for diseases like atrial fibrillation are growing trendier. By automating key indicators such as the RR interval and Electrocardiogram (ECG) analysis, AI-based applications enhance diagnostic accuracy and facilitate timely interventions, ultimately reducing cardiovascular disease-related morbidity and mortality (Acharya et al., 2020). This problem-free integration of AI within automation is reflective of an overarching movement towards efficiency in biomedical engineering, with the massive potential that exists for AI to push the design process to new heights of sophistication and reliability. On top of this, synergies created due to hybrid manufacturing systems, i.e., the union of traditional as well as additive methods of manufacturing, are reflective of the growing trend of utilization of AI within biomedical engineering. This integration of technologies not only enhances production capability but also allows devices to be customized to address individual patient requirements. The integration of wearable and Internet of Things (IoT) medical devices into this framework extends further the possibility of personalized medicine. AI is able to analyze real-time information from these devices, delivering information regarding patient health and sensing patterns that must be addressed by a doctor. This kind of system facilitates proactive care, as it provides an opportunity for patients to be given early alerts concerning alarming trends in their health parameters, hence improving treatment regimen adherence and overall health monitoring. As such technologies advance, integration potential of AI into design and manufacturing will revolutionize the whole face of biomedicine, towards more effective and patient-specific treatments (Browne et al., 2025) (Figure 10.8).

10.3.3. Case Studies of AI Implementation

In the rapidly evolving world of biomedical engineering, artificial intelligence (AI) in case studies shows its potential for transformation across a broad spectrum of applications. A prime example is the role of AI algorithms in the evaluation of medical imaging, as deep learning models increase diagnostic precision. Such computer solutions are capable of quickly scrutinizing large collections of imaging data, early symptoms of disease such as cancer being identified, often outperforming the diagnostic skills of human clinicians. The implications are great because not only are detection levels increased within these systems but also workload is minimized for healthcare professionals so they can spend time attending to patients rather than wasting it on image analysis. In line with this, the case studies point to the imperative of interdisciplinary cooperation among engineers, data scientists, and clinicians in the cutting through of the complex landscape of AI implementation in healthcare. Yet another intriguing use of AI exists within the context of 4D printing, where advances go beyond conventional static shape into adaptive structures that are capable of responding to environmental stimuli. This technology includes smart materials with programmable properties, which contribute to the improvement of medical device functions. For instance, AI calculations enhance the design automation process through the ability to predict material behavior under varying conditions, leading to optimized designs tailored for specific therapeutic use. These developments enable researchers to create adaptive prosthetics and implants capable of making real-time adjustments, greatly improving the outcome for the patient. By studying these case studies, researchers reveal the impact of synergizing AI with emerging technologies, showing a paradigm shift towards optimized and tailored healthcare solutions in the biomedical area. The fusion of AI with IoT-connected medical devices also emphasizes the movement towards enhanced connectivity and data-based decision-making in biomedical engineering. Wearable health monitoring systems with artificial intelligence capabilities continuously collect and analyze patient information, providing actionable insights that facilitate proactive management of healthcare. Case studies indicate that when employed along with predictive analytics, the devices are able to identify looming healthcare crises before they happen, enabling timely intervention. Moreover, data obtained from such IoT devices can be fed back into AI models, facilitating ongoing tuning of algorithms and an ongoing learning and improvement process in patient care strategies. This convergence illustrates how AI implementation case studies are not isolated incidents but more reflective of an overall trend towards more intelligent, responsive healthcare systems and are a pivotal part of continued trends and emerging technologies in biomedical engineering.

10.4. HYBRID MANUFACTURING SYSTEMS

The terrain in biomedical engineering is additionally dominated by new production techniques that combine traditional and advanced technology, with Hybrid Manufacturing Systems playing a leading role. Hybrid Manufacturing Systems combine additive and subtractive techniques to attain intricate geometries and precise parts essential in medical application. For instance, integrating traditional machining with 3D printing technologies enables the creation of molds that can easily adapt to various materials, thereby enhancing implant and prosthetic customization. The flexibility is crucial, particularly for personalized medicine, where unique patient needs must be met. The span of Hybrid Manufacturing Systems' capabilities is not only beneficial for attaining production effectiveness but also sustains through waste minimization, thus corresponding to the broader objectives of ongoing biomedical engineering initiatives (Dehghanghadikolaei et al., 2019). Furthermore, integration of Hybrid Manufacturing Systems greatly expands the scope of smart materials and 4D printing technologies in biomedical applications. These new devices enable the fabrication of materials that respond dynamically to external stimuli, which further necessitates the improvement of medical device performance. Shape-changing implants or drug delivery systems adjusting can, for example, be realized through special control by hybrid methods. This not only makes the devices more effective but also provides a path toward developing wearable technologies interacting with patients' biological signals. Therefore, the combination of Hybrid Manufacturing Systems and 4D printing is a phenomenal union of technology with the capacity to revolutionize treatment protocols, patient care, and overall healthcare provision (Ewart et al., 2019). In addition, the application of AI in design automation supports Hybrid Manufacturing Systems in optimizing the efficacy and efficiency of biomedical production. By employing AI algorithms, designers can automate additive and subtractive manufacturing to an extent that they can foresee regions of possible failure and enhance product functionality according to input from data-driven. Such coordination thus allows for quick iteration of prototypes, which is essential in the fast-paced biomedical sector. The adaptability of Hybrid Manufacturing Systems is also maximized when it comes to the fabrication of parts that are incorporated into Internet of Things (IoT) medical devices on a daily basis. With these devices becoming more dependent on interrelated data, the accuracy provided by hybrid methods guarantees them to be customized to address the unique, changing necessities of patients in real-time, ultimately leading to more responsive and individualized healthcare settings (Dehghanghadikolaei et al., 2019).

10.4.1. Definition and Components of Hybrid Systems

In the rapidly evolving field of biomedical engineering, hybrid systems become relevant as an emergent field of learning and practice. By combining a number of technologies and methodologies, hybrid systems are able to effectively tackle the complex problems to healthcare. These systems integrate traditional manufacturing processes with new technologies such as additive manufacturing, also known as 3D printing, which has a vital contribution to the designing and production of medical implants and devices. Besides, industry 4.0 initiated a blend of intelligent manufacturing systems and information technology in hybrid systems, which allows for improved efficiency in production and decentralization. This interconnectedness not only enhances design customization but also minimizes material waste, a paradigm changes in biomedical device development that is more efficient and sustainable (Dehghanghadikolaei et al., 2019). One vital feature of hybrid systems is the potential for artificial intelligence (AI) integration with design automation. This convergence supports rapid prototyping and streamlines manufacturing procedures and hence allows engineers to create extremely complex shapes and structures for use in medical implants and devices. These are particularly relevant in bioprinting, where personalized solutions are critical for individual patient cases. The use of AI algorithms here can predict material performance and manufacturability, making production phases even more streamlined. In addition, the smart systems can learn adaptively from ongoing processes, and this enhances general operational performance and reduces time to market. Thus, utilization of AI not only facilitates additive manufacturing but also boosts the hybrid systems potential to innovate in biomedical engineering technology, which ensures personalized care to patients (Hussein et al., 2012). Another typical feature of hybrid systems is their integration with wearable devices and Internet of Things (IoT) healthcare equipment. The integration is a futuristic approach towards patient monitoring and healthcare delivery by enabling real-time capture and analysis of data. Hybrid systems that incorporate these features in the right manner can lead to predictive healthcare solutions that maximize treatment algorithms based on a patient's individual data. For instance, smart materials in wearables are designed to respond dynamically to physiological activity, thereby enhancing user experience and therapeutic results. The potential for synergy in such hybrid systems not only facilitates patient engagement but also allows for a new generation of personalized care, revolutionizing the approach to healthcare in the 21st century. This macroscopic perspective of the hybrid systems is a consideration of their potential for redesign in transforming biomedical engineering (Dehghanghadikolaei et al., 2019; Hussein et al., 2012) (Figure 10.9).

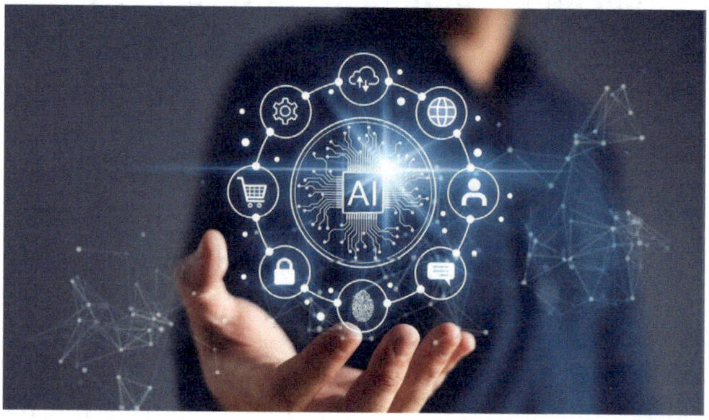

Figure 10.9. A critical component of hybrid systems lies in their capability to merge artificial intelligence (AI) with design automation.

Source: https://imageio.forbes.com/specials-images/imageserve/66fcdc589e002dcb85799ece/0x0.jpg?format=jpg&height=900&width=1600&fit=bounds.

10.4.2. Advantages Over Traditional Manufacturing

Innovation in manufacturing technology has transformed the sector of biomedical engineering with their unique benefits that supersede the implementation of standard methods. A notable example is additive manufacturing, also known as 3D printing. Additive manufacturing provides the capability to produce complex geometries that are difficult, if not impossible, to replicate using the traditional methods of fabrication. Not only does this technology make production easier, but it also reduces waste of materials because it builds products layer by layer as opposed to cutting off excess material. In terms of customization, additive manufacturing caters to patient-specific needs to create customized medical implants and devices. The Fourth Industrial Revolution's improvement of productive production and rapid prototyping is enhanced through the use of additive manufacturing as cited by Dehghanghadikolaei et al. (2019). This trend supports the prospect of creating tailored solutions with greater emphasis on personalized medicine in biomedical engineering. Application of cutting-edge technologies such as AI and smart materials differentiates contemporary manufacturing processes from the traditional ones. Productivity is improved by design automation using AI by making the design process more efficient and optimizing material usage to save costs on production. Besides, the emergence of smart materials capable of dynamically adapting to environmental stimulation offers unprecedented opportunity for innovation in biomedical devices. Combined with technologies like 4D printing, these materials can provide functionality that self-adjusts to specific physiological conditions and hence enhances the effectiveness of medical treatment. As elaborated by Chia et al. (2015), 3D printing has not only emerged to manufacture implants but also intricate scaffolds for tissue engineering and drug delivery systems, a revolutionary shift in manufacturing technology. This coming together of emerging technologies ensures that biomedical engineering is headed for a future with improved device performance and versatility. Furthermore, the synergetic interface between hybrid manufacturing systems and wearable as well as IoT medical devices is another historic breakthrough in the field. Hybrid systems that combine the additive and subtractive modes of manufacturing utilize the best characteristics of both approaches to create more complicated and tougher medical devices. This not only ensures accuracy but also the scalability of production. Additionally, the connectivity of wearable technologies with IoT gadgets enables real-time monitoring of patients and data collection, which can be used to tweak treatments in real time. This capability is consistent with the trends described by Dehghanghadikolaei et al. (2019) and Chia et al. (2015), as the technologies enable the development of patient-centered solutions that respond to individual health needs. With such innovations, biomedical engineering continues to advance with improved quality of care that could not have been achieved by traditional manufacturing.

10.4.3. Applications in Medical Device Production

New material science technology is revolutionizing medical device manufacturing, particularly with the introduction of 4D printing and intelligent materials. This technology leverages responsive and adaptive properties that are a characteristic of electroactive and photonic polymers, which integrate seamlessly into various applications. By using such new-generation materials, designers can design medical devices that not only adapt to shifting physiological states but also extend functionality and user experience. Notably, the integration offers the potential for the creation of smart systems within medical textiles and wearable technology, which enables innovation in assistive healthcare through, for instance, smart bandages responding to wound and vital sign alterations. As the demand for personalized and responsive medical solutions has grown, so too has the focus on 4D printing with smart materials indicated a significant shift towards creating personal health products and services, thus highlighting an encouraging path in biomedical engineering (Oliver et al., 2009). Artificial intelligence (AI) has already begun to alter the manner in which conventional approaches are executed in the design and manufacturing processes of medical devices, enhancing efficiency and accuracy. AI-powered automated design functionality can not only make aesthetics optimal but also the functionality of medical devices, saving time-to-market and reducing human error. The automation enables fast prototype creation so that various iterations can be test-checked quickly, thus optimizing designs before mass production. AI-powered predictive analytics enable intelligence on user behavior and device performance, enabling an instant feedback loop for constant improvement. With the integration of these technologies, their application in the production of medical devices is a revolutionary step towards meeting the mounting healthcare demands, particularly in designing user-friendly, very functional devices with real-time data collection and monitoring functions, thus reflecting the current trends in biomedical engineering (Ewart et al., 2019). The study on hybrid manufacturing systems also reflects the current trends in biomedical engineering, particularly in enhancing the production of medical devices. These systems integrate additive and subtractive manufacturing technologies in order to allow production of complex geometries that are traditionally required in medical devices. One example is the integration of conventional machining with 3D printing, which not only reduces the cost of manufacturing but also enhances the material properties of the finished products. These systems have tremendous potential for producing intricate medical components with improved surface finish and geometric precision with the capability of accommodating a broad range of materials from polymers to metals. Hybrid manufacturing techniques can facilitate rapid production of prototypes, such as injection molding inserts, significantly streamlining the designing and testing phase in medical device development. As a result, this new method is a significant part of altering manufacturing practices responsive to the demands of the medical field (Oliver et al., 2009) (Figure 10.10).

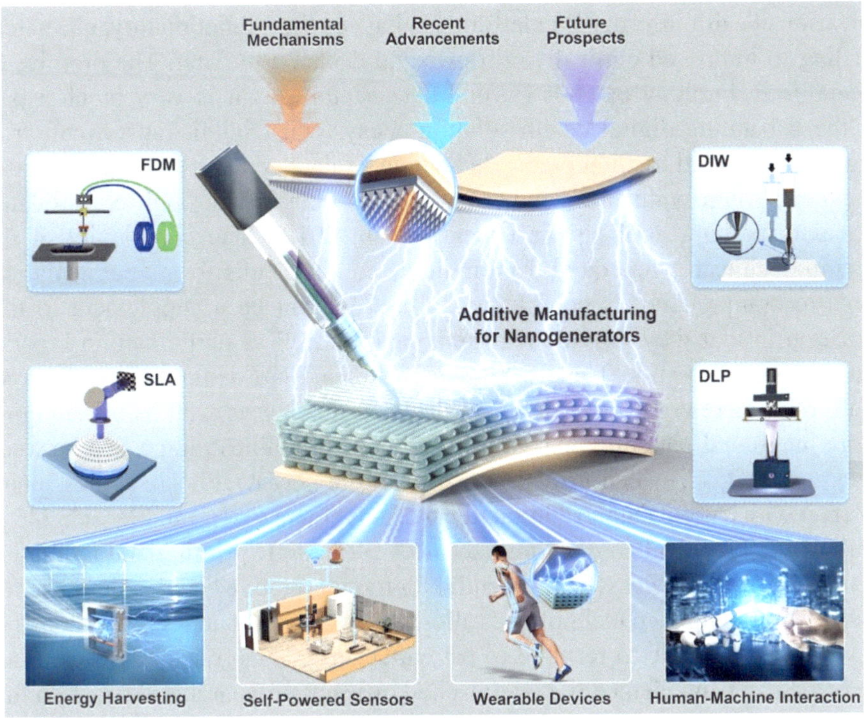

Figure 10.10. The exploration of hybrid manufacturing systems further exemplifies the current trends in biomedical engineering, particularly their role in enhancing medical device production.

Source: https://media.springernature.com/lw1200/springer-static/image/art%3A10.1007%2Fs40820-025-01874-2/MediaObjects/40820_2025_1874_Fig1_HTML.jpg.

10.5. INTEGRATION OF WEARABLE TECHNOLOGY

Improved wearable technology is a groundbreaking revolution in the discipline of biomedical engineering with tremendous potential to enhance health monitoring and patient care. This has evolved from basic fitness monitors to sophisticated wearable devices with the capability of in-depth physiological monitoring and data interpretation. Specifically, the integration of wearable sensors allows easy and discreet capture of health data, essential to the treatment of acute and chronic diseases. As outlined in current research, this innovation to pervasive monitoring of health heralds the shift towards more preventative and personalized healthcare, consistent with the wave for predictive and participatory medicine (Perez et al., 2015). Furthermore, the ability of such devices to connect to various health informatics platforms enhances their functionality, ultimately leading to improved clinical workflows and decision-making. The promise of wearable technology extends beyond data capture, as it is very much a part of the expanding digital health solution ecosystem. Digital transformation in healthcare has led to an appreciable amount of data generated through various channels, where valuable insights have to be obtained through consolidated machine learning applications (Arcuri et al., 2018). The complexity of the data in healthcare, generated from multiple sources, calls for potent analytical tools to comprehend its complexity. Wearables can be a supplement to this situation in that they provide real-time data, as well as participate in broader data fusion processes. That is aggregating data from a number of different platforms, thereby enriching clinical decision-making as well as encouraging more integrated patient management methods. Wearables plug a gap between data and insights, which provokes a shift in the way healthcare professionals interact with patient data. Additionally, the convergence of wearable technology with new biomedical engineering advances such as 4D printing and intelligent materials better showcases the potential for transformative health solutions. The intersection of the two technologies allows the creation of adaptive, customized devices that are able to respond to patient-specific situations and needs. Such convergence can enhance the comfort and efficacy of wearable devices so that they are easily part of daily life while maximizing their health-monitoring capabilities. Furthermore, as machine learning and AI programming improve in managing big data, their convergence with wearables can not only push the boundaries of personal health monitoring but also foresee and prevent health crises through continuous data interpretation and immediate results. Therefore, the integration of these technologies not only transforms patient treatment but also supports the establishment of a data-driven sustainable healthcare system, capable of addressing future challenges (Arcuri et al., 2018; Perez et al., 2015).

10.5.1. Overview of Wearable Medical Devices

Technological advancements in recent years have brought with them wide opportunities for massive innovations in the area of wearable medical devices, illustrating an intersection of health and engineering. Integrating smart materials and 4D printing techniques has initiated the development of adaptive, multipurpose products with the capability to customize itself according to the physiological requirements of the users. These wearable devices utilize dynamic properties-controllable electro-active polymers and bio-responsive hydrogels to enhance user experience and convenience. For instance, in assistive healthcare, smart bandages with sensors are able to monitor healing of wounds and transmit real-time data to healthcare professionals, enabling personalized interventions.

This new material function in increasing functionality is a window to the wearable devices of the future that are proactive rather than supportive in health care management (Oliver et al., 2009). Artificial intelligence (AI) incorporation into wearable medical technology development is another paradigm shift in biomedical engineering. AI technologies can process vast amounts of data that have been collected using various sensors embedded in wearable devices and provide insights that are used for customized healthcare plans. Other technologies also enable the quantified self-movement because people can track measures such as heart rate, physical activity, and sleep using the devices.

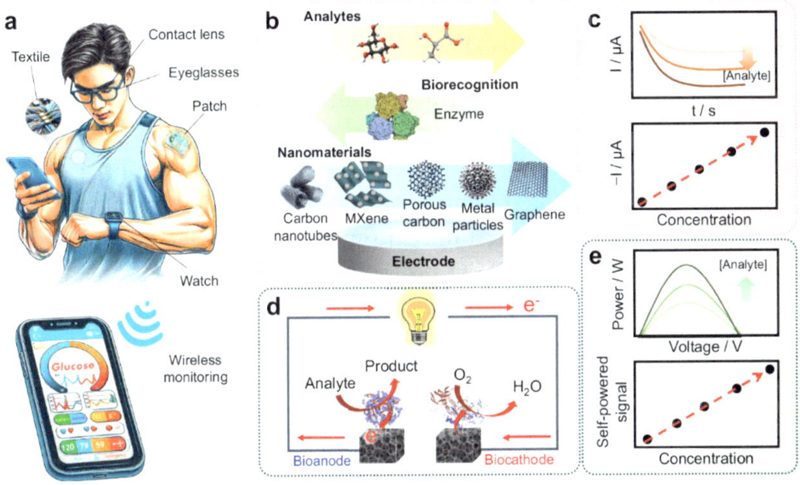

Figure 10.11. The integration of smart materials and 4D printing techniques has catalyzed the development of adaptive, multifunctional products that can respond to the users' physiological needs.

Source: https://media.springernature.com/full/springer-static/image/art%3A10.1038%2Fs43246-024-00557-6/MediaObjects/43246_2024_557_Fig1_HTML.png.

However, there is a limitation in concentrating on physiological data alone without considering social and environmental contexts of individuals' lives. A comprehensive view, referred to as 360 Quantified Self, encourages integration of sensor data with social networks and lifestyle indicators insight. The whole picture enhances care and comprehension of individual health enormously, facilitating vastly improved patient outcomes through increasingly personalized interventions (Haddadi et al., 2015). As wearable medical devices continue to evolve, their potential to monitor health in real time and aggregate data quickly increases, bringing on an era of preventive healthcare management. By leveraging emerging technologies such as IoT and hybrid manufacturing systems, producers can develop products that not only capture and analyze health data and provide actionable feedback to users in real time. Such products can facilitate on-time interventions, reduce hospital visits, and curb health care spending, thus making the entire health system more efficient. With ongoing R&D of wireless communication technologies, uninterrupted connectivity of wearable devices to healthcare systems is now achievable, enhancing care delivery process convenience and accessibility to patients. This innovation points to the potential of wearable medical devices playing a key role in revolutionizing healthcare delivery and management in the days ahead (Figure 10.11).

10.5.2. Data Collection and Patient Monitoring

With the progress of healthcare towards more accessible and personalized care, the gathering of data and observation of patients are essential to better patient outcomes. Integration of telemedicine systems without gaps allows healthcare services to be taken up in a more refined way where monitoring and sharing of information is enabled in real time. Portals like those developed by the INTERREG IIIB ARCHIMED project deploy cutting-edge technology to provide essential services such as telecollaboration and teleconsultation. It is especially vital in rural and remote areas where traditional access to medical care is limited. Notably, the effectiveness of the system also depends on its ability to distribute a variety of data—ranging from life-sustaining biosignals to diagnostic imaging—over an assortment of communication channels, such that medical practitioners can offer immediate interventions and treatment to risk populations (Androulidakis et al., 2011). In addition, the use of Wireless Body Area Networks (WBAN) is a great leap in remote patient monitoring, particularly in developing healthcare systems. In Benin, the establishment of the National Integrated Patient Monitoring Network (RNIMP) demonstrates the potential of technology to bear upon vast healthcare challenges. Not only does this new approach aim to improve patient care, but it also maximizes the reach and efficiency of nursing staff. By imitating Technocenter functionality and providing a seamless flow of physiological information, the RNIMP is an exemplar of how data acquisition can have tangible value to healthcare delivery. As these systems evolve, interoperability and compliance with safety and performance regulations are becoming increasingly significant to support patient confidence and efficacy in remote monitoring solutions (Ahouandjinou et al., 2020). Emergence of new technologies for patient monitoring as well as information collection is also underscored by growing utilization and significance of wearable devices as well as Internet of Things (IoT) solutions in the medical sector. These assist in ongoing observation of well-being and enable patients to become pro-active towards maintaining their health. By collecting comprehensive health data, wearable technology not only provides individual health data but also contributes to comprehensive sets of data that can inform public health initiatives. Moreover, artificial intelligence integration facilitates predictive analysis to allow healthcare professionals to anticipate patient needs and trends. This combination of real-time data gathering and AI-facilitated intelligence is paving the way for more responsive healthcare environments that anticipate patient conditions, eventually leading to improved health outcomes and patient satisfaction (Figure 10.12).

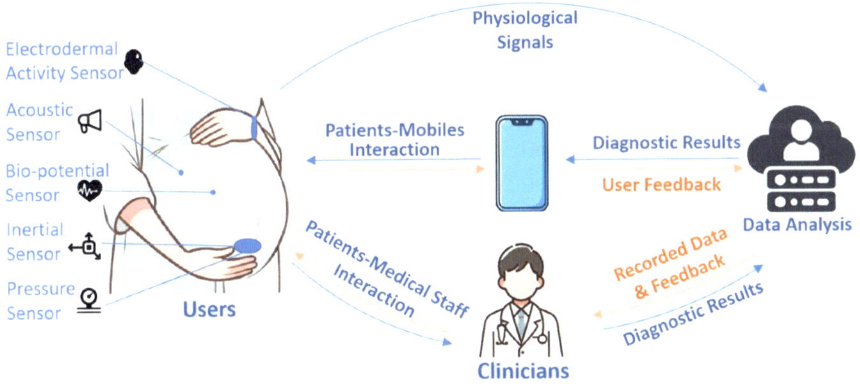

Figure 10.12. By collecting vast amounts of health data, wearable devices not only provide insights into individual health metrics but also contribute to larger datasets that can inform public health initiatives.

Source: https://www.mdpi.com/sensors/sensors-24-06426/article_deploy/html/images/sensors-24-06426-g001.png.

10.5.3. Impact on Chronic Disease Management

The landscape of chronic disease management has been transformed with the advent of advanced biomedical technologies. The meeting of wearables with ambient health monitoring systems allowed real-time data capture and analysis to radically redefine patient engagement strategies. Patients are now proactively engaged to track their health condition, with treatment plans tailored around real-time data rather than sporadic clinical visits. This shift to ongoing monitoring of an individual's health allows for early intervention in disease and improved management of chronic conditions since healthcare providers can identify trends and abnormalities in patient data. As noted in recent studies, the ability to integrate pervasive sensing technology into current health informatics infrastructure enhances the ability to tailor therapy and interventions based on patients' unique needs (Perez et al., 2015). The advent of the quantified self-phenomenon, spearheaded by wearable technologies, has also redefined the management of chronic illnesses. With technologies tracking various aspects of health—sleeping patterns to steps taken—people are able to understand their health situation in great detail. While the technologies yield vast amounts of data on physiological states, their usefulness is limited until contextual data such as social environment or lifestyle are considered. Current advancements suggest that medicine can potentially require a deeper insight, achieved by integrating social media information and wearable device knowledge. Such a 360° understanding allows a more personal insight into a patients health, facilitating more holistic approach to chronic disease management. This integration is a significant shift from existing methods of monitoring, ultimately culminating in the better life quality of the patient (Haddadi et al., 2015). With chronic diseases placing healthcare systems increasingly under siege, new technologies signal the path to sustainable approaches. Developments in 4D printing and intelligent materials open up new doors to the design of individually customized medical devices that adapt dynamically to patient needs. Furthermore, the use of artificial intelligence in design automation enhances medical interventions' efficacy and effectiveness. With the automation of design protocols, medical engineers can create customized solutions targeting directly the unique characteristics of chronic patients. In parallel, hybrid manufacturing systems bring with them a novel paradigm with the capability to combine the manufacturing and patient-specific requirements harmoniously. With increased pervasiveness, the collective impact of these technologies on chronic disease management will be astonishing, an era in which treatment is more personalized, timely, and effective (Perez et al., 2015).

10.6. INTERNET OF THINGS (IOT) IN HEALTHCARE

The rapid rate of technology innovation in healthcare is becoming more dominated by the convergence of the Internet of Things (IoT), which has enormous potential to enhance patient monitoring, treatment outcomes, and overall healthcare delivery. By installing sensors and networked devices on standard medical equipment, healthcare workers can gather and measure large amounts of real-time data, leading to improved clinical decision-making and personalized patient care. Such data-oriented model is pivotal in addressing long-standing weaknesses that are present in conventional health care systems. It allows not only remote monitoring and immediate notification in case of patient emergencies but also aids in preventive care, thereby improving the quality of healthcare. Also, the intersection of IoT with emerging technologies such as artificial intelligence, referenced in the UN Sustainable Development Goals, provides a new way to increase healthcare accessibility and equity globally (Farooq et al., 2017). Aside from enhancing patient engagement, IoT integration advantages healthcare providers by generating operational efficiencies that can significantly reduce costs. Through the utilization of connected devices, hospitals are able to track usage of equipment, manage levels of inventory, and streamline workflows, all of which ultimately lead to a responsive health ecosystem. This connectedness of technology results in a data-driven environment in which healthcare professionals can see trends and overcome systemic inefficiencies. Furthermore, the integration of IoT and 5G technology allows for low-latency, high-speed communication required for the exchange of data in real-time, a basis upon which telemedicine and remote surgery are improved.

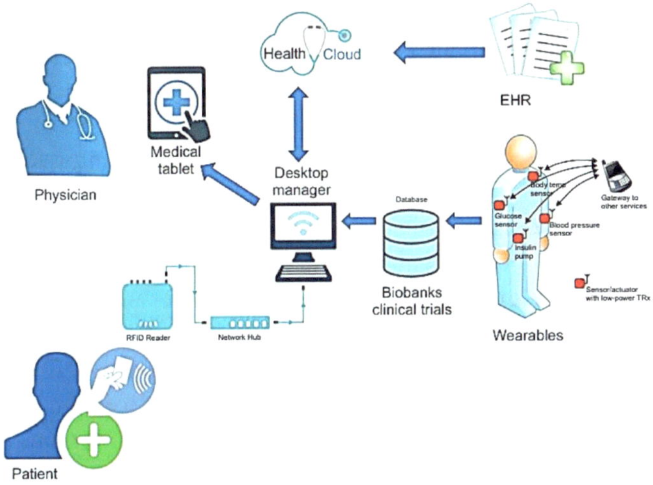

Figure 10.13. By embedding sensors and connected devices within everyday medical equipment, healthcare providers can gather and analyze vast amounts of real-time data, leading to more informed clinical decisions and personalized patient care.

Source: https://www.mdpi.com/electronics/electronics-12-02050/article_deploy/html/images/electronics-12-02050-g001.png.

This ability is very useful for urban as well as rural settings, since specialist services may be unavailable. This innovation will have its place among the big picture of expanding healthcare accessibility, as penned by the trends in biomedical engineering (Guan et al., 2015). The essence of IoT in healthcare lies in being able to fill the need for offering a sustainable and long-term framework. Smart devices and sensors require a reliable source of power, so there is considerable interest in energy harvesting solutions that can sustain their use. Wireless energy harvesting (WEH) contains potential solutions for powering IoT devices using ambient sources of energy. WEH not only extends device lifespan but also guarantees the self-sustenance of a networked healthcare system. With the extended growth of IoT to industries like smart hospitals and personalized wearable devices, the inclusion of efficient WEH systems will be imperative. Research in this sector is crucial to overcoming technical challenges, thus ensuring that the inherent potential of IoT can be tapped maximally in redefining healthcare systems worldwide (Guan et al., 2015) (Figure 10.13).

10.6.1. Definition and Functionality of IoT

Advances in technology in biomedical engineering have consistently highlighted the significance of the Internet of Things (IoT) with respect to health monitoring and patient care. IoT facilitates seamless communication between medical devices and systems, supporting real-time data analysis and processing. Interconnectedness enables healthcare providers to monitor physiological parameters and vital signs remotely, improving patient care and reducing hospital stay. These skills are particularly relevant in settings where medical personnel access is limited or during urgent interventions. Application of IoT in healthcare not only enhances easier monitoring of patients but also enhances the efficacy of health intervention initiatives since it provides data-driven information to clinical staff, thus enabling them to provide more informed decision-making processes that have a huge impact on patient outcomes. Furthermore, the application of IoT is not just about observation but also about a complete infrastructure to receive, transmit, and process information. Through the use of technologies such as Wireless Body Area Networks (WBANs), medical devices can exchange vital information efficiently, which is crucial during emergencies or with chronic patients who require continuous monitoring. For instance, National Integrated Network for Patient Monitoring (RNIMP) specific to the Beninese healthcare system demonstrates how IoT applies in the solution of critical health problems like the effective utilization of resources and enhanced patient safety (Ahouandjinou et al., 2020). The network facilitates remote access to health information, which enables healthcare providers to offer on-time interventions and help patient autonomy without reducing the quality of care. Thus, IoT application in biomedical engineering is a central infrastructure that is promoting innovation and efficiency. On the front of new technologies, the integration of IoT with other technologies such as additive manufacturing and smart materials is particularly significant. Smart materials with adaptive properties can be integrated with IoT systems to create responsive medical devices with response to environmental stimuli. Moreover, additive manufacturing optimizes the customization of medical devices in a way that they can be designed for the unique requirements of single patients and kept at optimal functioning (Dehghanghadikolaei et al., 2019). Such synergy between IoT and advanced manufacturing technologies propels a next generation of smart healthcare solutions not only to address existing healthcare challenges but also to enable future opportunities. Through the exploitation of the complete potential of these synergistic technologies, the discipline of biomedical engineering can expect to achieve unprecedented strides in personalized medicine, where treatment is not merely more effective but also more efficient and accessible than ever.

10.6.2. Benefits of IoT in Patient Care

The internet of things (IoT) role has transformed the development of healthcare technologies significantly, causing a paradigm shift in patient care. This connected system of devices allows patients to be monitored in real time, leading to accurate diagnosis and timely intervention. Implementation of IoT within the healthcare system allows for the capture and analysis of huge amounts of data that reflect individual patient behavior and physiological status. For instance, wearables that monitor vital signs can notify healthcare workers about anomalies to ensure prompt intervention is made prior to worsening patient's condition. Additionally, the integration of context information—such as environmental conditions with health information—serves to enhance the effectiveness of health interventions, thereby reducing neglect or response delay in treatment (Jung et al., 2017). With the evolution of proactive patient care, IoT effectively enhances overall patient quality of life through individualized treatment regimens responsive to their unique health needs. Not only does the future of healthcare involve real-time monitoring of patients, with IoT, but also more expansive aspects of medication management. The use of smart medication dispensers connected to IoT can significantly lower the risk of medication errors while at the same time guaranteeing patient adherence, particularly with the elderly or chronic disease patients. Such technologies not only eliminate the myth surrounding medication timing but can also feedback pertinent information to healthcare providers in the event of skipped or wrongly taken doses. Furthermore, there is growing interest in the potential for reuse of IoT technologies for medicines dispensed, with an ability to build a huge public health return on investment while minimizing environmental wastage (Donyai et al., 2020). With the integration of advanced technologies and pharmacy practice, stakeholders have the ability to build a more efficient and sustainable system of health, in the end leading to improved patient outcomes and management of resources. The disruptive influence of IoT on patient care is exemplified in the shape of sophisticated systems for predicting health crises such as falls among elderly patients. Traditional approaches to monitoring patient well-being did not incorporate multifactorial conditions and therefore translated to inadequacies in fall prediction systems that revolved around physiological parameters alone. However, through the integration of IoT sensors that gather contextual data in the form of environmental data and behavioral data, healthcare professionals are able to design more holistic prevention programs (Jung et al., 2017). This is not only easier to do than traditional fall detection, but it also empowers patients and caregivers with usable information, thereby providing a sense of autonomy for vulnerable individuals. As medicine continues to advance toward embracing IoT, personalized patient care becomes the focal point with anticipatory safety precautions being put into action to achieve maximum safety and foster overall well-being. Through these technologies, IoT solidifies itself as a cornerstone of modern biomedical engineering (Figure 10.14).

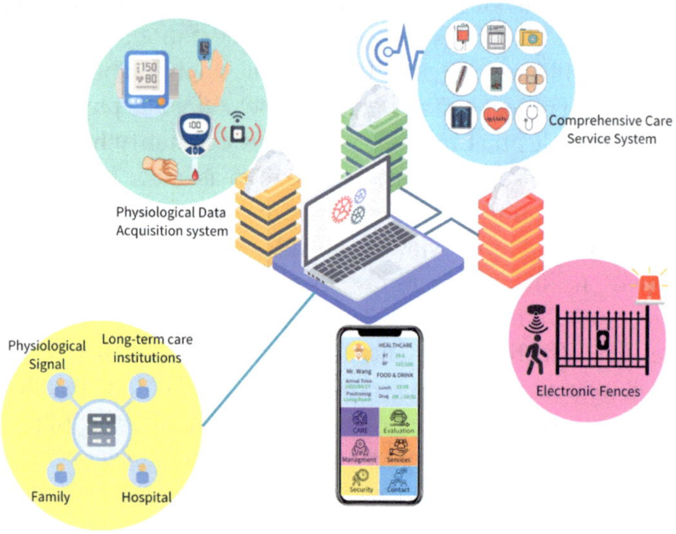

Figure 10.14. The integration of IoT in healthcare enables the collection and analysis of vast amounts of data that reflect individual patient behaviors and physiological states.

Source: https://www.mdpi.com/sensors/sensors-23-05913/article_deploy/html/images/sensors-23-05913-g001.png.

10.6.3. Challenges and Security Concerns

The integration of new technologies into biomedical engineering, such as AI-aided design automation and the application of 4D printing and smart materials, presents unique challenges to address. The new technologies increase the performance and agility of medical devices but also raise security concerns. Using AI to design medical devices creates unintentional vulnerabilities unless properly regulated or under surveillance. Big data networks that work with real-time patient information, especially in combination with IoT devices, are susceptible to cyber threats. This reality will require tighter data security measures, and a profound understanding of how these connections might be exploited, ultimately bringing ethical considerations to the forefront. The experience of these problems is essential in order to make progress matter without compromising the safety of patients or security of data. Within the hybrid manufacturing system model, with conventional and advanced technology both being utilized, the production complexity introduces further security issues. Collaboration between industry and academia, as New Hampshire's University Research and Industry plan illustrates, highlights the need for securing successful partnerships that innovate while maintaining robust security provisions. Having strong guidelines and frameworks is what allows these complexities to be managed because more sophisticated manufacturing techniques have the unwitting effect of creating more zones of weakness. Ensuring workers are thoroughly well-versed in the strengths and weaknesses of new technology, as well as strict industry standards, is the key. A profound understanding of ethical practice, supported by responsible research and innovation, can guide the successful management of such issues, allowing for secure progress in the biomedical sciences. With wearable and IoT medical devices, the many benefits they bring are integrated with substantial security concerns that must be addressed. Data privacy is a fundamental issue in this situation, as individual health information collected and exchanged by such devices can be targeted by cyber-attacks. Research ethics must catch up with these technologies, and transparency and user consent must be on top. As is cited in the neuro-ICT research, adopting a paradigm of discourse ethics in addressing problems in the world of biomedicine is able to enhance ethical regulation and foster trust in such new systems (Akintoye et al., 2019). It is also able to indicate the general necessity of strong regulatory measures protecting individuals' rights as well as promoting innovation. Balancing technological innovation with security measures will be crucial in guaranteeing the sustainability and success of wearable health technologies in improving patient outcomes.

10.7. CONCLUSION

The convergence of cutting-edge technologies in biomedical engineering represents a period characterized by improvement and innovation in healthcare delivery. While these technologies continue to evolve, 4D printing and smart materials take the forefront in such revolution. By integrating the time dimensions into traditional 3D printing procedures, 4D printing enables the creation of dynamic structures that can react to environmental changes, thereby enhancing the performance of medical devices and implants. The use of smart materials also allows for the development of responsive biomaterials that can interact with biological systems in real time, hence enhancing the rate of successful treatments and personalized medicine. These advances represent a shift towards more human-oriented healthcare experience that not only addresses immediate medical needs but also anticipates future issues in treating patients. Artificial intelligence (AI) and machine learning are emerging as strong drivers in streamlining design processes in biomedical engineering. AI enhances productivity by automating complex design processes, which stimulates rapid innovation. For instance, AI systems can search huge datasets to identify patterns employed in device design, reducing design cycles by a great extent. This allows clinicians and engineers to create tailored solutions that improve patient care with meticulous customization. Moreover, the integration of AI with hybrid manufacturing systems offers the capacity to switch between analog and digital methods of fabrication easily, with the potential to get even more agile and scalable in production. With such smart systems going mainstream, they are pointing towards a scenario where biomedical engineers can spend more time focusing on problem-solving and innovation, which in turn will lead to revolutionary healthcare breakthroughs. The adoption of wearable and IoT medical devices into the health infrastructure is a revolution towards anticipatory patient management and monitoring. These technologies allow for the continuous gathering of health data, which is critical to preventive as well as personalized medicine protocols. Recent advances in pervasive healthcare highlight the demand for unobtrusive health monitoring systems that are capable of monitoring and responding to health incidents in real-time. As discussed in the literature, such systems have the potential to revolutionize chronic disease care and enhance clinical outcomes through data-driven decision-making (Perez et al., 2015). In addition, with advancing diagnostic procedures for diseases like Atrial Fibrillation, incorporating effective monitoring services will be capable of significantly reducing patient morbidity and mortality rates (Acharya et al., 2020). Overall, these trends paint a positive vision for biomedical engineering, fundamentally transforming the delivery and reception of health services.

10.7.1. Summary of Key Trends and Technologies

Among the rapidly evolving field of biomedical engineering, one of the most significant trends to emerge is the application of 4D printing, a technology that shares revolutionary potential beyond traditional 3D manufacturing. 4D printing relies upon the concept wherein materials are able to change their shape and function upon exposure to some external stimulus such as heat or moisture. This new approach can be used to fabricate dynamic implants and devices that can sense the physiological conditions of the human body and optimize the effectiveness of medical treatments. Furthermore, smart materials that respond to environmental stimuli can have the capability to revolutionize tissue engineering by allowing for the creation of responsive flexible scaffolds that mimic the performance of natural tissue. With ongoing research in the characteristics and applications of high-tech materials, the integration of 4D printing will come to reshape the paradigm of biomedicine solutions, leading to improved patient-specific healthcare outcomes (Chia et al., 2015). AI has begun to play an important role in automation procedures for biomedical engineering design, streamlining workflows and augmenting innovation. Through the use of machine learning algorithms, scientists are able to process complicated biological information in order to streamline the design of medical devices and treatment plans at an unprecedented level of efficiency. This combined use of AI streamlines time-consuming processes, permitting engineers to concentrate on refinement and innovation and thus greatly accelerating the development process. Apart from this, artificial intelligence-based simulations can predict outcomes and duplicate diverse design scenarios without the need to employ large physical models, reducing costs and time-to-market for new biomedical devices. As artificial intelligence and biomedical engineering continue to develop, it is expected to offer sophisticated solutions coping with divergent patient needs and contributing to the establishment of personalized medicine (Matsunaga et al., 2015). The other emerging trend that mirrors the trend of integration in biomedical engineering is the integration of hybrid manufacturing systems. Hybrid systems integrate additive and subtractive manufacturing techniques to create complex structures that leverage both precise machining and intricate 3D printing capabilities. This double-pronged approach allows developers to create custom implants and devices that not only function but also are tuned to the individual anatomical details of specific patients. The systems can also be readily interfaced with wearable and IoT medical devices to provide real-time health monitoring and data collection. These advances provide the means to a future where preventive medicine and individualized treatment become more readily available so that practitioners can make informed decisions based on extensive analysis of data and consultation with integrated medical systems (Chia et al., 2015).

10.7.2. Future Directions in Biomedical Engineering

New technologies in biomedical engineering have tremendous potential to revolutionize traditional medical procedures to a large extent. The development of 4D printing and smart materials is a revolution that allows for the creation of dynamic structures that can change form or function in response to environmental input. This capability promises new dimensions for the fabrication of personalized medical implants and devices that can be optimized to meet the individual patients' needs, enhancing recovery outcomes.

The introduction of these newer materials to clinical applications has the potential not only to improve biocompatibility but to allow the creation of systems that can respond intelligently to physiological parameters, thereby reducing the frequency of complications. With a growing need for customized medicine, it is imperative that scientists and clinicians start exploring how 4D printing can be utilized effectively in conjunction with other emerging technologies in order to overcome the challenges of contemporary medicine (Biros et al., 2016). Artificial intelligence (AI) is quickly becoming the centerpiece of biomedical engineering, most notably in design and automation areas. The application of AI algorithms permits the optimization and analysis of complex biomedical systems, enabling engineers to create more efficient and innovative solutions. This revolution enables one to cut the time required to design and test new medical devices down to a very low level, speeding up the pace of technological advancement.

Moreover, AI technology design automation can lead to greater accuracy in forecasting and simulation, ultimately to safer and more efficient medical devices. As scientists use AI increasingly, the partnership between automated processes and innovative design can transform product development operations, thus emphasizing the requirements of continuous multidisciplinary collaboration within the field (Nagle et al., 1996). The convergence of hybrid manufacturing systems with wearable and IoT medical devices heralds a new era in patient care management. By combining traditional manufacturing strategies with modern digital fabrication technologies, engineers can design more complex and individualized medical devices, which are increasingly interconnected through the Internet of Things (IoT).

This connectivity allows for real-time data collection and analysis, making proactive management of chronic disease possible and enhancing patient activation. Additionally, the incorporation of intelligent technology into wearable devices offers round-the-clock monitoring of health status, enabling early treatment. With growth in these manufacturing systems, it is essential to address problems with regard to data security as well as device compatibility, so that new developments in biomedical engineering not only advance patient care quality but are also compatible with safety and effectiveness in an increasingly digitizing healthcare system (Biros et al., 2016).

10.7.3. Importance of Continued Innovation

Biomedical engineering continues to advance with the necessity for groundbreaking innovations that advance in line with the medical needs of the present. The field is enabled by technologies such as 4D printing and intelligent materials that not only enhance the efficiency of medical devices but offer tailored solutions according to a patient's unique needs. Innovation strategy also includes integrating advanced materials and adaptive systems sensitive to environmental cues, thereby transforming the treatment protocols. While healthcare systems are transitioning toward enhancing healthcare as personalized medicine, ongoing technology development demonstrates a key trend in biomedical engineering that emphasizes the importance of ongoing innovation in order to remain competitive and effectively respond to diverse medical needs. Hence, the sheer pursuit of development and research in the domain is the epitome of keeping pace with technology advancements and clinical needs with a view to improved patient care. Further, design automation employing artificial intelligence (AI) is also a new paradigm for the biomedical engineering sector. Continual advancement of AI technologies enables engineers to automate complex design procedures, enhancing accuracy and efficiency in the development of products. Through the application of machine learning techniques, biomedical engineers can analyze large sets of data to identify patterns and predict device behavior and thus speed up the innovation cycle. These advancements not only ease the design process but also provide new opportunities for the creation of sophisticated medical devices with more functions. As there is mounting pressure to accelerate development, the strategic application of AI not only optimizes existing process but also generates novel ideas that challenge conventional methodology. This merger of AI and design underlines the necessity of continuous innovation in the establishment of a more responsive and agile biomedical engineering sector. Lastly, the emergence of hybrid manufacturing systems is the pinnacle of the shift toward continuous innovation within biomedical engineering. This hybrid process combines traditional manufacturing techniques with sophisticated additive procedures to offer unprecedented flexibility and precision in the creation of medical devices. With industries wanting increased manufacturing efficiency and the removal of waste, hybrid processes allow device personalization and meet evolving market needs. In addition, the interconnection of these systems with wearable and Internet of Things (IoT) medical devices is transforming the monitor and therapy models of patients. Having the ability to tap into real-time data from connected devices accelerates the product development feedback loop and, as a result, helps build a more responsive healthcare system. Hence, the commitment to continued innovation in manufacturing and device integration is essential for the advancement of biomedical engineering and overall quality of care.

REFERENCES

1. Abels, A. A., Pereira, A. O., Andrade, A., Akbulut, Y., Almeida, R., Amirabdollahian, F., Atkins, M., et al. (2014). Bridging the gap between robotic technology and health care. https://core.ac.uk/download/42391924.pdf (accessed on 14th October 2025).
2. Acharya, U. R., Ciaccio, E. J., & Faust, O. (2020). A review of atrial fibrillation detection methods as a service. https://core.ac.uk/download/322489443.pdf (accessed on 14th October 2025).
3. Ahouandjinou, M. H., Houessouvo, R. C., Jossou, T. R., Medenou, D., et al. (2020). New intelligent network approach for monitoring physiological parameters: The case of Benin. https://core.ac.uk/download/305119894.pdf (accessed on 14th October 2025).
4. Akintoye, S., Fothergill, B. T., Guerrero, M., Knight, J., et al. (2019). Beyond research ethics: Dialogues in neuro-ICT research. https://core.ac.uk/download/228188834.pdf (accessed on 14th October 2025).
5. Andreu Perez, J., Ip, H., Leff, D., Yang, G., et al. (2015). From wearable sensors to smart implants–Towards pervasive and personalized healthcare.
6. Androulidakis, A., Bracale, U., Konnis, G., Koutsouris, D., et al. (2011). A feasibility study for the provision of electronic healthcare tools and services in areas of Greece, Cyprus and Italy. https://core.ac.uk/download/16664902.pdf (accessed on 14th October 2025).
7. Arcuri, A., Rector, A. L., Wood, A. M., Glas, A. S., Kulis, B., Cortes, C., Sammut, C., et al. (2018). Beyond volume: The impact of complex healthcare data on the machine learning pipeline. http://arxiv.org/abs/1706.01513 (accessed on 14th October 2025).
8. Baranwal, J., Barse, B., Fais, A., Delogu, G., & Kumar, A. (2022). Biopolymer: A sustainable material for food and medical applications. *Polymers, 14*, 983–983. https://doi.org/10.3390/polym14050983 (accessed on 14th October 2025).
9. Biros, G., Bungartz, H., Corones, J., Cramer, J., et al. (2016). Research and education in computational science and engineering. https://core.ac.uk/download/148025463.pdf (accessed on 14th October 2025).
10. Bizopoulos, P., & Koutsouris, D. (2021). Deep learning in cardiology. http://arxiv.org/abs/1902.11122 (accessed on 14th October 2025).
11. Browne, T. D., Gilmore, J. S., & Heller, T. S. (2025). Technology transfer–A selected bibliography. https://core.ac.uk/download/pdf/85235519.pdf (accessed on 14th October 2025).

12. Chia, H. N., & Wu, B. M. (2015). Recent advances in 3D printing of biomaterials. https://core.ac.uk/download/323078409.pdf (accessed on 14th October 2025).

13. Chou, T. K. A., Demaine, E. D., Deshpande, A. R., Lang, R. J., Paik, J. K., Pellegrino, S., et al. (2019). Assembly of advanced materials into 3D functional structures by methods inspired by origami and kirigami: A review. https://core.ac.uk/download/160738838.pdf (accessed on 14th October 2025).

14. Das, N., & Yip, M. (2017). Robot autonomy for surgery. http://arxiv.org/abs/1707.03080 (accessed on 14th October 2025).

15. De Geyter, N., Desmet, T., Dubruel, P., Leys, C., et al. (2009). Nonthermal plasma technology as a versatile strategy for polymeric biomaterials surface modification: A review. https://core.ac.uk/download/55837365.pdf (accessed on 14th October 2025).

16. Debackere, K., Monard, E., Raspoet, D., Ratinckx, E., et al. (2025). Technologie en innovatie in Vlaanderen: Prioriteiten. https://core.ac.uk/download/pdf/6468460.pdf (accessed on 14th October 2025).

17. Dehghanghadikolaei, A., Emamian, S. S., Fotovvati, B., Gisario, A., et al. (2019). The potential of additive manufacturing in the smart factory industrial 4.0: A review. https://core.ac.uk/download/231748826.pdf (accessed on 14th October 2025).

18. Donyai, P., Hui, T. K. L., McCrindle, R., Mohammed, A., et al. (2020). Enhancing pharmaceutical packaging through a technology ecosystem to facilitate the reuse of medicines and reduce medicinal waste. https://core.ac.uk/download/305108990.pdf (accessed on 14th October 2025).

19. Ewart, P. (2019). A comparison of processing techniques for producing prototype injection molding inserts. https://core.ac.uk/download/322841895.pdf (accessed on 14th October 2025).

20. Farooq, S., Imran, M. A., Latif, S., Qadir, J., et al. (2017). How 5G wireless (and concomitant technologies) will revolutionize healthcare? https://core.ac.uk/download/143476480.pdf (accessed on 14th October 2025).

21. Fluitman, J. (1996). Microsystems technology: Objectives. https://core.ac.uk/download/pdf/11453403.pdf (accessed on 14th October 2025).

22. Goldenberg, A., Hoffman, M. M., Leskovec, J., Nguyen, T., et al. (2018). Machine learning for integrating data in biology and medicine: Principles, practice, and opportunities. http://arxiv.org/abs/1807.00123 (accessed on 14th October 2025).

23. Guan, Y. L., Kamalinejad, P., Leung, V. C. M., Mahapatra, C., et al. (2015). Wireless energy harvesting for Internet of Things. https://core.ac.uk/download/30611147.pdf (accessed on 14th October 2025).

24. Haddadi, H., Mejova, Y., Ofli, F., Srivastava, M., et al. (2015). 360 quantified self. https://core.ac.uk/download/159074769.pdf (accessed on 14th October 2025).

25. Hussein, H., Mohd. Hashim, S. Z., Salim, N., Shamsir, M., et al. (2012). Educating the educators: Incorporating bioinformatics into biological science education in Malaysia. https://core.ac.uk/download/11778588.pdf (accessed on 14th October 2025).

26. Jung, T. P., Litvan, I., & Rajagopalan, R. (2017). Fall prediction and prevention systems: Recent trends, challenges, and future research directions. https://core.ac.uk/download/323065612.pdf (accessed on 14th October 2025).

27. Matsunaga, N., & Sullivan, R. (2015). Image processing for the extraction of nutritional information from food labels. https://core.ac.uk/download/72853103.pdf (accessed on 14th October 2025).

28. N/A. (2006). *Review of EU, National and Regional Innovation Drivers.* https://core.ac.uk/download/30624497.pdf (accessed on 14th October 2025).

29. N/A. (2016). *New Hampshire University Research and Industry Plan: A Roadmap for Collaboration and Innovation.* https://core.ac.uk/download/215517669.pdf (accessed on 14th October 2025).

30. N/A. (2025). *2011 Strategic Roadmap for Australian Research Infrastructure.* https://core.ac.uk/download/pdf/30672610.pdf (accessed on 14th October 2025).

31. Nagle, E. (1996). The new knowledge environment: Quality initiatives in health sciences libraries. https://core.ac.uk/download/4817382.pdf (accessed on 14th October 2025).

INDEX

C

D

E

F

G

H

N

O

S

T